Endovascular Venous Surgery

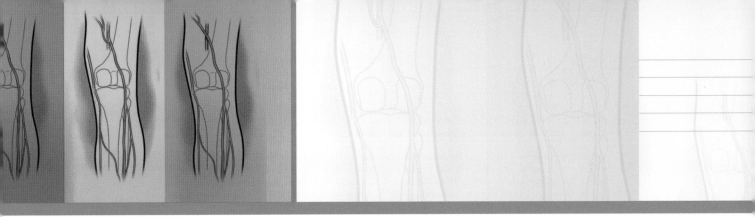

ATLAS OF
Endovascular
Venous Surgery

Jose I. Almeida, MD, FACS, RPVI, RVT

Founder, Miami Vein Center
Voluntary Associate Professor of Surgery
University of Miami—Jackson Memorial Hospital
Miami, Florida

ELSEVIER
SAUNDERS

1600 John F. Kennedy Blvd.
Ste 1800
Philadelphia, PA 19103-2899

ATLAS OF ENDOVASCULAR VENOUS SURGERY   ISBN: 978-1-4377-1790-7

Library of Congress Cataloging-in-Publication Data
Atlas of endovascular venous surgery / [edited by] Jose I. Almeida.
    p. ; cm.
  Includes bibliographical references and index.
  ISBN 978-1-4377-1790-7 (hardcover : alk. paper)
  I. Almeida, Jose I.
  [DNLM: 1. Vascular Diseases—surgery—Atlases. 2. Endovascular Procedures—methods—Atlases. 3. Veins—surgery—Atlases. WG 17]
  LC classification not assigned
  617.4′1300223—dc23

                                                                            2011030544

Acquisitions Editor: Judith A. Fletcher
Developmental Editor: Joanie Milnes
Publishing Services Manager: Patricia Tannian
Senior Project Manager: Claire Kramer
Designer: Louis Forgione

Printed in China

Last digit is the print number: 9 8 7 6 5 4 3 2 1

To my father, Jose Almeida, MD, who died on April 16, 2009. My father served as the chief physician for the CIA-trained force of Cuban exiles whose unsuccessful attempt to overthrow the Cuban government of Fidel Castro is now known as the Bay of Pigs Invasion. After release from his 2-year incarceration as a Political prisoner of Cuba, my father went on to train at the renowned Menninger School of Psychiatry in Topeka, Kansas. The school became the hub for training professionals in the biopsychosocial approach and represented the center of a psychiatric education revolution. He practiced psychiatry in West Palm Beach, Florida, until he died at home from multiple sclerosis at the age of 75.

To the memory of Robert Zeppa, MD, Chairman of Surgery at the University of Miami-Jackson Memorial Hospital, under whom I received my general surgery residency training. His untimely death left a void in surgical education.

To my wife, Yvette Angela Almeida, for her strong support of my surgical academic endeavors.

Jose I. Almeida, MD, FACS, RPVI, RVT
Founder, Miami Vein Center
Voluntary Associate Professor of Surgery
University of Miami—Jackson Memorial Hospital
Miami, Florida
Venous Anatomy
Noninvasive Testing
Endovenous Thermal Ablation of Saphenous Reflux
Radiofrequency Thermal Ablation
Laser Thermal Ablation
Chemical Ablation
Treatment of Perforating Veins
Ambulatory Phlebectomy
Endovenous Approach to Recurrent Varicose Veins
Thromboembolic Disease
Iliofemoral Venous Occlusive Disease

Vittorio P. Antonacci, MD
Director, Charlotte Radiology Vein and Vascular Center
Charlotte Radiology
Interventional Radiologist
Carolinas Medical Center and Levine Children's Hospital
Charlotte, North Carolina
Venous Malformations

James F. Benenati, MD
Director, Peripheral Vascular Laboratory
Baptist Cardiac and Vascular Institute
Clinical Associate, Professor of Radiology
University of South Florida College of Medicine
Tampa, Florida
Pelvic Congestion Syndrome and Ovarian Vein Reflux

Ronald Bush, MD
Assistant Clinical Professor of Surgery
Department of Surgery
Medical College of Ohio
Toledo, Ohio
Treatment of Venous Ulcers

Antonios P. Gasparis, MD, RVT, FACS
Associate Professor of Surgery
Director, Stony Brook Vein Center
Department of Surgery
Stony Brook University Medical Center
Stony Brook, New York
Endovenous Thrombectomy and Thrombolysis
Postthrombotic Syndrome

Peter Gloviczki, MD
Joe M. and Ruth Roberts Professor of Surgery
Division of Vascular and Endovascular Surgery
Mayo Clinic
Rochester, Minnesota
Evidence-Based Summary of Guidelines from the American
Venous Forum and the Society for Vascular Surgery

Barry T. Katzen, MD
Clinical Professor
Radiology and Surgery
Associate Dean for Clinical Affairs for Baptist Health
Florida International University Herbert Wertheim College
of Medicine
Founder and Medical Director
Baptist Cardiac and Vascular Institute
Miami, Florida
Venous Malformations

Nicos Labropoulos, MD
Professor of Surgery and Radiology
Director, Vascular Laboratory
Department of Surgery
Stony Brook University Medical Center
Stony Brook, New York
Venous Pathophysiology
Endovenous Thrombectomy and Thrombolysis
Postthrombotic Syndrome

Timothy K. Liem, MD, FACS
Associate Professor of Surgery
Vice-Chairman, Department of Surgery
Oregon Health & Science University
Portland, Oregon
Thromboembolic Disease
Endovenous Placement of Inferior Vena Caval Filter

Edward G. Mackay, MD
Private Practice
Palm Harbor, Florida
Treatment of Spider Telangiectasias

Rafael D. Malgor, MD, RPVI
Vascular Surgery 0+5 Resident
Division of Vascular Surgery
Department of Surgery
Stony Brook University Medical Center
Stony Brook, New York
Venous Pathophysiology
Endovenous Thrombectomy and Thrombolysis
Postthrombotic Syndrome

Mark H. Meissner, MD
Professor of Surgery
Department of Surgery
University of Washington
Seattle, Washington
Evidence-Based Summary of Guidelines from the American
Venous Forum and the Society for Vascular Surgery

Carolyn E. Munschauer
Research Coordinator
Venous Institute of Buffalo
Buffalo, New York
Severity Scoring and Measuring Outcomes

Constantino S. Peña, MD
Department of Radiology
University of South Florida
Tampa, Florida
Medical Director of Vascular Imaging
Baptist Cardiac and Vascular Institute
Miami, Florida
Pelvic Congestion Syndrome and Ovarian Vein Reflux
Endovenous Management of Central and Upper Extremity
Veins
Venous Malformations

Michael A. Vasquez, MD, FACS, RVT
The Venous Institute of Buffalo
State University of New York at Buffalo
Department of Surgery
DeGraff Memorial Hospital
North Tonawanda, New York
Severity Scoring and Outcomes Measurement

FOREWORD

I am pleased, as Chairman of the University of Miami Daughtry Family Department of Surgery, to write this foreword for the first edition of the *Atlas of Endovascular Venous Surgery* for Dr. Almeida, who is one of our own.

The Department of Surgery at the University of Miami Miller School of Medicine is composed of 17 divisions that provide primary, secondary, tertiary, and quaternary surgical care at Jackson Memorial Hospital, one of the busiest hospitals in North America, and at the University of Miami Hospital. With more than 560 staff members, the department's mission is to provide high-quality clinical care with compassion, world-class medical education, and cutting-edge research. Dr. Almeida finished as chief resident in surgery in 1996 at the University of Miami and then went on to complete his fellowship in vascular surgery at the University of Missouri–Columbia. After returning to Miami in 1998 and practicing open and endovascular arterial surgery for 5 years, he decided to focus his efforts on the emerging field of endovascular venous surgery.

The field of endovascular venous surgery commenced about 12 years ago; it really originated as we know it today when the first-generation radiofrequency ablation catheter garnered approval from the United States Food and Drug Administration (FDA) and became commercially available to doctors for the treatment of saphenous vein incompetence. Shortly thereafter, in 2002, an 810-nm wavelength endovenous laser was approved by the FDA for saphenous vein ablation. Before this, surgeons were usually performing surgical saphenectomy (high ligation of the saphenofemoral junction with stripping of the greater saphenous vein) in hospital operating rooms. In the mid-to-late 1990s, surgical saphenectomy began to gain popularity in the office environment with tumescent anesthesia. Dr. Almeida was an early adopter of these technologies and has played a major role in shifting superficial venous care from the hospital into the office setting.

Dr. Almeida's efforts have culminated in a large educational commitment to others interested in venous disease. He is course director of the International Vein Congress, now the largest dedicated venous meeting in the world, which is held annually in Miami. He has authored more than 20 peer-reviewed journal articles, 30 textbook chapters, and 40 non–peer-reviewed articles in endovascular venous surgery, and he has given more than 500 formal lectures on the subject around the globe. He has been principal investigator in 10 clinical trials funded through industry-sponsored grants. He holds two patents on endovascular venous medical devices. He has been appointed chairman to three important committees at the American Venous Forum.

Dr. Almeida has had a voluntary faculty appointment at the University of Miami for more than 10 years and has worked closely with the University of Miami Division of Vascular Surgery. Currently, the focus of their joint efforts is on femoro-ilio-caval endovascular and open reconstructions for patients with advanced chronic venous insufficiency who have venous ulceration. We look forward to having this seminal publication available to our residents and students in the departmental library.

Alan S. Livingstone, MD
Lucille and DeWitt Daughtry Professor and Chairman
Chief, Division of Surgery Oncology
Daughtry Family Department of Surgery
University of Miami Miller School of Medicine
Chief of Surgical Services, Jackson Memorial Hospital

P R E F A C E

*"This book was conceived as a well illustrated
technical guide for the endovascular surgical
management of venous diseases. ... our efforts
will be realized if the book proves helpful to any
physician committed to treating patients with
venous disease."*

Although this first edition of the *Atlas of Endovascular Venous Surgery* is set up as a
text atlas, I hope that it will grow into a definitive evidence-based reference not only
for vascular surgeons, but also for all physicians who treat venous disease. Currently,
the best evidence-based reference of venous disorders is the *Handbook of Venous Disorders: Guidelines of the American Venous Forum,* edited by Peter Gloviczki, MD. This
first edition of the *Atlas of Endovascular Venous Surgery* should serve as a nice com-
panion to the *Handbook of Venous Disorders* because it beautifully illustrates the technical aspects of endovenous vascular surgery through full-color illustrations, photographs,
and radiologic (ultrasound, fluoroscopy with and without contrast venography, and
cross-sectional) images.

Never has the discipline of venous surgery been so exciting! Traditional open surgery
remains important in a select group of patients, but it has largely been supplanted by
ever-expanding endovascular options. Although we plan to increase the page content
for the second edition, a more comprehensive book, we decided that the length of this
edition is appropriate for most readers.

Readers increasingly use Web-based resources, and we are pleased that the current
book is bundled as a print and Web version. The Web version contains all the references and will be updated as needed with new relevant references selected from sources
such as the *Journal of Vascular Surgery* and the *Journal of Vascular and Endovascular
Surgery.* It also contains video presentations.

All this work would not have been possible without the assistance of many others.
I was greatly assisted by the hard work and diligence of the authors who prepared the
chapters that make up about 50% of this book. Realizing the demands of this task, I
selected recognized experts and limited their contributions so that they could focus on
this endeavor. We were rewarded by excellent contributions.

A special recognition goes to the beautiful artistic renderings prepared by Tiffany Davanzo. Her illustrations really make the technical details of the procedures self-explanatory.

Finally, we appreciate the assistance of many individuals at Elsevier who tolerated our demands for excellence and then exceeded them. Judy Fletcher served as the Publishing Director and Joanie Milnes as the Developmental Editor. Their efforts, combined with those of many other copy editors, artists, and printers, helped to assemble this final product.

Jose I. Almeida, MD, FACS, RPVI, RVT

CONTENTS

ATLAS OF
Endovascular Venous Surgery

CHAPTER 1

Venous Anatomy

Jose I. Almeida

HISTORICAL BACKGROUND

Chronic venous diseases (CVDs) include a spectrum of clinical findings ranging from spider telangiectasias and varicose veins to debilitating venous ulceration. Varicose veins without skin changes are present in about 20% of the general population, and they are slightly more frequent in women.

References to varicose veins are found in early Egyptian and Greek writings and confirm that venous disease was recognized in ancient times. A votive tablet in the National Museum in Athens showing a man holding an enlarged leg with a varicose vein is frequently featured in many historical writings regarding venous disease.

The venous system originates at the capillary level and progressively increases in size as the conduits move proximally toward the heart. The venules are the smallest structures, and the vena cava is the largest. It is critical that all endovascular venous surgeons understand the anatomic relationships between the thoracic, abdominal, and extremity venous systems; especially from the anatomic standpoint (Fig. 1-1). Veins of the lower extremities are the most germane to this book and are divided into three systems: deep, superficial, and perforating. Lower extremity veins are located in two compartments: deep and superficial. The deep compartment is bounded by the muscular fascia. The superficial compartment is bounded below by the muscular fascia and above by the dermis. The term *perforating veins* is reserved for veins that perforate the muscular fascia and connect superficial veins with deep veins. The term *communicating veins* is used to describe veins that connect with other veins of the same compartment.

VENOUS SYSTEM OVERVIEW

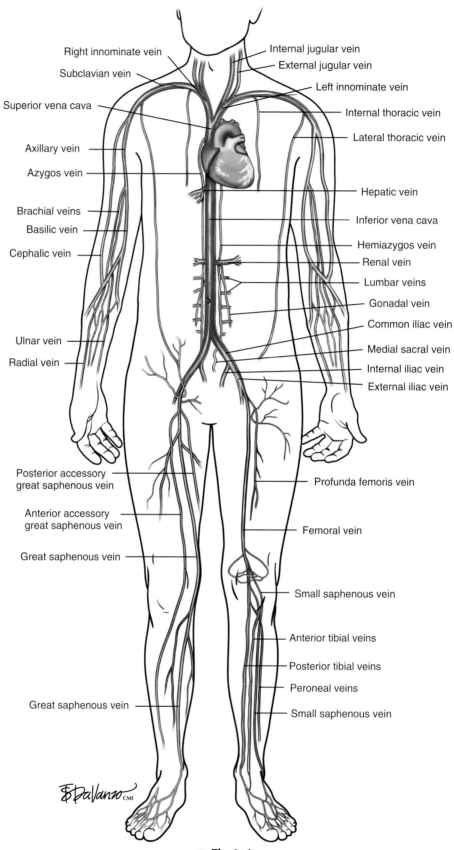

Right innominate vein

Subclavian vein

Superior vena cava

Axillary vein

Azygos vein

Brachial veins

Basilic vein

Cephalic vein

Ulnar vein

Radial vein

Posterior accessory
great saphenous vein

Anterior accessory
great saphenous vein

Great saphenous vein

Great saphenous vein

Internal jugular vein

External jugular vein

Left innominate vein

Internal thoracic vein

Lateral thoracic vein

Hepatic vein

Inferior vena cava

Hemiazygos vein

Renal vein

Lumbar veins

Gonadal vein

Common iliac vein

Medial sacral vein

Internal iliac vein

External iliac vein

Profunda femoris vein

Femoral vein

Small saphenous vein

Anterior tibial veins

Posterior tibial veins

Peroneal veins

Small saphenous vein

■ Fig 1-1

The vein wall is composed of three layers: intima, media, and adventitia. Notably, the muscular tunica media is much thinner than on the pressurized arterial side of the circulation. Venous valves are an extension of the intimal layer, have a bicuspid structure, and support unidirectional flow (Fig. 1-2).

Surgeons interested in performing thermal or chemical ablation therapy of the great saphenous vein (GSV) and its related structures must have a good understanding of the saphenous canal. The importance of the saphenous canal in relation to B-mode ultrasound anatomy is

VENOUS STRUCTURE

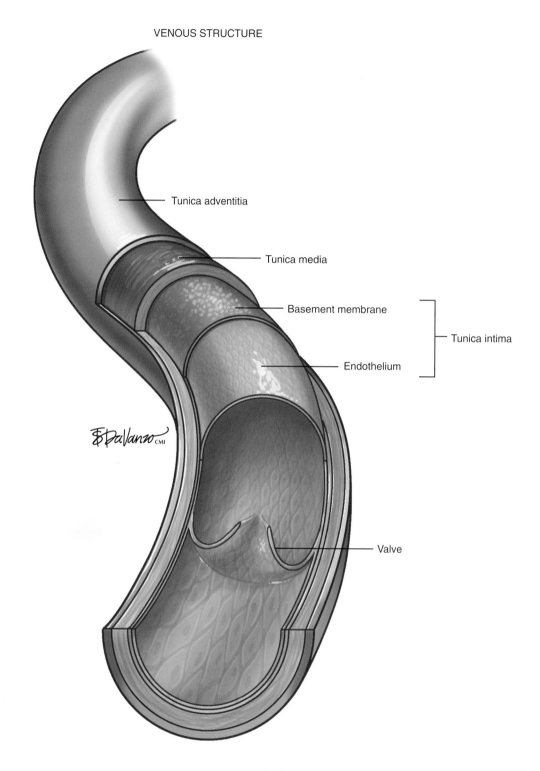

Tunica adventitia

Tunica media

Basement membrane

Tunica intima

Endothelium

Valve

■ **Fig 1–2**

discussed in more detail in Chapter 2. A cross section of the saphenous canal (Fig. 1-3) depicts many of the critical relationships referable to GSV treatment—the most important is how it courses atop the muscular fascia in a quasi-envelope called the *saphenous fascia*. The saphenous fascia is the portion of the membranous layer of the subcutaneous tissue that overlies the saphenous veins. Veins coursing parallel to the saphenous canal are termed *accessory veins*, whereas those coursing oblique to the canal are referred to as *circumflex veins*. Compressible structures superficial to the muscular fascia are potential targets for treatment; however, treating those structures deep to the muscular fascia may lead to a disastrous outcome. Noncompressible structures generally represent major arteries. Perforating veins must pierce the muscular fascia as they drain blood from the superficial to deep systems.

As diagnostic and therapeutic options for venous disorders expanded, the nomenclature proposed in 2002 by the International Interdisciplinary Committee[1] required revision. The nomenclature was extended and further refined,[2] taking into account recent improvements in ultrasound and clinical surgical anatomy. The term *great saphenous vein* should be used instead of terms such as *long saphenous vein, greater saphenous vein,* or *internal saphenous vein.* The LSV abbreviation, used to describe both the *long saphenous vein* and *lesser saphenous vein,* was clearly problematic. For this reason these terms have been eliminated. Similarly, the term *small saphenous vein,* abbreviated as SSV, should be used instead of the terms *short, external,* or *lesser saphenous vein.*

The GSV originates at the medial foot and receives deep pedal tributaries as it courses to the medial malleolus. From the medial ankle, the GSV ascends anteromedially within the calf and continues a medial course to the knee and into the thigh. The termination point of the GSV into the common femoral vein is a confluence called the *saphenofemoral junction* (SFJ) (Fig. 1-4).

SAPHENOUS CANAL CROSS SECTION

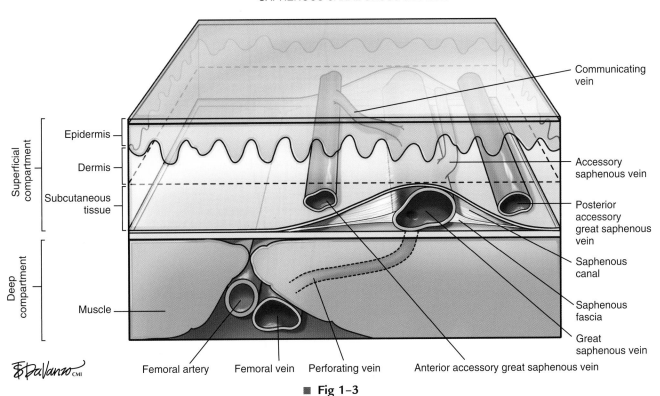

■ **Fig 1–3**

SUPERFICIAL VENOUS ANATOMY (ANTERIOR)

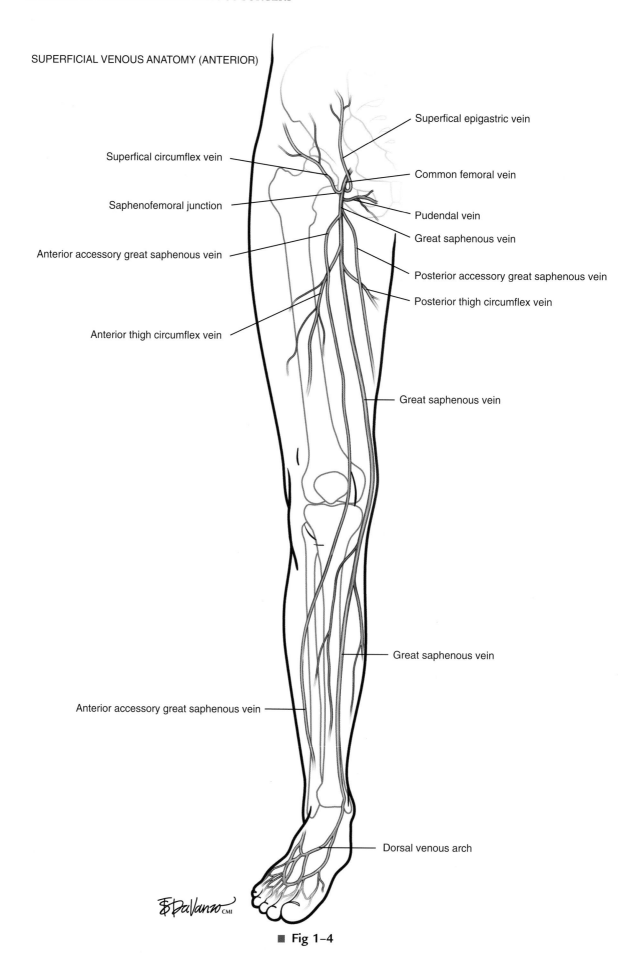

Superfical epigastric vein

Superfical circumflex vein

Common femoral vein

Saphenofemoral junction

Pudendal vein

Great saphenous vein

Anterior accessory great saphenous vein

Posterior accessory great saphenous vein

Posterior thigh circumflex vein

Anterior thigh circumflex vein

Great saphenous vein

Great saphenous vein

Anterior accessory great saphenous vein

Dorsal venous arch

■ Fig 1–4

The terminal valve of the GSV is located within the junction itself. A subterminal valve can often be identified approximately 1 cm distal to the terminal valve. From the upper calf to the groin, the GSV is usually contained within the saphenous compartment. Visualization of this fascial envelope is an important landmark in identifying the GSV with duplex ultrasound. The saphenous compartment is bounded superficially by a hyperechoic saphenous fascia and deeply by the muscular fascia of the limb.

At the groin, the GSV drains blood from the external pudendal, superficial epigastric, and external circumflex iliac veins just before it enters the common femoral vein confluence. As in all human anatomy, variations are crucial to recognize to guide the correct diagnosis and treatment. Historically, the GSV has been reported to be duplicated in the thigh in as many as 20% of subjects. However, recent examinations have demonstrated that true duplication, with two veins within one saphenous compartment, occurs in less than 1% of cases. Large extrafascial veins, which are termed *accessory saphenous veins*, can run parallel to the GSV and take on the characteristics of duplicated veins.

The accessory saphenous veins are venous segments that ascend in a plane parallel to the saphenous veins. They may be anterior, posterior, or superficial to the main trunk. The term *anterior accessory great saphenous vein* (AAGSV) describes any venous segment ascending parallel to the GSV and located anteriorly, both in the leg and in the thigh. The term *posterior accessory great saphenous vein* (PAGSV) is consistent with any venous segment ascending parallel to the GSV and located posteriorly, both in the leg and in the thigh. The leg segment corresponds to the popular terms *Leonardo's vein* or *posterior arch vein*. The term *superficial accessory great saphenous vein* (SAGSV) is considered to be any venous segment ascending parallel to the GSV and located just superficial to the saphenous fascia, both in the leg and in the thigh.

Circumflex veins by definition drain into the GSV from an oblique direction. The posterior thigh circumflex vein (PTCV) is present in virtually every case; however, the anterior thigh circumflex vein (ATCV) is less common.

The small saphenous vein (SSV) originates in the lateral foot and passes posterolaterally in the lower calf. The SSV lies above the deep fascia in the midline as it reaches the upper calf, where it pierces the two heads of the gastrocnemius muscle and courses cephalad until it enters the popliteal space. In approximately two thirds of patients, the SSV drains entirely into the popliteal vein just above the knee at the saphenopopliteal junction (SPJ). In as many as one third of patients, the cranial extension of the SSV drains into a posterior medial tributary of the GSV or directly into the GSV (vein of Giacomini) or into the femoral vein via a thigh perforating vein.

In variant drainage, a standard SPJ may or may not be present. The SSV is truly duplicated in 4% of cases; most often this is segmental and primarily involves the midportion of the vein (Fig. 1-5).

SUPERFICIAL VENOUS ANATOMY (POSTERIOR)

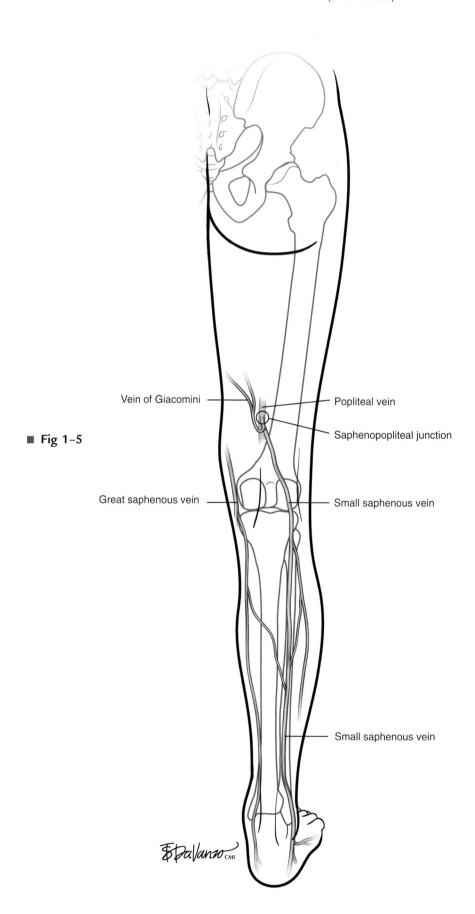

Vein of Giacomini

Popliteal vein

Saphenopopliteal junction

■ Fig 1–5

Great saphenous vein

Small saphenous vein

Small saphenous vein

PERFORATING VEINS

Identifying perforating veins based on the original descriptions of investigators (i.e., Cockett, Sherman, Dodd) is falling into disfavor. Descriptive terms based on topography, which designate the anatomic location, have become the contemporary approach. Perforating veins pass through defects in the deep fascia to connect deep and superficial veins of the calf or thigh. Venous valves prevent reflux of blood from the deep veins into the superficial system. Perforating veins may connect the GSV to the deep system at the femoral, posterior tibial, gastrocnemius, and soleal vein levels. Located between the ankle and the knee are perforating veins formerly known as Cockett's perforators that connect the posterior tibial venous system with the PAGSV of the calf (a.k.a., posterior arch vein) (Fig. 1-6).

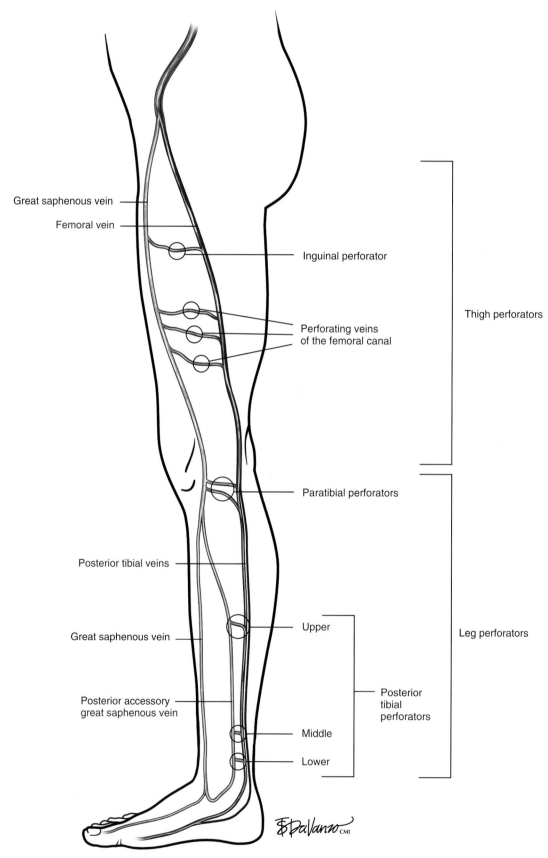

Great saphenous vein

Femoral vein

Inguinal perforator

Perforating veins of the femoral canal

Thigh perforators

Paratibial perforators

Posterior tibial veins

Great saphenous vein

Upper

Leg perforators

Posterior accessory great saphenous vein

Posterior tibial perforators

Middle

Lower

■ Fig 1–6

Deep Veins

Below the knee, there are six named axial veins that are generally paired and are located on either side of a corresponding named artery. The names of the three pairs of deep veins in the leg are the anterior tibial, posterior tibial, and peroneal veins. In addition, venous sinusoids within the deep calf muscle coalesce to form the nonaxial soleal and gastrocnemius venous plexi, which ultimately drain into the peroneal veins at the level of the midcalf. In the lower popliteal space, the anterior and posterior tibial veins join with the peroneal veins to become the popliteal vein.

At the upper margin of the popliteal fossa, above the adductor canal, the femoral vein originates from the popliteal vein. The "superficial femoral vein" terminology was clearly problematic and has been abandoned since the femoral vein is a deep structure. The deep femoral vein (profunda femoris) drains the deep muscles of the lateral thigh, communicates with the popliteal vein, and serves as a critical collateral vessel in cases where the femoral vein occludes with thrombus. The common femoral vein runs from the confluence of the femoral vein and the deep femoral vein to the external iliac vein at the level of the inguinal ligament (Figs. 1-7 and 1-8).

Above the inguinal ligament, the external iliac vein represents the final common pathway of lower extremity venous drainage. The external iliac vein is joined by the internal iliac vein (hypogastric), which drains pelvic blood to form the common iliac vein. The union of the right and left common iliac veins forms the inferior vena cava (IVC) at about the level of the fourth lumbar vertebrae.

The IVC continues the journey in a cephalad direction as it leaves the pelvis, enters the abdomen, and terminates in the thoracic cavity. In the abdomen, the IVC picks up paired lumbar veins, the right gonadal vein, the right and left renal veins, and the entire hepatic venous drainage (right, middle, and left hepatics). The IVC is joined by the superior vena cava (SVC), the azygos vein, and the coronary sinus as all four structures empty into the right atrium of the heart.

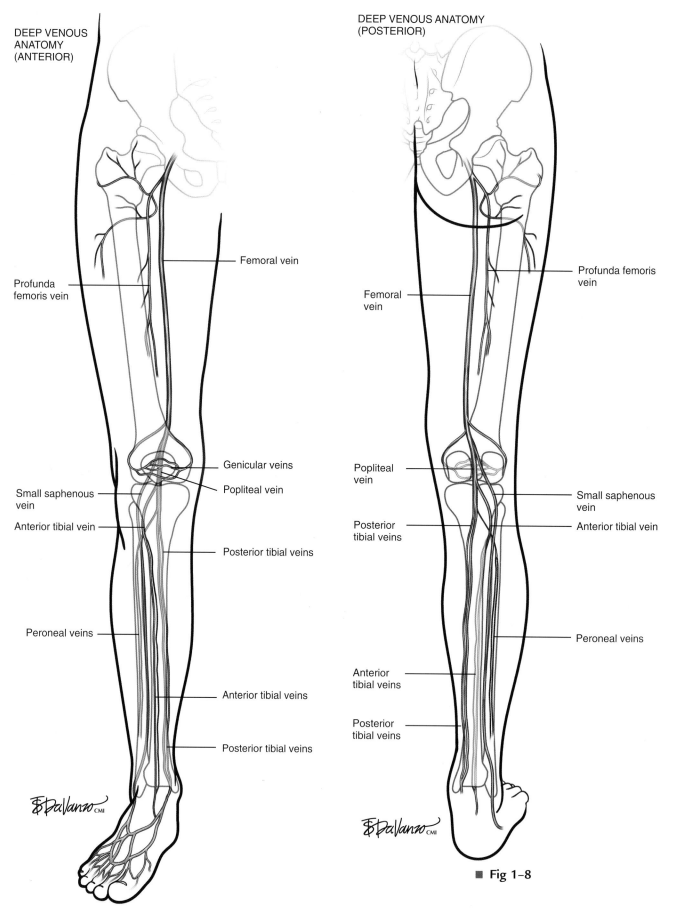

DEEP VENOUS
ANATOMY
(ANTERIOR)

Profunda
femoris vein

Femoral vein

Genicular veins

Popliteal vein

Small saphenous
vein

Anterior tibial vein

Posterior tibial veins

Peroneal veins

Anterior tibial veins

Posterior tibial veins

■ Fig 1–7

DEEP VENOUS ANATOMY
(POSTERIOR)

Profunda femoris
vein

Femoral
vein

Popliteal
vein

Small saphenous
vein

Posterior
tibial veins

Anterior tibial vein

Peroneal veins

Anterior
tibial veins

Posterior
tibial veins

■ Fig 1–8

Upper Extremity Veins

Venous blood from the hand drains into the forearm via the deep radial and ulnar veins and the superficial cephalic and basilic veins. In the upper arm, deep drainage from the paired brachial veins enters the axillary vein at the shoulder. The axillary vein also drains the superficial tissues via the cephalic vein—which enters the deltopectoral groove—and the basilic veins of the medial arm. The subclavian vein is protected by the clavicle as it carries upper extremity blood from the axillary vein. The subclavian vein then picks up drainage from the head and neck via the jugular veins and ultimately empties into the innominate veins of the thoracic cavity. Right and left innominate veins drain into the SVC and enter the right atrium of the heart. The SVC also receives venous blood from the azygos system, which drains the thoracic cage via intercostal veins and ultimately enters the SVC (Fig. 1-9).

UPPER EXTREMITY VENOUS ANATOMY

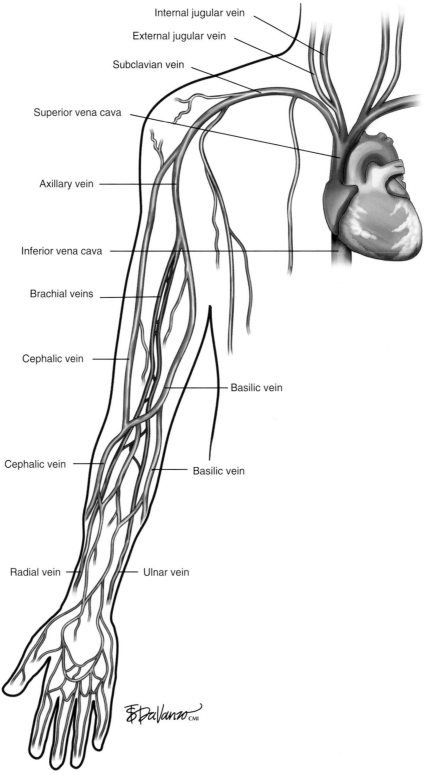

■ Fig 1–9

Lower Extremity Nerves

The posterior division of the femoral nerve provides sensory fibers to the inner surface of the leg (saphenous nerve), to the quadriceps muscles (muscular branches), and to the hip and knee joints. The saphenous nerve descends beneath the sartorius muscle, winding around its posterior edge and exiting at the adductor canal. The infrapatellar branch pierces the sartorius muscle and courses anteriorly to the infrapatellar region. The descending branch passes down the medial aspect of the leg juxtaposed to the great saphenous vein and here is at highest risk for injury from thermal ablation procedures. At the lower third of the leg, it divides into two branches: one of the branches of the descending portion of the saphenous nerve courses along the medial border of the tibia and ends at the ankle, whereas the other branch passes anterior to the ankle and is distributed to the medial aspect of the foot, sometimes reaching as far as the metatarso-phalangeal joint of the great toe (Fig. 1-10).

The most interesting issue referable to surgical work in the popliteal space is clearly the neuroanatomy. The sciatic nerve descends the posterior thigh and divides into the tibial and

NERVES OF THE LEG (ANTERIOR)

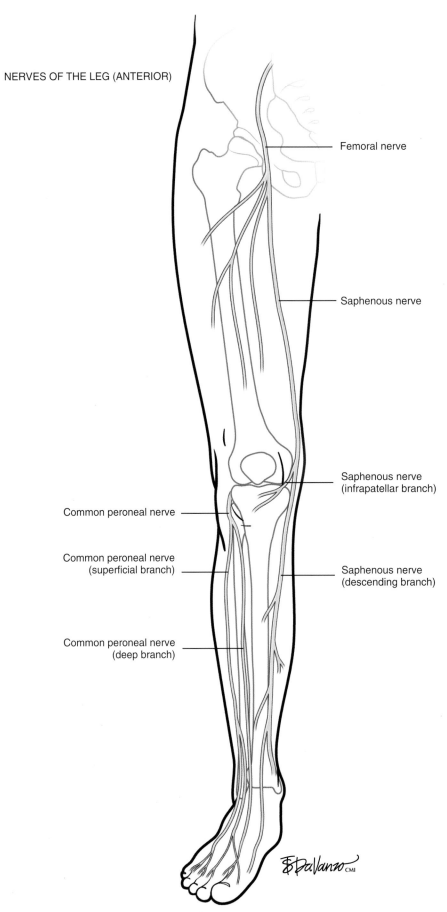

Femoral nerve

Saphenous nerve

Saphenous nerve
(infrapatellar branch)

Common peroneal nerve

Common peroneal nerve
(superficial branch)

Saphenous nerve
(descending branch)

Common peroneal nerve
(deep branch)

■ Fig 1–10

common peroneal nerves in the popliteal area (Fig. 1-11). The exact location of this division can range several centimeters proximally or several centimeters distally. The tibial nerve continues its descent to the ankle, and its innervation mostly affects motor function. The common peroneal nerve, however, divides near the zone of the head of the fibula, into deep and superficial branches. The common peroneal nerve courses anteriorly around the fibula, taking a sharp turn as it rounds the fibular neck to enter the anterior compartment. Because of the sharp turn, the nerve is more tethered than the superficial branch; immediately below the fibular head, the deep peroneal nerve lies on the anterior cortex of the fibula for a distance of 3 to 4 cm. The deep peroneal nerve innervates the dorsiflexors of the leg and, when injured, results in the dramatic foot drop. The tissues innervated by the superficial peroneal nerve provide only sensory information for interpretation in the brain.

There is a natural flare at the midcalf level where the inferior border of the medial and lateral heads of the gastrocnemius muscles is located. The sural nerve is a sensory nerve, which innervates the skin of the posterolateral aspect of the distal third of leg, the lateral malleolus, along the lateral side of the foot and little toe.

NERVES OF THE LEG (POSTERIOR)

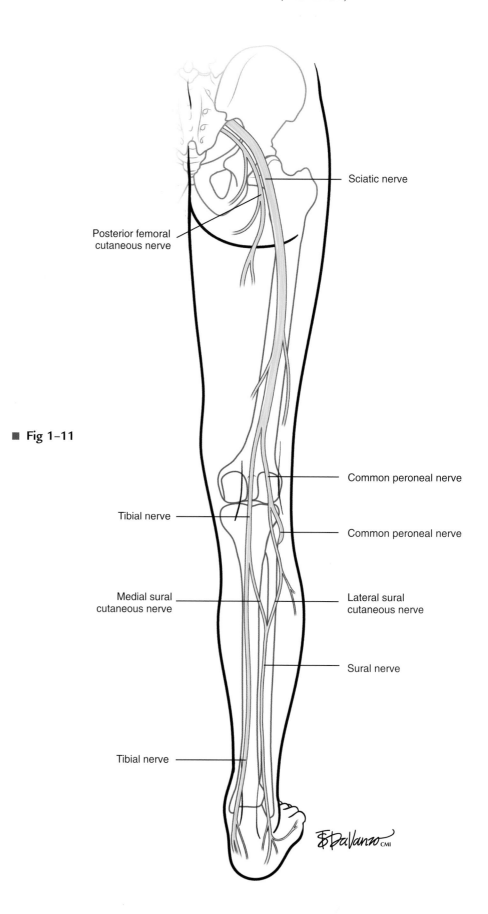

Sciatic nerve

Posterior femoral
cutaneous nerve

■ **Fig 1–11**

Common peroneal nerve

Tibial nerve

Common peroneal nerve

Medial sural
cutaneous nerve

Lateral sural
cutaneous nerve

Sural nerve

Tibial nerve

The sural nerve is formed by the union of the medial sural cutaneous nerve (MSCN) and the lateral sural cutaneous nerve (LSCN). When viewed from the posterior position, the sural nerve is arranged like the letter "Y" in most persons. The MSCN is a branch of the tibial nerve, and the LSCN originates from the common peroneal nerve. The site of union is usually in the lower third of the leg or just below the ankle.[3] The SSV travels in proximity to the sural nerve in the lower leg, where the nerve is joined at the midline. Where the gastrocnemius muscle bellies become prominent in the upper calf, the sural nerve is separated into the MSCN and LSCN. Therefore the SSV in the upper calf is distanced from the sural nerve, making this segment safer for thermal ablation

As stated earlier, B-mode ultrasound has made it possible to develop an accurate diagnosis and treatment plan for patients with venous disease. The main reference point of the ultrasound examination is at the inguinal crease where the GSV empties into the CFV. In the first cross section of Figure 1-12, one can study the saphenofemoral junction as it looks using B-mode (gray scale) ultrasound.

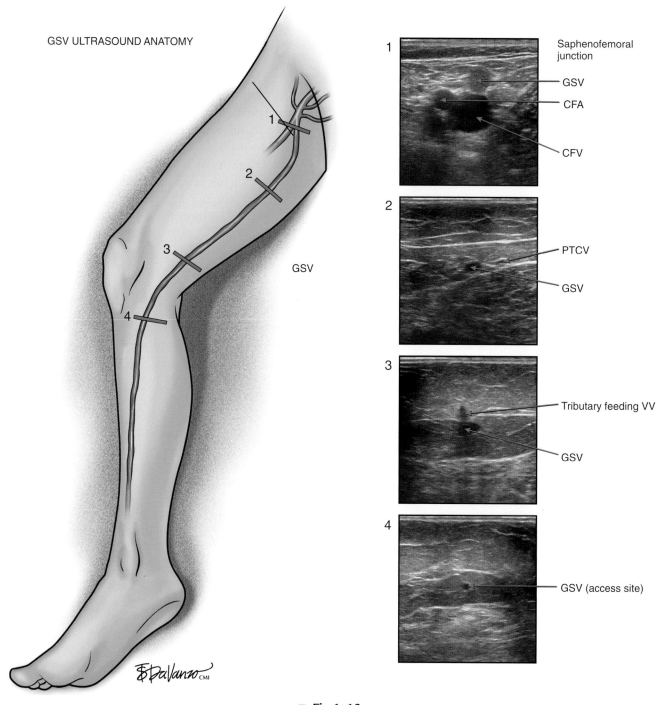

GSV ULTRASOUND ANATOMY

GSV

1 Saphenofemoral junction

GSV

CFA

CFV

2 PTCV

GSV

3 Tributary feeding VV

GSV

4 GSV (access site)

■ Fig 1–12

ETIOLOGY AND NATURAL HISTORY OF DISEASE

Early theories were based on the belief that varicose veins resulted from the effects of venous hypertension secondary to valvular incompetence at the saphenofemoral or saphenopopliteal junction resulting in retrograde flow of blood down a hydrostatic pressure gradient. Unfortunately, there is little evidence of a constitutive valvular abnormality in primary venous disease. The theories do not explain why truncal varicosities are often found below competent valves, why normal valves are often seen between variceal segments, or why venous dilation often precedes valvular incompetence.[4,5] Rather than being initiated at the saphenofemoral junction, both detailed studies of surgical specimens and ultrasound observation suggest that primary valvular incompetence is a multicentric process that develops simultaneously in discontinuous venous segments.[6]

Histologic and ultrastructural studies of varicose saphenous veins have found hypertrophy of the vein wall with increased collagen content,[7] together with disruption of the orderly arrangements of smooth muscle cells and elastin fibers.[8,9] Cultures of smooth muscle cells from varicose saphenous veins have demonstrated disturbed collagen synthesis, overproduction of collagen type I, and reduced synthesis of collagen type III.[10] Because collagen type I is thought to confer rigidity and collagen type III to confer distensibility to tissues, such changes could contribute to the weakness and reduced elasticity of varicose veins. A complicating factor is the heterogeneity of the varicose vein wall; hypertrophic segments can alternate with thinner atrophic segments with fewer smooth muscle cells and reduced extracellular matrix.

Despite advances in our understanding of varicose veins, the underlying etiology remains elusive. Varicose veins demonstrate diverse histologic abnormalities, including irregular thickening of the intima, fibrosis between the intima and adventitia, atrophy and disruption of elastic fibers, thickening of individual collagen fibers, and disorganization of the muscular layers in varicosed tributaries.[11-15] Varicose veins have increased collagen with a decrease in smooth muscle and elastin content.[16,17] Most recent evidence suggests that such changes in the vein wall precede the development of reflux.[18,19] The exact cause of primary valvular incompetence in superficial veins remains unknown. However, valvular incompetence is thought to result as a phenomenon secondary to dilatation of weakened vein walls, with enlargement of the valve ring preventing adaptation of the leaflets.[17] Interestingly, studies suggest the strength of the valves is far greater than the strength of the venous wall.[19]

PEARLS AND PITFALLS

Successful treatment is predicated on an accurate diagnosis. In the field of endovascular venous surgery, the key to diagnostic accuracy is a thorough understanding of venous anatomy.

REFERENCES

1. Caggiati A, Bergan JJ, Gloviczki P, et al. International Interdisciplinary Consensus Committee on Venous Anatomical Terminology. Nomenclature of the veins of the lower limbs: an international interdisciplinary consensus statement. J Vasc Surg 2002;36:416-422.
2. Caggiati A, Bergan JJ, Gloviczki P, et al. International Interdisciplinary Consensus Committee on Venous Anatomical Terminology. Nomenclature of the veins of the lower limb: extensions, refinements, and clinical application. J Vasc Surg 2005;41:719-724.

3. Mahakkanukrauh P, Chomsung R. Anatomical variations of the sural nerve. Clin Anat 2002;15:263-266.
4. Alexander CJ. The theoretical basis of varicose vein formation. Med J Aust 1972;1:258-261.
5. Cotton LT. Varicose veins. Gross anatomy and development. Br J Surg 1961;48:589-597.
6. Labropoulos N, Giannoukas AD, Delis K, et al. Where does venous reflux start? J Vasc Surg 1997;26:736-742.
7. Travers JP, Brookes CE, Evans J, et al. Assessment of wall structure and composition of varicose veins with reference to collagen, elastin and smooth muscle content. Eur J Vasc Endovasc Surg 1996;11:230-237.
8. Porto LC, Ferreira MA, Costa AM, et al. Immunolabeling of type IV collagen, laminin, and alpha-smooth muscle actin cells in the intima of normal and varicose saphenous veins. Angiology 1998;49:391-398.
9. Wali MA, Eid RA. Changes of elastic and collagen fibers in varicose veins. Int Angiol 2002;21:337-343.
10. Sansilvestri-Morel P, Rupin A, Badier-Commander C, et al. Imbalance in the synthesis of collagen type I and collagen type III in smooth muscle cells derived from human varicose veins. J Vasc Res 2001;38:560-568.
11. Ascher E, Jacob T, Hingorani A, et al. Expression of molecular mediators of apoptosis and their role in the pathogenesis of lower-extremity varicose veins. J Vasc Surg 2001;33: 1080-1086.
12. Bouissou H, Julian M, Pieraggi MT, et al. Vein morphology. Phlebology 1988;3(suppl 1):1-11.
13. Jones GT, Solomon C, Moaveni A, et al. Venous morphology predicts class of chronic venous insufficiency. Eur J Vasc Endovasc Surg 1999;18:349-354.
14. Lowell RC, Gloviczki P, Miller VM. In vitro evaluation of endothelial and smooth muscle function of primary varicose veins. J Vasc Surg 1992;16:679-686.
15. Porto LC, Azizi MA, Pelajo-Machado M, et al. Elastic fibers in saphenous varicose veins. Angiology 2002;53:131-140.
16. Travers JP, Brookes CE, Evans J, et al. Assessment of wall structure and composition of varicose veins with reference to collagen, elastin and smooth muscle content. Eur J Vasc Endovasc Surg 1996;11:230-237.
17. Gandhi RH, Irizarry E, Nackman GB, et al. Analysis of the connective tissue matrix and proteolytic activity of primary varicose veins. J Vasc Surg 1993;18:814-820.
18. Rose SS, Ahmed A. Some thoughts on the aetiology of varicose veins. J Cardiovasc Surg 1986;27:534-543.
19. Cotton LT. Varicose veins. Gross anatomy and development. Br J Surg 1961;48:589-597.

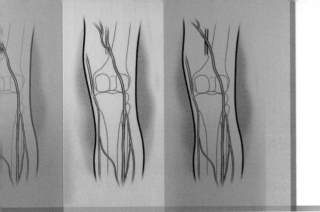

CHAPTER 2

Noninvasive Testing

Jose I. Almeida

HISTORICAL BACKGROUND

Of the 25 million Americans with venous disease, approximately 7 million exhibit serious symptoms such as edema, skin changes, and venous ulcers. One million seek formal medical advice annually. Of these, 80% of venous patients are managed conservatively with observation, leg elevation, and support stockings, while the remainder are treated surgically with vein stripping or endovenous ablation. With the development of safe, less traumatic, and effective endovenous techniques for venous insufficiency, most venous surgeons acknowledge that more patients will seek treatment, and physicians will be more inclined to move from conservative therapy to surgical therapy.

Physiologic testing is used to identify, grade, and follow venous insufficiency and to define deep venous thrombosis (DVT). Since more patients will be presenting for therapy because of improved outcomes with endovenous techniques over traditional surgery, physiologic testing will take on increasing importance. For purposes of this chapter, physiologic testing includes the various plethysmography devices and color flow duplex imaging. The goal of these studies is to provide accurate information describing the hemodynamic or anatomic characteristics of the patient with chronic venous insufficiency, precluding the need for invasive studies[2] (Fig. 2-1).[1]

ETIOLOGY AND NATURAL HISTORY OF DISEASE

The venous system in the lower extremities is composed of three interconnected parts: the deep system, the perforating system, and the superficial system. In healthy veins, blood flows toward the right side of the heart (i.e., upward) and from the superficial system to the deep system (i.e., inward), driven by the venous muscular pump and unidirectional valves. Lower extremity muscle compartments contract during ambulation; this contraction compresses the deep veins, producing a pumping action, which propels blood upward toward the right side of the heart. Transient pressures in the deep system have been recorded as high as 5 atmospheres (atm) during strenuous lower extremity exertion. This pumping action secondary to ambulation has the effect of reducing pressure within the superficial system (Figs. 2-2 and 2-3).

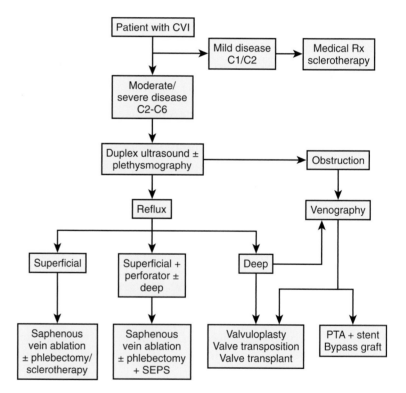

■ **Fig 2–1** Flowchart of chronic venous insufficiency.

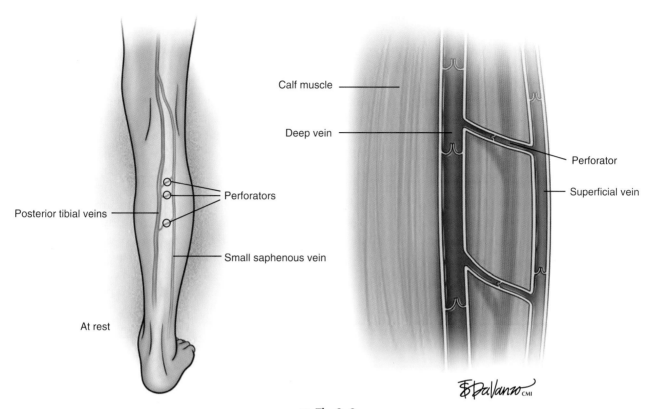

Calf muscle

Deep vein

Perforator

Superficial vein

Posterior tibial veins

Perforators

Small saphenous vein

At rest

■ **Fig 2-2**

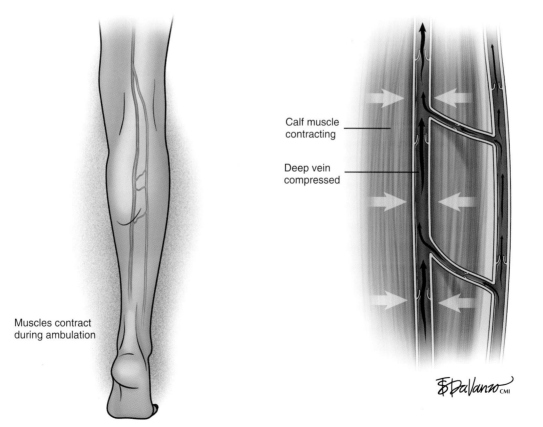

Calf muscle
contracting

Deep vein
compressed

Muscles contract
during ambulation

■ **Fig 2-3**

All three venous systems of the lower extremity are subjected to hydrostatic pressure. A fluid column has weight and can produce a pressure gradient. In an individual who has a height of 6 feet, the distance from the level of the right atrium to the ankle is 120 cm and produces a hydrostatic pressure of approximately 90 mm Hg (Fig. 2-4). Deep veins can withstand elevated pressure because the fascia in which they exist limits dilation. In contrast, the superficial system, surrounded by fat and elastic skin, is constructed for low pressure; therefore, elevated pressure in the superficial system can produce dilation, elongation, and valve failure. Dilation increases the diameter of the veins and elongation causes them to be more tortuous.

Because of valve failure, supraphysiologic pressure develops in the superficial venous system and venous dilation ensues (other theories suggest that it is the vein wall that fails with subsequent loss of valvular coaptation). With dilation and multiple valve failure, venous blood will flow in the direction of the pressure gradient, which is downward and outward. This flow direction is directly opposite physiologic flow (i.e., upward and inward). The early result is varicose veins and telangiectasia, which are visible on the skin surface. Symptoms of early or mild superficial venous incompetence produce low-level pain, edema, burning, throbbing, and leg cramping. As the disease progresses, patients can develop venous stasis changes that can lead to debilitating severe soft tissue ulceration. On the basis of hemodynamics and clinical experience, symptoms can improve dramatically on elimination of high pressure or flow in diseased superficial venous channels.

INSTRUMENTATION

Plethysmography

To understand lower extremity venous hemodynamics, venous pressure measurements by dorsal foot vein cannulation can be instructive. The cannula tubing is connected to a fluid column. With the subject standing erect, the fluid column will rise to the level of the right atrium. This is due to the fact that right atrial pressure is near zero and, therefore, the dorsal foot vein pressure at the cannulation site is almost entirely based on the subject's hydrostatic blood column (the subject's blood and the fluid in the column have nearly the same *specific weight*). When the subject is asked to perform repeated ankle flexion, the fluid column drops to between 50% and 60% of its resting height. This simulates walking and the reduction in superficial venous pressure secondary to the ambulatory venous pump. In subjects with venous insufficiency, the fluid column will not drop to normal levels. If a subject's fluid column falls to normal levels during occlusion of the superficial system, the observer knows the deep system is intact and the superficial system is incompetent. If the fluid column remains elevated with exclusion of the superficial system, the

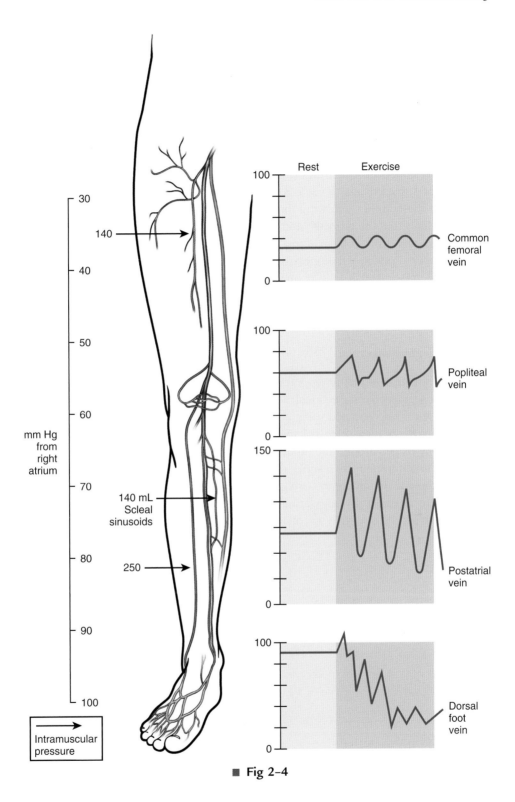

■ Fig 2–4

observer knows the deep system is incompetent. Physiologic venous testing is based on these principles (Fig. 2-5).

Plethysmographs are devices that measure volume change. During the past 50 years, plethysmographs have been developed and used clinically that employ completely different principles. Descriptions of four plethysmographs are given next.

Impedance Plethysmograph

The impedance plethysmograph (IPG) is based on a fundamental principle of electronics, which states that voltage (V) across a segment is equal to the impedance (Z) of the segment multiplied by the current (I) flowing through the segment ($V = Z \times I$). It is possible to isolate a portion of a limb (e.g., thigh, calf) and subject the limb segment to a standard and known current while measuring the voltage across the segment. Blood, subcutaneous tissue, and even bone v impedance. In practice, the operator places circular electrodes around the segment of interest, generally the proximal calf, and connects the electrodes to the electrical console. The subject is asked to perform a series of maneuvers, and outputs from the device are recorded. This method has been used with success by some investigators in the assessment of DVT and venous insufficiency.

Straingauge Plethysmograph

A straingauge plethysmograph (SGP) measures circumference of a limb segment, which is related to segment cross-sectional area. Cross-sectional area multiplied by length equals volume. The device is constructed using a small hollow elastic tube filled with mercury and an electrical circuit capable of measuring voltage across the tubing length. The tube containing the mercury is carefully placed around the limb segment of interest and connected to the electric circuit. The subject is asked to perform a series of maneuvers and outputs from the device are recorded. As the limb segment circumference is changed secondary to venous blood volume, the length of the elastic tube changes. By measuring circumference as a function of time, venous blood volume as a function of time may be measured.

Photoplethysmograph

Photoplethysmographs (PPGs) are not true plethysmographs because they measure cutaneous microvasculature. PPG instrumentation includes a surface transducer, which is taped to the lower leg just above the medial malleolus and connected to an electrical circuit. The electrical circuit excites the transducer and records and interprets the returning signal. The PPG transducer is designed with an infrared light emitting diode and a photosensor. The transducer transmits light to the skin, which is both scattered and absorbed by the tissue in the illuminated field. Blood is more opaque than surrounding tissue and therefore attenuates the reflected signal more than other tissue in the field. The intensity of reflected light is reduced with more blood in the field. If the electrical circuit filters the higher frequency arterial pulsations, it is possible to register a signal, which qualitatively corresponds to venous volume in the segment of interest.

Air Plethysmograph

An air bladder (cuff) is connected to a console via a single rubber tube, and any change in limb volume is measured by a pressure change within the bladder. If limb volume increases, the bladder volume will decrease, but the bladder pressure will increase. An air plethysmograph (APG) is able to detect changes in venous limb volume secondary to various patient maneuvers. The APG is used in the clinical assessment of venous insufficiency and DVT. The use of the APG

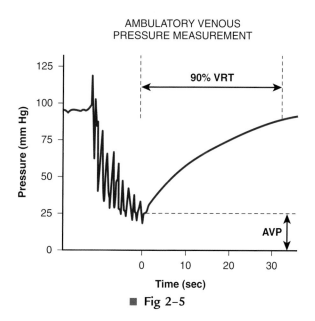

■ Fig 2–5

is based on the use of air bladders, which are devices similar to standard blood pressure cuffs. Physiologic parameters related to chronic venous disease such as chronic obstruction, valvular reflux, calf muscle pump function, and venous hypertension can be measured (Figs. 2-6 and 2-7).

Plethysmography for Venous Insufficiency

Venous insufficiency is characterized by misdirected flow between the three venous systems of the lower extremity. When the patient is supine, the venous pressure in the lower extremities is slightly above right atrial pressure (about 0 mm Hg). In the erect position, the lower extremity venous pressure increases due to the hydrostatic column of blood extending from the right atrium to the segment of interest. Because veins are compliant, venous blood volume in the segment of interest increases. This volume increase is displayed on a graph from which measurements may be taken.

First, the patient is supine, and outflow testing identifies obstruction and the degree of superficial collateralization. Next, the patient is asked to stand, and the filling rate of the veins by

■ Fig 2–6

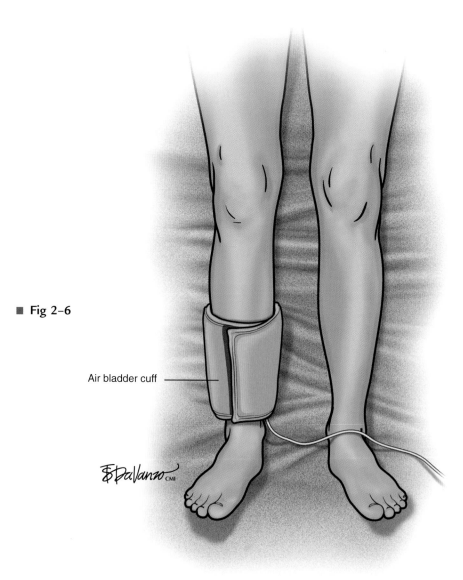

Air bladder cuff

Supine position

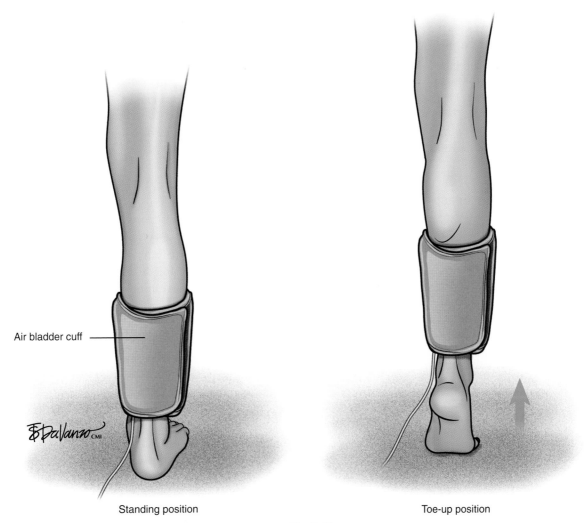

Air bladder cuff

Standing position

Toe-up position

■ **Fig 2–7**

reflux through incompetent valves is measured. The patient is then asked to perform a toe-up exercise, and the calf muscle pump function is measured as an ejection fraction. Finally, the patient performs 10 toe-ups quickly, and a noninvasive measure of ambulatory venous pressure is completed.

Venous Filling Index

Briefly, venous filling index (VFI) is the venous filling index that represents the average filling rate of the veins to 90% of the total venous volume (VV) after first being emptied by gravity. VFI does not rely on the calf muscle pump for complete vein emptying. Ejection fraction (EF) represents the efficiency of the calf muscle pump and is analogous to left ventricular ejection fraction used in cardiology. Residual volume fraction (RVF) is proportional to the invasively measured ambulatory venous pressure, which is a global measurement related to severity of disease. It is important to recognize that VFI measures thigh-to-calf reflux only. Perforator reflux has no effect on VFI, nor does reflux isolated to either the calf or the thigh.

The patient must help in obtaining a clean VFI trace by standing up smoothly and without bumping the cuff. Remind the patient to relax the leg muscles and keep the knee slightly bent to prevent popliteal entrapment.

Ejection Fraction

The EF test consists of three steps. First, the patient applies equal weight on both legs. Next, the patient does his or her best toe-up effort using both legs equally and without supporting his or her weight on the support frame, which is used only for balance. The patient remains in the toe-up position for several seconds until the ejection volume is stable (plateau). Finally, the patient returns to the resting position by removing his or her weight from the test leg with the toe just touching the floor. The veins will quickly refill.

Patients with poor outflow (deep vein obstruction) will take longer to expel calf blood with the single toe-up movement. If the patient were to perform the toe-up exercise quickly, less blood would be ejected past the obstructed vein and the calf pump would appear less effective.

The possible causes of poor calf muscle pump are (1) non–venous-related problems, including arthritis, ankylosis, and neurologic deficit (whatever prevents the patient from performing a good toe-up movement); (2) proximal obstruction that prevents blood from quickly exiting the calf veins; (3) incompetent calf perforator veins that shunt blood from the deep to the superficial system within the calf; and (4) calf varicosities that retain a large venous volume not expelled with calf muscle contraction.

Residual Volume Fraction

Before beginning the RVF test, one should be certain that VFI testing is completed. The exercise hyperemia resulting from the 10 toe-ups will almost certainly increase VFI and may be mistaken as reflux. The 10 toe-ups are performed similarly to the single toe-up in the EF test, but they are done quickly, approximately one per second. After that, the veins are allowed to refill while the patient stands in the resting position (all weight on the nontested leg). Finally, the patient is returned to the supine position with the operator holding the heel/ankle of the test leg up at 45 degrees with the knee slightly bent. This position is held until an ending baseline is reached. The ending baseline (after the RVF test) may be higher or lower than the baseline value at the beginning of the VFI test.

Recently, the RVF test has been modified by having the patient walk on a treadmill. Walking is no longer simulated by the 10 toe-up movements and the effect of the calf pump is a more accurate reflection of ambulating. Treadmill testing better shows the subtle differences in calf pump function found with the use of compression stockings. The toe-up movement may be such an overpowering use of the calf pump that the effect of compression stockings is overwhelmed and unnoticed.

DEEP VENOUS THROMBOSIS BY PLETHYSMOGRAPHY

The deep venous system is not only a conduit for returning blood to the right side of the heart but is also a storage or capacitant system. This means its volume changes rapidly relative to pressure. If one examines a vein at low pressure, the walls are nearly fully collapsed and only a small flow channel is present. It takes very little increase in internal fluid pressure to expand the flow channel of a vein. Finally, if there is obstruction in a segment of deep vein, despite rich venous collateral channels, venous pressure distal to the obstruction will increase. Examination by plethysmography makes use of these two principles (i.e., volume change with increased pressure and resistance).

Typically, a plethysmograph transducer is placed at the calf or distal thigh with the patient lying supine on a table. In the case of APG, the transducer is an air bladder inflated to 5 mm Hg; in the case of PPG, the transducer is a light-emitting diode. Proximal to the transducer, a method of rapidly occluding the deep system must be used. For all transducers, this can be a thigh cuff inflated rapidly by hand bulb or automatic inflator.

With the transducer recording a stable venous signal at 5 mm/s chart speed, the pressure in the proximal occluding cuff is rapidly elevated to 50 mm Hg. The transducer is measuring absolute levels of volume. With the increased pressure in the proximal cuff, venous blood in the deep system cannot pass under the cuff until the venous pressure reaches approximately occluding cuff pressure. This increase in venous pressure (i.e., pooling) develops because the proximal cuff does not obstruct the arterial inflow. After about 20 to 40 seconds, pressure in the distal venous system reaches the pressure in the occluding cuff and venous volume reaches a plateau. Once the plateau has been reached, the operator rapidly releases the pressure in the occluding cuff. The pooled venous blood can then return to the right side of the heart via the larger veins upstream. Two measures of venous hemodynamics are taken during this test. First, there is the volume increase from the baseline to the plateau. This is known as *segmental venous capacitance* and represents the blood storage capacity of the segment vein. This is generally quoted in millimeters of deflection or milliliters if the system is calibrated to volume. The second measurement is the slope of the volume-time curve immediately after the pressure in the occluding cuff is released. This is known as *maximum venous outflow* (MVO) and represents resistance to blood flow in the deep system. This may be quoted in millimeters of deflection per second or milliliters per second if the system is calibrated to volume.

This technique has been largely replaced by duplex ultrasound, which is much more sensitive and specific for the detection of DVT.

CONTINUOUS-WAVE DOPPLER

Continuous-wave (CW) Doppler instruments are widely available, relatively inexpensive, and used extensively to rapidly investigate the peripheral vascular system. CW Doppler measurements can be used independently or, as mentioned earlier, combined with measurements from a plethysmograph.

Deep Venous Thrombosis

With the patient standing, the points of interest include the common femoral vein at the inguinal ligament, the popliteal vein at the popliteal fossa, and the posterior tibial vein just behind the medial malleolus. With the pencil-like probe positioned toward the venous flow and at 60 degrees to the flow streamline, the target velocity is optimized. The fact that a velocity is identified means the vein is patent at the target level, and this is the first of three major diagnostic criteria. The second diagnostic criterion is associated with the spontaneous and phasic nature of the signal. When veins are not obstructed proximal to the target vein, the local pressure is low and local velocity changes as a function of respiration. Low-pressure veins collapse and local velocity is often reduced to zero shortly after inspiration. This is due to the fact that when the diaphragm moves down on inspiration, pressure in the closed abdominal cavity increases and collapses veins at low pressure. With proximal obstruction, this phasic velocity is disturbed and becomes continuous. The third criterion is associated with velocity response secondary to distal compression. When veins are unobstructed proximal to the target and compression is performed distally, the local velocity will increase in response to compression. In a high resistance proximal venous system, distal compression will not evoke increased velocity.

If a subject demonstrates at the femoral, popliteal, and posterior tibial veins good velocity signals that are phasic with respiration and augment with distal compression, the chance of DVT involving the iliac, common femoral, femoral, or popliteal veins is very low. DVT limited to the calf veins is more problematic due to vein duplication at this level.

Venous Insufficiency

The main use of CW Doppler signal in venous insufficiency is in assessing reflux in the major deep veins of the lower extremity (common femoral, femoral, and popliteal veins). This procedure is most effectively performed with the subject standing. To the extent possible, weight should be shifted to the contralateral leg. A bidirectional CW Doppler signal with a stereo audio signal and printout is recommended. For venous work, an ultrasound frequency range of 5 to 7 MHz is suggested. Unlike duplex ultrasound, with CW Doppler signal the exact path of the target vein is not well defined. Therefore, in practice the operator will have to manually adjust the probe angle to obtain the maximum signal (audio level and velocity level). The concept is quite simple; target veins are assessed for reversal of flow velocity after rapid manual limb compression and release. The more reversal, the more reflux there is. In terms of diagnostic criteria, a normal vein demonstrates no evidence of reflux when this technique is used. Flow reversal can be assessed both by audio signal and by examination of velocity-versus-time printouts.

DUPLEX ULTRASOUND

Duplex ultrasound has become the gold standard in the diagnosis of both DVTs and venous insufficiency and has replaced the use of venous plethysmographs, CW Dopplers signals, and contrast venography. Power color pulsed-wave Doppler signals with high-resolution B-mode imaging characterize state-of-the-art duplex ultrasound.

Deep Venous System

The examination should be performed on a flat examining table in which the patient's lower extremities are placed in the dependent position at approximately 15 degrees. This slight angle dilates the deep system, which makes the identification of veins easier and improves the velocity signals. Deep vein interrogation from the level of the inguinal ligament to the ankle should include the common femoral, femoral, popliteal, and tibial veins. The deep femoral vein should also be included, especially in cases where femoral vein thrombosis has been identified.

The evaluation begins at the groin using gray-scale imaging. Usually seen are the common femoral vein, common femoral artery, and great saphenous vein (GSV), forming a "Mickey Mouse image." We have found keeping the lateral (arterial) structures on the left side of the screen for both the right and left leg to be helpful. This requires that the technologist rotate the linear array probe 180 degrees when moving from the right to the left leg. The marker on the probe should be oriented to the lateral aspect of the leg. With this orientation, Mickey's face is the common femoral vein and is the larger and lower of the three structures. The common femoral artery forms Mickey's right ear, and the GSV forms Mickey's left ear. As the probe is moved distally, the GSV will disappear, and the common femoral artery will divide into the superficial femoral artery and the deep femoral artery. As the probe continues distally, the technologist should focus on keeping the superficial femoral artery and the femoral vein in clear view. The popliteal artery and the popliteal vein are difficult to visualize in the adductor canal; therefore, these structures are identified from behind by placing the probe in the popliteal crease. In the calf, the duplicated posterior tibial and peroneal veins with their associated single arteries can be viewed from a medial approach as they travel between the muscle bellies. Similarly, the gastrocnemius and soleus veins are identified; however, they are located within the muscular bellies. In general, the anterior tibial veins are not interrogated because they are rarely pathologic (Fig 2-8).

With the probe, the technologist can compress the vein in the short axis view. The ability to fully compress the vein walls—and obliterate the venous lumen momentarily—confirms vein patency and absence of thrombus formation (Fig. 2-9). If the technologist identifies thrombus, the next step is to determine its age. Acute thrombi are characterized by vein dilatation and noncompressible echolucent material, while chronic thrombi take on a speckled, hyperechoic ultrasonic appearance.

If the evaluated system from the common femoral vein through the tibial veins is compressible and no evidence of thrombus formation is seen, the study is considered negative for DVT. The technologist may use the Doppler portion of the duplex system in the long-axis view to verify artery versus vein and determine flow direction. Color Doppler signals, power Doppler signals, compression maneuvers, and respiratory maneuvers can be used to supplement this procedure if necessary. Normal veins have spontaneous flow, which is phasic with respiration.

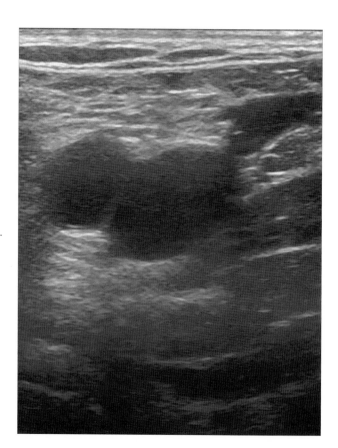

■ **Fig 2–8** Mickey Mouse image.

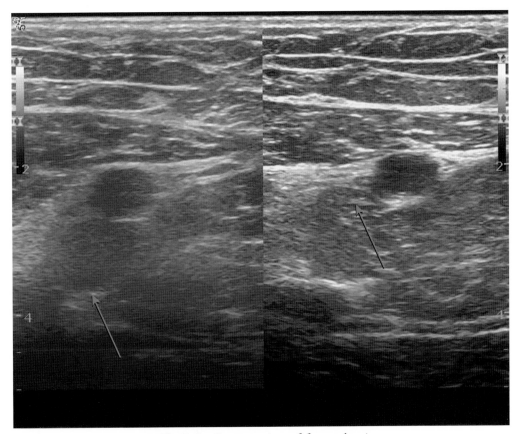

■ **Fig 2–9** Compression of femoral vein.

Superficial Venous System

For superficial venous studies, patients are examined in the erect position. The patient is asked to rotate the leg of interest to expose the medial surface of the lower extremity from the groin to the ankle. To the extent possible, weight should be shifted from the leg of interest to relax the musculature. A standing stool with arm support may be necessary.

Once positioned, the technician begins at the groin and produces the Mickey Mouse landmark described earlier. Starting from the three-vessel image in the transverse view, the probe descends down the leg following the course of the GSV. The normal GSV extends from the saphenofemoral junction to the ankle and is enveloped by superficial fascia above and muscular fascia below. Diameter measurements are recorded in millimeters, and the presence of reflux (positive or negative) is documented at the saphenofemoral junction, midthigh, and below knee. If reflux is present, the duration of retrograde flow in seconds is also documented.

Reflux is determined at locations of interest using the following technique.[2] The technologist adjusts the color box of the Duplex system in the measurement location. The velocity scale is adjusted (maximum 25 cm/s). While a signal is being obtained, the technologist compresses the calf (below the probe) in a brisk manner. The vein highlighted in the color box should demonstrate an increase in velocity toward the heart with compression. On release, the vein should demonstrate no velocity or minimal velocity away from the heart. We have found that reflux (venous flow away from the heart after release) lasting between 0.5 to 2.0 seconds is mild. Reflux is severe if present longer than 2.0 seconds.

The same evaluation is repeated posteriorly for the small saphenous vein (SSV). This vein originates in the distal calf and can terminate in the upper thigh. We access this vessel with ultrasound by rotating the subject to expose the back of the legs. We identify the SSV at the distal calf and advance over the course of the SSV. Multiple levels may be assessed; however, we generally record a characteristic SSV diameter (in millimeters) and assess reflux in the most diseased location (Fig. 2-10).

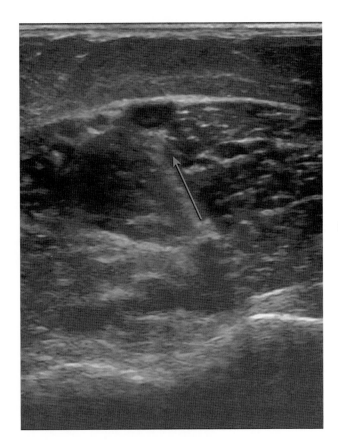

■ **Fig 2–10** Small saphenous vein.

It is important to note that there are variations in superficial venous anatomy. For example, the GSV may be quite small and complemented by an anterior accessory saphenous vein, which may be competent or incompetent. Further, the GSV may be duplicated in portions of its course. It is worth repeating that these variations are common and must be known and anticipated by the technologist if a comprehensive report is to be generated.

The lower extremity has some common perforators that play significant roles in venous insufficiency. Hunterian perforating veins are located in the midthigh. Dodd perforating veins are located at the distal thigh. The Boyd perforating vein is located below the level of the popliteal fossa. Finally, Cockett No. 1, 2, and 3 perforating veins are located between the ankle and the lower calf, respectively. This assessment must also be part of this work-up. If present, perforators should be assessed regarding diameter, degree of reflux, and extension to other superficial structures.

Duplex ultrasound is not only diagnostic but also plays crucial roles in endovenous ablation, ultrasound-guided sclerotherapy, and monitoring the success of vein closure procedures (Figs. 2-11 through 2-17).

Text continued on p. 46

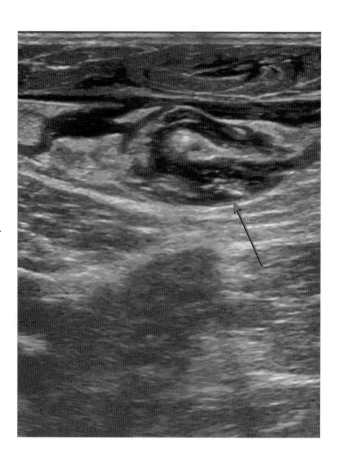

■ **Fig 2–11** Perivenous tumescent anesthesia.

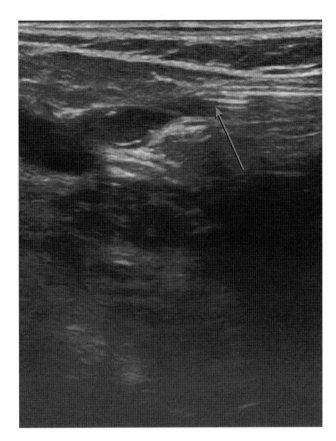

■ **Fig 2–12** Position of radiofrequency catheter at saphenofemoral junction.

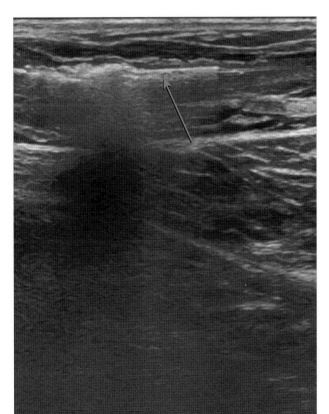

■ **Fig 2–13** Steam bubble formation during endovenous laser.

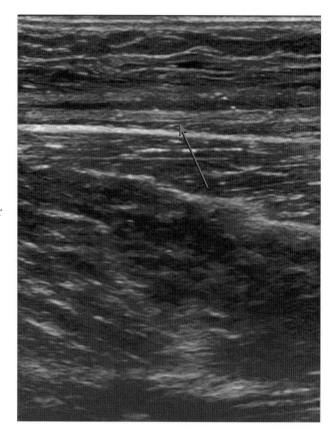

■ **Fig 2-14** Thick vein walls after radiofrequency ablation of great saphenous vein (GSV).

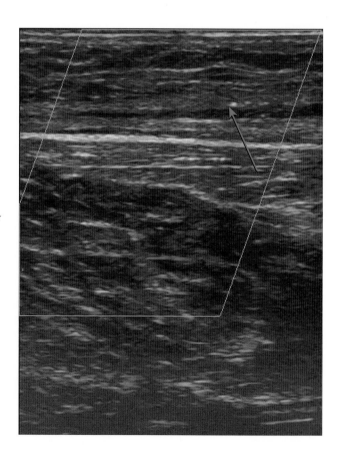

■ **Fig 2-15** No flow in saphenous vein by color flow duplex imaging (CFDI).

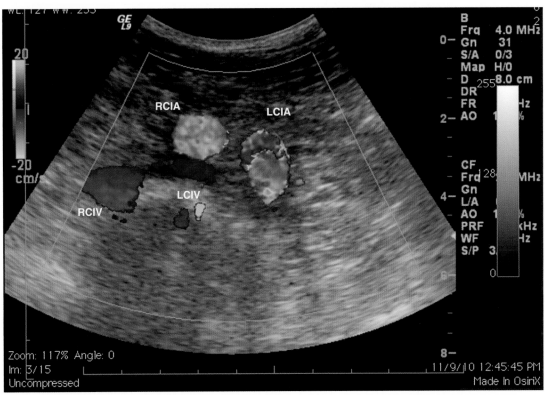

■ **Fig 2–16** Ultrasound image of left common iliac vein compression from overlying right common iliac artery (RCIA). *LCIA,* Left common iliac artery; *LCIV,* left common iliac vein; *RCIV,* right common iliac vein.

MIAMI VEIN CENTER
NON-INVASIVE VENOUS EVALUATION

NAME:_____ DATE:_____ MED. REC#:_____

SEX: M/F DOB:___/___/___AGE:_____   ATTENDING PHY: **Jose I. Almeida, M.D. FACS**

HISTORY:_____

PREVIOUS DVT:_____ PULM EMBOLI: _____ ANTICOAGULANTS:_____IVC FILTER:_____

New Patients

RIGHT CEAP: 0 1 2 3 4 5 6				**LEFT** CEAP: 0 1 2 3 4 5 6			
Right	**Reflux +/−**	**Flow:** **C = cont** **P = phasic**	**Size** **(mm)**	**Left**	**Reflux +/−**	**Flow:** **C = cont** **P = phasic**	**Size** **(mm)**
CIV				CIV			
EIV				EIV			
CFV				CFV			
PFV				PFV			
FV				FV			
POP				POP			
PT				PT			
PERO				PERO			

Follow-up Patients

RIGHT AND **LEFT**: There is patency, phasicity, and augmentation of CFV, SFV, DFV, and popliteal vein. All vessels are fully compressible in transverse view. The tibials are well visualized and patent.

Comments:

_____

ULTRASOUND MACHINE: GE-9/GE-e   TECHNOLOGIST:_____ DATE:_____

PHYSICIAN:_____

Revised 2/2010

A

■ **Fig 2–17 A,** Documentation of deep veins.

MIAMI VEIN CENTER
SUPERFICIAL VEIN MAPPING

Name:	Date:___/___/___
DOB____/_____/_____	Patient ID#
Indications:	

Right Reflux	+/−	Reflux Duration (sec)		Left Reflux	+/−	Reflux Duration (sec)
GSV						
AASV						
Other						
SSV						

	D (mm)				D (mm)	
	GSV	AASV			GSV	AASV
SFJ						
MT						
BK						
SSV						
Perforators						
Tributaries						

Comments:
Ultrasound Machine: GE-9 / GE-E   Technologist:

Revised 10/4/2010

B

■ **Fig 2–17, cont'd B,** Documentation of superficial vein mapping.

REFERENCES

1. Marston WA. PPG, APG, duplex: which noninvasive tests are most appropriate for the management of patients with chronic venous insufficiency? Semin Vasc Surg 2002;15: 13-20.
2. Raines JK, Almeida JI. Role of physiologic testing in venous disorders. In: Bergan JJ. The Vein Book. San Diego: Elsevier; 2007:47-55.

CHAPTER 3

Venous Pathophysiology

Rafael D. Malgor and Nicos Labropoulos

ETIOLOGY AND NATURAL HISTORY OF DISEASE

Primary Venous Disease

Primary venous disease affects two-thirds of patients with chronic venous disease (CVD). The most accepted theory is based on increased venous hydrostatic pressure transmitted to the vein wall, causing smooth muscle relaxation, endothelial damage, and extracellular matrix degradation with subsequent vein wall weakening and wall dilatation.[1] It has also been suggested that valve damage may occur because of local inflammation.[2] Leukocyte migration, plasma-granulocyte activation, and increased activity of metalloproteinases causing degradation of the valve leaflets support that theory.[2,3] Figure 3-1 summarizes the pathophysiologic pathways of CVD.

Superficial veins are most commonly involved in primary CVD, followed by perforators and deep veins.[4] It has been shown that reflux starts in superficial veins in more than 80% of the patients. In the early stages of CVD, reflux is found in the great saphenous vein (GSV) and its tributaries without almost any junctional involvement (Fig. 3-2). This is followed by reflux in the small saphenous vein (SSV) system (Fig. 3-3) and nonsaphenous veins (Fig. 3-4). Patients with competent saphenous, perforators, and deep veins may also present tributary reflux in 10%, with the GSV tributaries being affected in 65% of the cases.

Text continued on p. 52

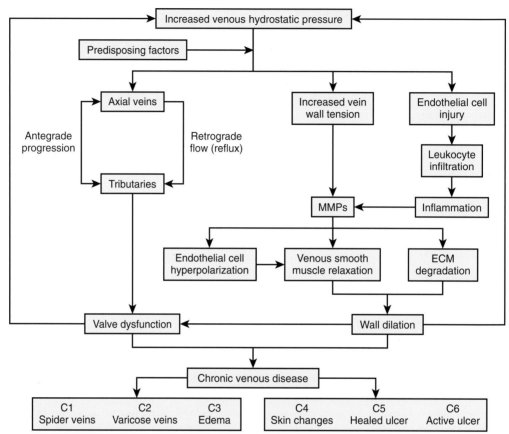

■ **Fig 3-1** Mechanisms of varicose vein formation. Increased hydrostatic pressure and wall tension in individuals with predisposing risk factors cause matrix metalloproteinase (MMPs) activation and changes in the endothelium and vascular smooth muscle function. In addition, leukocyte wall infiltration and inflammation activate MMPs and lead to extracellular matrix (ECM) degradation, venous wall weakening, and wall/valve fibrosis. Although a possible mechanism may involve primary valve insufficiency in both the axial and tributary veins, this likely represents a secondary event from primary venous wall changes and dilation. Persistent venous wall dilation and valvular dysfunction lead to increased hydrostatic pressure. MMP-mediated vein wall dilation with secondary valve dysfunction leads to chronic venous disease (CVD) and varicose vein formation. The early stages of CVD are maintained within the vasculature, leading to clinical signs of varicose veins, while more advanced CVD causes progression of chronic venous insufficiency affecting surrounding tissues and leading to skin changes and ulcer formation. *(From Raffetto JD, Khalil RA. Mechanisms of varicose vein formation: valve dysfunction and wall dilation. Phlebology 2008;23:85-98.)*

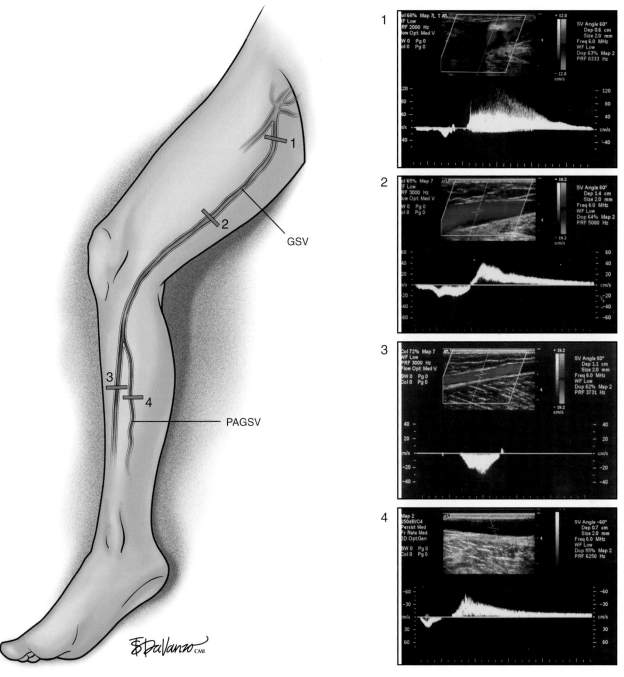

■ **Fig 3-2** Great saphenous vein (GSV) reflux from saphenofemoral junction to upper calf and the posterior accessory calf vein. The below knee segment of GSV is normal.

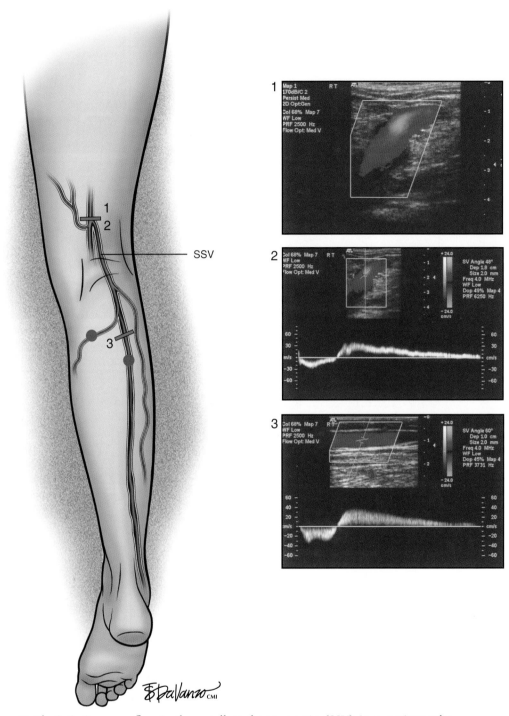

■ **Fig 3-3** Severe reflux in the small saphenous vein (SSV) in a patient who presented with CEAP classes 1 through 4, itching, and pain during prolonged standing. Reflux was also found in two tributaries and two perforator veins (*red dots*).

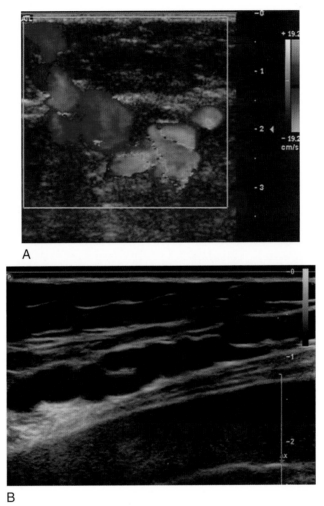

■ **Fig 3–4** Nonsaphenous vein reflux. **A,** Vulvar vein reflux in a female patient with a history of three pregnancies. The veins from this region are very tortuous and extend in a nonpredicted manner in the extremity. **B,** Sciatic nerve vein reflux giving rise to popliteal fossa varicosities that emerge in the posterolateral calf.

Isolated primary deep vein reflux is rare. It may present as either segmental or axial reflux extending from the femoral vein in the thigh to the below-knee popliteal vein. The most frequent location of primary deep vein reflux is the common femoral vein, followed by the femoral and popliteal veins[5] (Fig. 3-5). Because most deep venous reflux is deemed to be caused by superficial venous reflux propagation, both common femoral and femoral vein reflux are associated with GSV incompetence and popliteal vein reflux is associated with SSV and/or gastrocnemial vein incompetence[5] (Fig. 3-6). In addition, deep vein reflux has a shorter duration compared with superficial venous reflux. Association between deep and superficial venous reflux ranges from 5% to 38%.[5-8]

Perforator vein (PV) reflux in primary CVD always occurs in association with superficial vein reflux.[9] Essentially, PVs become incompetent secondary to either ascending extension of superficial vein reflux or descending propagation of the reflux in a reentry fashion (Fig. 3-7). Most often, PV reflux originates from the GSV system and renders the deep veins incompetent in 13% of the cases.[9] Deep vein reflux secondary to PV reflux is usually segmental and has a short duration.[9]

Text continued on p. 60

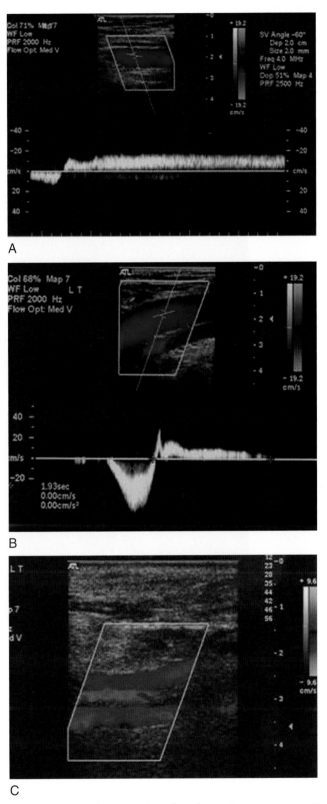

■ **Fig 3–5** Examples of postthrombotic reflux from three patients. **A,** Severe reflux in the femoral vein in a patient who had previous extensive deep venous thrombosis from the common femoral to calf veins. **B,** Popliteal vein reflux in a patient who presented with swelling and pain. **C,** Reflux in both posterior tibial veins, which have the same color as the artery in the middle.

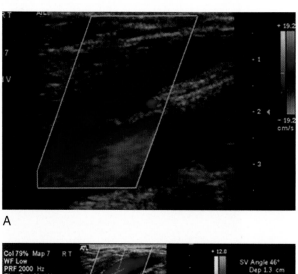

A

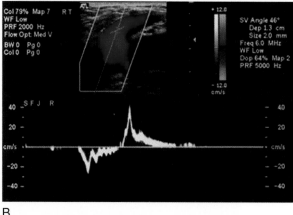

B

■ **Fig 3-6** Imaging of the saphenofemoral junction (SFJ). **A,** Cephalad flow is seen in the SFJ during distal compression. The saphenous vein has a normal diameter and is competent. **B,** SFJ reflux rendering the common femoral vein incompetent. In such cases in patients with primary chronic venous disease, correction of the saphenous reflux abolishes the common femoral vein reflux.

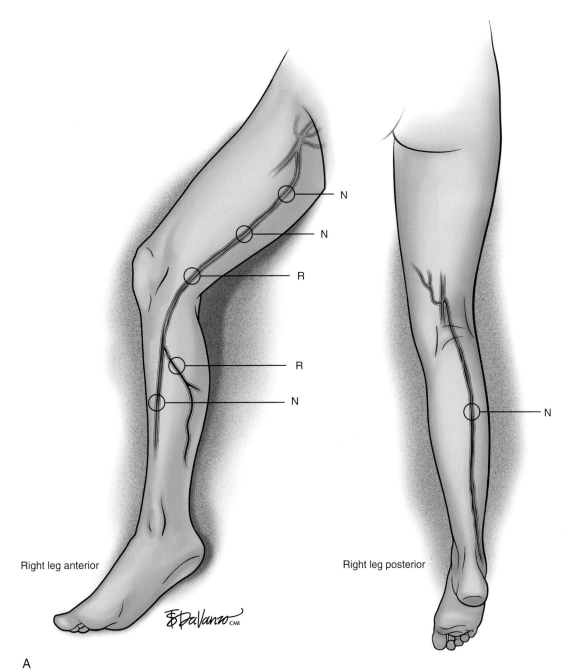

Right leg anterior

Right leg posterior

A

■ **Fig 3-7** Schematic drawing of the different patterns of perforator reflux development. **A** and **B,** Reflux developed in descending manner in a reentry perforator at the lower medial calf. *N,* Normal; *R,* reflux.

Continued

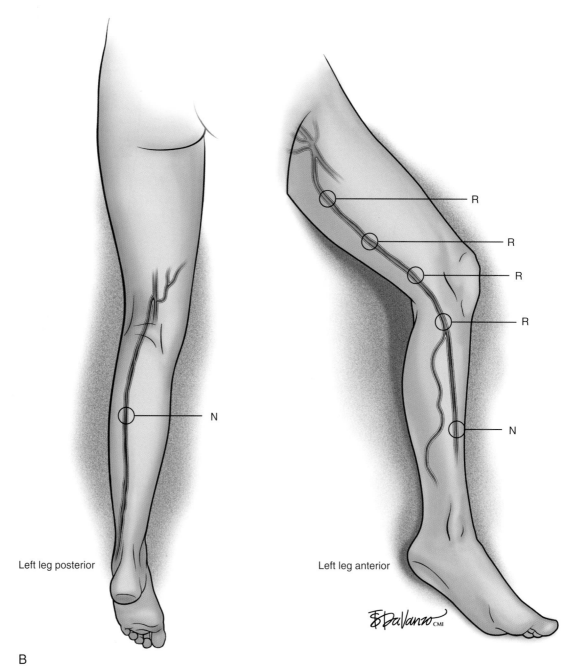

Left leg posterior

Left leg anterior

B

■ **Fig 3-7, cont'd** Schematic drawing of the different patterns of perforator reflux development. **A** and **B**, Reflux developed in descending manner in a reentry perforator at the lower medial calf. *N*, Normal; *R*, reflux.

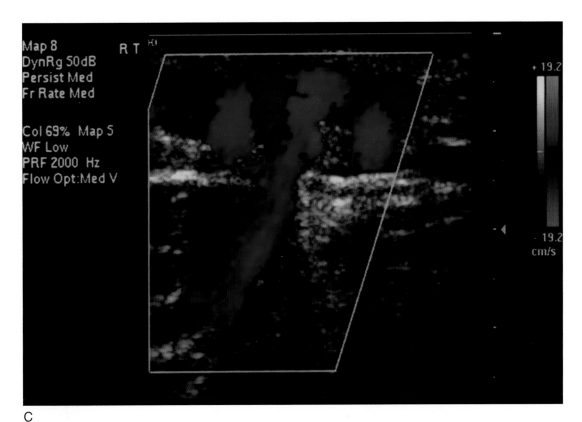

C

■ **Fig 3–7, cont'd   C,** Baseline ultrasound examination in a 53-year-old female patient with a long-standing history of chronic venous disease. On the right limb, she had great saphenous vein (GSV) reflux from the lower thigh to the upper calf and in the posterior calf accessory vein. On the left limb, she had reflux in the GSV from the saphenofemoral junction to the upper calf and the posterior accessory calf vein. There was no perforator vein reflux at this time.

Continued

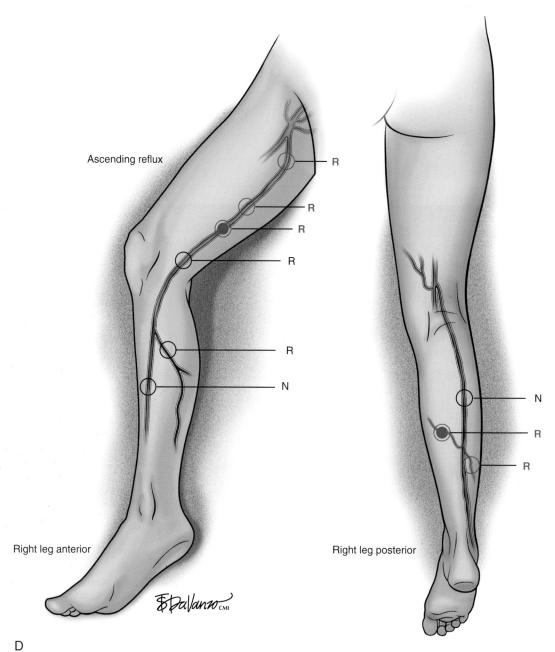

Ascending reflux

R

R

R

R

R

N

Right leg anterior

N

R

R

Right leg posterior

SDaVanzo CMI

D

■ **Fig 3–7, cont'd D** and **E,** During the second examination at 38 months on the right limb, the patient developed ascending reflux in the GSV, a perforator vein at the thigh, a new reflux site in a posterior calf tributary, and a midcalf perforator. On the left limb, she developed a reentry type of reflux in a medial perforator vein from the posterior calf accessory vein. She had worsening of her disease from CEAP class 2 to 3 in the right limb and from class 3 to 4A in the left limb. She also became symptomatic in the left limb, with aching and itching along the varicosities of medial calf. *N,* Normal; *R,* reflux. The *red dot* indicates reflux in a perforator vein. The *red letters* and *lines* indicate the new sites of reflux in the second examination.

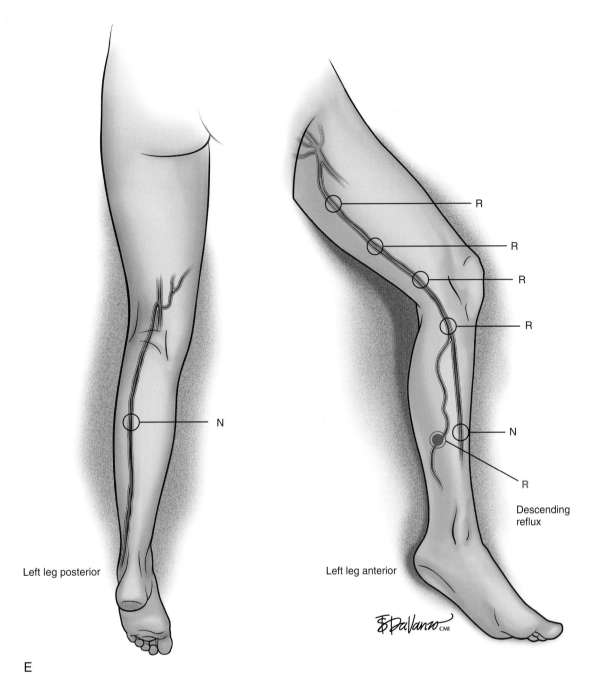

Left leg posterior

Left leg anterior

Descending reflux

E

■ **Fig 3-7, cont'd** For legend see opposite page.

Secondary Venous Disease

Secondary venous disease is caused by a thrombotic event or is secondary to trauma. The incidence of arteriovenous fistula (AVFs) as cause of secondary CVD is reduced compared with postthrombotic CVD (Fig. 3-8).

Most frequently, AVFs are created when both common femoral vessels are inadvertently punctured during endovascular procedures or secondary to penetrating or blunt traumatic injuries. Animal models based on AVF creation have been used to explain the findings of chronic venous disease.[10] Initially, lower resistance in the distal portion of the artery and pulsatile flow in the vein are noted. Venous hypertension supervenes, distending the veins and causing some degree of edema in the limb but no reflux. Subsequently, the valves are unable to appose what portends the reflux. Continuous venous hypertension and reflux entail valve atrophy and "arterialization" of the venous wall in the long term. In humans, the occurrence of CVD secondary to AVFs is rare and requires a long course to generate clinical impairment that frequently is devastating.

Deep venous thrombosis (DVT) is a result of stasis, endothelial damage, and/or hypercoagulable state. The predisposing factors for DVT and therefore secondary CVD are well established, including pregnancy, operations, immobilization, malignancy, trauma, and obesity. Patients who sustain inherited disorders (i.e., active protein C resistance, protein S and antithrombin III deficiency) are also prone to develop thromboembolic events.

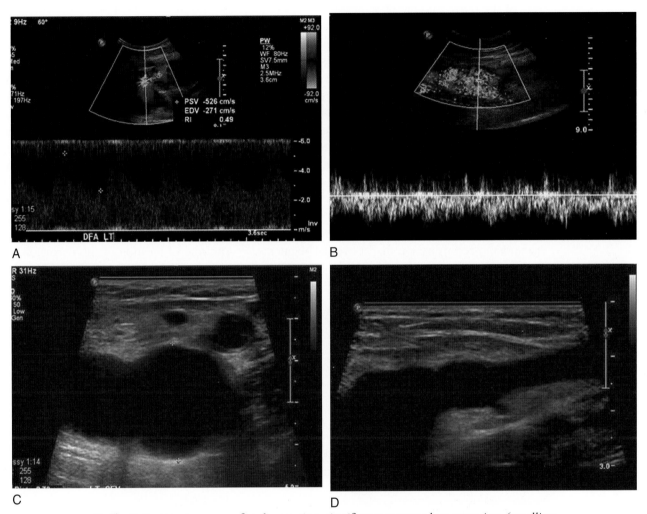

■ **Fig 3–8** Arteriovenous fistula causing significant venous hypertension (swelling of the entire limb, pain, and discoloration) in a male patient after a gunshot wound in the left groin. **A,** Fistula between the deep femoral artery and the common femoral vein. There are high velocities with a low resistance pattern. **B,** Waveform with turbulent flow in the common femoral vein proximal to the fistula. **C,** The common femoral vein is dilated (2.8 cm) due to the local high pressure. **D,** Dilatation of the saphenofemoral junction and the great saphenous vein with continuous reflux (not shown).

Regardless of the initial thrombi formation, the majority of the limbs evolve with thrombus resolution. Notably, only one-third of the patients with secondary CVD develop postthrombotic syndrome (PTS), which consists of signs and symptoms such as pain, edema, heaviness, and intolerance to efforts that may progress to skin changes and ulcers (Fig. 3-9). Often, patients with PTS have a combination of reflux and obstruction (Fig. 3-10). PTS represents the most severe manifestation of secondary CVD, carrying significant socioeconomic impact, and is discussed in Chapter 15.

At the other extreme of secondary CVD are patients who develop DVT with no symptoms. This specific group of patients may have a total silent course of the disease for decades, being diagnosed with DVT during postoperative screening ultrasound or for nonrelated diagnostic purposes. The incidence of PTS in this subset of patients is low.

The location of the DVT and its extent have been investigated. Involvement of at least one proximal deep vein segment was proposed as a mandatory condition for the development of CVD. Three anatomic and hemodynamic patterns are found following an episode of DVT, reflux, obstruction, or a combination of reflux and obstruction. In that scenario, reflux is caused by destruction of the valves secondary to inflammation. It has been hypothesized that leukocyte infiltration in the venous wall causes amplification and activation of metalloproteinases, leading to venous wall and valve damage.[1]

Failure in resolving an obstruction by either partial or complete recanalization of the thrombosed segment is found in less than 10% of cases.[11,12] Partial recanalization is known to have higher incidence of reflux than complete recanalized segments, and calf veins are more prone to undergo recanalization than proximal segments.[11,12] The role of location of the occlusion has

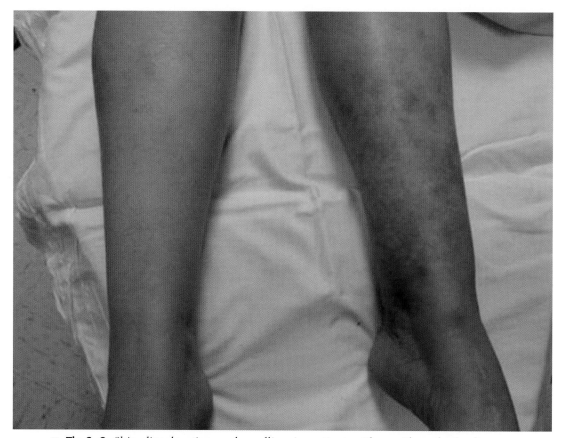

■ **Fig 3–9** Skin discoloration and swelling in patient with postthrombotic deep venous disease.

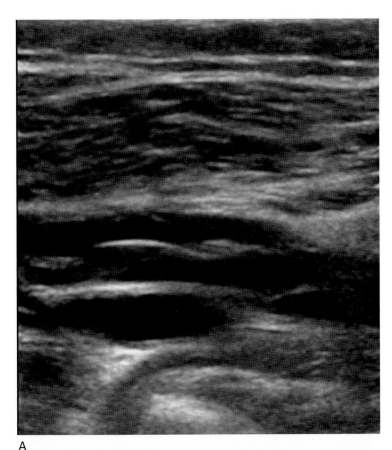

A

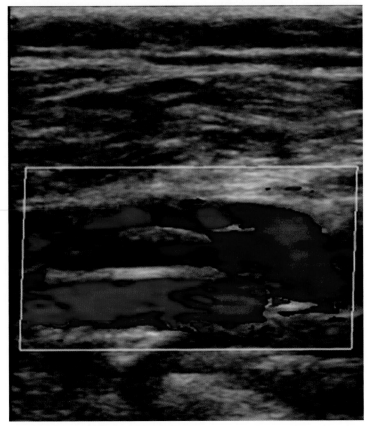

B

■ **Fig 3-10** Patient with leg edema and skin changes with partial recanalization of the popliteal vein. **A,** Synechiae are clearly seen in the lumen of the vein. **B,** Multiple flow channels are seen through the synechiae. Patients with reflux and obstruction are more likely to develop postthrombotic signs and symptoms.

been investigated. In a 1-year prospective study of 70 limbs, recanalization rate was lower in femoral veins, while all calf veins had complete recanalization. Finally, patients with reflux or obstruction present with milder changes and symptoms than those with both abnormalities. The presence of reflux and outflow obstruction in the same limb leads to higher rates of skin damage.[13,14]

Congenital

Congenital vascular malformations contribute to 1% to 3% of CVD. Pure venous malformations are rare and present as an isolated cluster of veins that abuts surrounding tissues, including soft tissue and bone. The most common congenital malformation involving veins is Klippel-Trenaunay, which is characterized by varicose veins, limb hypertrophy, and port-wine stains[15] (Fig. 3-11). Agenesis of valves and segments of the deep veins is rare but is known to cause CVD.[16]

Natural History

CVD slowly evolves over time and is classified based on its *c*linical (telangiectasias to skin damage), *e*tiologic (primary, secondary, or congenital), *a*natomic (superficial, deep, or perforators), and *p*athophysiologic (reflux, obstruction, or both) patterns, forming the acronym CEAP.[17] The clinical portion of the score is extensively used because of its simplicity, being cited as initial stages of CVD, including telangiectasias and varicose veins (C1-C2), and chronic venous insufficiency, including edema, skin changes, and ulcers (C3-C6).

Because the venous pressure increases in the lower extremity veins for hydrostatic reasons in during standing, it has been believed that reflux develops in a retrograde fashion. However, multiple studies have demonstrated that this is not true.[18-21] Predominantly, reflux starts from the saphenous veins and their tributaries and progresses proximally, distally, or in both directions.[22] In a longitudinal study of 116 limbs, progression of reflux occurred in 31. GSV and tributaries were the most common anatomic sites affected by reflux progression, followed by perforator veins. Seventeen limbs had extension of preexisting reflux in a proximal or distal direction, or both, and 14 limbs had reflux in a new segment that was independent of the preexisting site. Among patients with new signs or symptoms, documented reflux progression by duplex ultrasound was found in 53.8%, which was significantly higher than the 23.3% of patients without new symptoms ($p = .04$). Bernardini et al.[23] corroborated the findings that the reflux most frequently starts in the GSV and its tributaries, reporting progression of venous disease in 94% of the patients in a mean period of 4 years. Further evidence is provided by a recent study on wall characteristics[24] and interventional studies in which reflux in the saphenous vein was corrected after eliminating reflux in the saphenous tributaries.[25-27]

Secondary CVD was found to progress faster than primary CVD,[12] for reasons that are likely to be multivariate. The presence of reflux and obstruction aggravates the clinical status of patients, as shown in a study by Johnson et al.[13] In a cohort of 64 patients, overall progression of the CEAP clinical class occurred in 31.5%. Notably, secondary CVD CEAP class 4 to 6 was noted in 4% of the limbs at a 1-year period, increasing to 25% at 5-year follow-up.[14]

Prandoni et al. analyzed the data of 1626 consecutive patients and found that residual thrombosis, unknown origin, and thrombophilia are risk factors for recurrent DVT over a period of 10 years.[28] Long-term follow-up with duplex ultrasound in a prospective cohort of 153 patients with recurrent DVT showed increased risk of skin damage (C4-C6) in patients with previous recurrent ipsilateral DVT.[29]

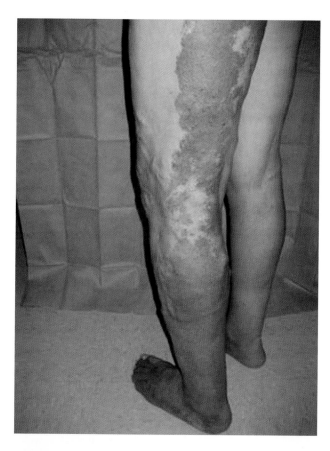

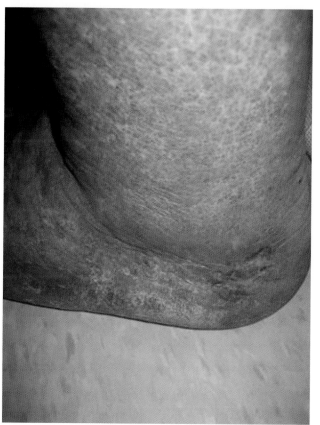

■ **Fig 3–11** Klippel-Trenaunay syndrome in a young female patient who presented with pain and ulceration. The left limb has the typical discoloration and enlargement seen in patients with this syndrome. There were no anomalies seen in the deep axial veins. Reflux was found in multiple superficial, perforator, and muscular veins.

An overview of clinical distribution (reflux, obstruction, or both), classification, and pathophysiology of CVD in consecutive patients attending a vascular clinic is shown in Figure 3-12. Most patients have primary vein reflux, which is most often found in the superficial veins and varicose veins. Skin damage is present in about one-third of the patients, while isolated deep vein reflux and obstruction are uncommon.[30]

PEARLS AND PITFALLS

A complete understanding of venous pathophysiology is essential to offer an adequate treatment for patients with CVD. The relationship between deep and superficial venous reflux, obesity, and dilated veins with no reflux deserves attention.

Obesity

An association between obesity and CVD has been identified. The role of obesity as a causative versus an aggravating factor remains debatable. It is known that obese patients have higher intraabdominal pressure compared with nonobese patients and have reduced distensibility of the veins that could explain the higher incidence of CVD. Van Rij and associates[31] reported an increased incidence of more severe CVD (CEAP 4-6) in obese patients than in nonobese patients. Interestingly, the authors concluded that obese patients have better venous calf muscle pump than nonobese patients. Sedentary behavior may explain the reduced effect of the pump to compensate reflux.

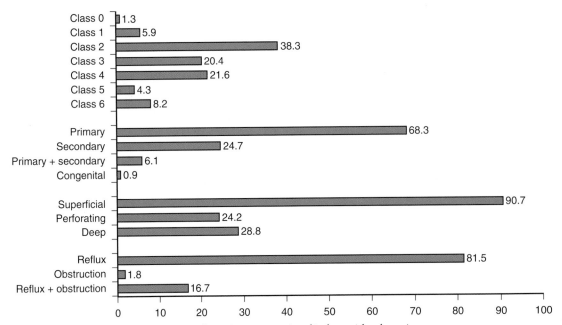

■ **Fig 3-12** Presentation of 1000 consecutive limbs with chronic venous disease (CVD) according to CEAP classification. In the anatomic classification, for simplicity only the overall contribution of each system is shown. This classification has allowed better communication and comparisons in the medical literature as chronic venous disease terminology is more specific and has been adopted worldwide.

Padberg and colleagues also reported a correlation between higher body mass index (BMI) and severity of the CVD[32] in a cohort of morbidly obese patients (BMI >40 kg/m²). Obese patients had longer mean ulcer healing time, up to 7 months. Notably, 62% of those patients had no anatomic evidence of reflux despite severe CVD changes.[32] Perhaps the disease in that subset of patients may be secondary to microcirculatory changes or even segmental venous hypertension associated with lymphatic drainage impairment. Therefore, a high level of suspicion should be raised when evaluating such patients because venous reflux may not be the cause of skin damage.

Effects of Superficial Vein Reflux on the Deep Veins

The role of superficial venous reflux as a causative factor for deep venous reflux has been investigated. Over the past three decades, selected patients with CVD who presented with deep venous reflux, advanced venous stasis, and skin damage have been subject to a multiple techniques to improve venous return, including valve transposition, repair, or even axillary vein transfer.[33]

Because isolated deep venous reflux is rare, the current concept of flow overload in the superficial venous system causing venous hypertension and valve dysfunction has been stated. Transmission of the reflux through perforators and saphenofemoral junctions is likely to explain deep venous reflux in association with superficial venous reflux.

Several authors have advocated treatment of superficial venous reflux instead of direct procedures to correct deep venous reflux. Walsh et al.[6] performed GSV stripping in 29 limbs with primary CVD, including only CEAP classes 1 through 3, and achieved success abolishing femoral vein reflux in 93% of the cases. In a similar subset of patients including only CEAP classes 1 through 3, Sales et al.[8] achieved hemodynamic normalization of the deep veins in 94% of the patients. However, at the other extreme of the disease presentation, Padberg et al.[34] treated 11 limbs with active ulcers and obtained hemodynamic success in only 27%. All perforators were ligated and GSV stripping was performed. Nonetheless, the patients did improve, and the ulcers healed with no recurrence at mean 16-month follow-up. Ciostek et al. analyzed photoplethysmography and duplex ultrasound reflux parameters following GSV ablation in 11 patients with secondary CVI and found no statistically significant improvement in deep venous reflux.[35]

The rationale for treating superficial venous reflux before any deep venous intervention is based on clinical and hemodynamic findings. Patients with superficial reflux associated with deep venous reflux present with milder deep vein impairment than do patients with isolated axial deep venous reflux, suggesting propagation and therefore response to a secondary mechanism as seen in study of 152 limbs.[5] In addition, deep vein reflux is abolished in patients with initial disease after saphenous vein interruption, corroborating the former mechanism of superficial venous reflux propagation.[6,8] Hemodynamic results may be compromised in patients with skin damage or secondary CVD due to prolonged inflammatory changes and more severe dilation of the deep veins.

FIVE SALIENT REFERENCES

Labropoulos N, Gasparis AP, Tassiopoulos AK. Prospective evaluation of the clinical deterioration in post-thrombotic limbs. J Vasc Surg 2009;50:826-830.

Labropoulos N, Jen J, Jen H, et al. Recurrent deep vein thrombosis: long-term incidence and natural history. Ann Surg 2010;251:749-753.

Labropoulos N, Leon L, Kwon S, et al. Study of the venous reflux progression. J Vasc Surg 2005;41:291-295.

Prandoni P, Noventa F, Ghiarduzzi A, et al. The risk of recurrent venous thromboembolism after discontinuing anticoagulation in patients with acute proximal deep vein thrombosis or pulmonary embolism. A prospective cohort study in 1,626 patients. Haematologica 2007;92:199-205.

Raffetto JD, Khalil RA. Mechanisms of varicose vein formation: valve dysfunction and wall dilation. Phlebology 2008;23:85-98.

REFERENCES

1. Raffetto JD, Khalil RA. Mechanisms of varicose vein formation: valve dysfunction and wall dilation. Phlebology 2008;23:85-98.

2. Coleridge Smith PD, Thomas P, et al. Causes of venous ulceration: a new hypothesis. Br Med J 1988;296:1726-1727.

3. Raffetto JD, Qiao X, Koledova VV, et al. Prolonged increases in vein wall tension increase matrix metalloproteinases and decrease constriction in rat vena cava: potential implications in varicose veins. J Vasc Surg 2008;48:447-456.

4. Labropoulos N, Leon L, Kwon S, et al. Study of the venous reflux progression. J Vasc Surg 2005;41:291-295.

5. Labropoulos N, Tassiopoulos AK, Kang SS, et al. Prevalence of deep venous reflux in patients with primary superficial vein incompetence. J Vasc Surg 2000;32:663-668.

6. Walsh JC, Bergan JJ, Beeman S, et al. Femoral venous reflux abolished by greater saphenous vein stripping. Ann Vasc Surg 1994;8:566-570.

7. Puggioni A, Lurie F, Kistner RL, et al. How often is deep venous reflux eliminated after saphenous vein ablation? J Vasc Surg 2003;38:517-521.

8. Sales CM, Bilof ML, Petrillo KA, et al. Correction of lower extremity deep venous incompetence by ablation of superficial venous reflux. Ann Vasc Surg 1996;10:186-189.

9. Labropoulos N, Tassiopoulos AK, Bhatti AF, et al. Development of reflux in the perforator veins in limbs with primary venous disease. J Vasc Surg 2006;43:558-562.

10. Bergan JJ, Pascarella L, Schmid-Schonbein GW. Pathogenesis of primary chronic venous disease: Insights from animal models of venous hypertension. J Vasc Surg 2008;47: 183-192.

11. Yamaki T, Nozaki M. Patterns of venous insufficiency after an acute deep vein thrombosis. J Am Coll Surg 2005;201:231-238.

12. Labropoulos N, Gasparis AP, Pefanis D, et al. Secondary chronic venous disease progresses faster than primary. J Vasc Surg 2009;49:704-710.

13. Johnson BF, Manzo RA, Bergelin RO, et al. Relationship between changes in the deep venous system and the development of the postthrombotic syndrome after an acute episode of lower limb deep vein thrombosis: a one- to six-year follow-up. J Vasc Surg 1995;21:307-312; discussion 313.

14. Labropoulos N, Gasparis AP, Tassiopoulos AK. Prospective evaluation of the clinical deterioration in post-thrombotic limbs. J Vasc Surg 2009;50:826-830.

15. Lee BB, Bergan J, Gloviczki P, et al. Diagnosis and treatment of venous malformations Consensus Document of the International Union of Phlebology (IUP)-2009. Int Angiol 2009;28:434-451.

16. Gloviczki P, Duncan A, Kalra M, et al. Vascular malformations: an update. Perspect Vasc Surg Endovasc Ther 2009;21:133-148.

17. Eklof B, Rutherford RB, Bergan JJ, et al. Revision of the CEAP classification for chronic venous disorders: consensus statement. J Vasc Surg 2004;40:1248-1252.

18. Labropoulos N, Delis K, Nicolaides AN, et al. The role of the distribution and anatomic extent of reflux in the development of signs and symptoms in chronic venous insufficiency. J Vasc Surg 1996;23:504-510.

19. Caggiati A, Rosi C, Heyn R, et al. Age-related variations of varicose veins anatomy. J Vasc Surg 2006;44:1291-1295.

20. Pittaluga P, Chastane S, Rea B, et al. Classification of saphenous refluxes: implications for treatment. Phlebology 2008;23:2-9.

21. Garcia-Gimeno M, Rodriguez-Camarero S, Tagarro-Villalba S, et al. Duplex mapping of 2036 primary varicose veins. J Vasc Surg 2009;49:681-689.
22. Labropoulos N, Giannoukas AD, Delis K, et al. Where does venous reflux start? J Vasc Surg 1997;26:736-742.
23. Bernardini E, De Rango P, Piccioli R, et al. Development of primary superficial venous insufficiency: the ascending theory. Observational and hemodynamic data from a 9-year experience. Ann Vasc Surg 2010;24:709-720.
24. Labropoulos N, Kokkosis AA, Spentzouris G, et al. The distribution and significance of varicosities in the saphenous trunks. J Vasc Surg 2010;51:96-103.
25. Labropoulos N, Leon L, Engelhorn CA, et al. Sapheno-femoral junction reflux in patients with a normal saphenous trunk. Eur J Vasc Endovasc Surg 2004;28:595-599.
26. Pittaluga P, Chastanet S, Rea B, et al. Midterm results of the surgical treatment of varices by phlebectomy with conservation of a refluxing saphenous vein. J Vasc Surg 2009;50: 107-118.
27. Pittaluga P, Chastanet S, Locret T, et al. The effect of isolated phlebectomy on reflux and diameter of the great saphenous vein: a prospective study. Eur J Vasc Endovasc Surg 2010;40:122-128.
28. Prandoni P, Noventa F, Ghirarduzzi A, et al. The risk of recurrent venous thromboembolism after discontinuing anticoagulation in patients with acute proximal deep vein thrombosis or pulmonary embolism. A prospective cohort study in 1,626 patients. Haematologica 2007;92:199-205.
29. Labropoulos N, Jen J, Jen H, et al. Recurrent deep vein thrombosis: long-term incidence and natural history. Ann Surg 2010;251:749-753.
30. Labropoulos N. Hemodynamic changes according to the CEAP classification. Phlebolymphology 2003;40:125-129.
31. van Rij AM, De Alwis CS, et al. Obesity and impaired venous function. Eur J Vasc Endovasc Surg 2008;35:739-744.
32. Padberg F Jr, Cerveira JJ, Lal BK, et al. Does severe venous insufficiency have a different etiology in the morbidly obese? Is it venous? J Vasc Surg 2003;37:79-85.
33. Raju S. Venous insufficiency of the lower limb and stasis ulceration. Changing concepts and management. Ann Surg 1983;197:688-697.
34. Padberg FT Jr, Pappas PJ, Araki CT, et al. Hemodynamic and clinical improvement after superficial vein ablation in primary combined venous insufficiency with ulceration. J Vasc Surg 1996;24:711-718.
35. Ciostek P, Michalak J, Noszczyk W. Improvement in deep vein haemodynamics following surgery for varicose veins. Eur J Vasc Endovasc Surg 2004;28:473-478.

CHAPTER 4

Endovenous Thermal Ablation of Saphenous Reflux

Jose I. Almeida

HISTORICAL BACKGROUND

Treatment of this disorder has evolved from sclerotherapy to open radical surgery to the use of sophisticated technology such as laser, radiofrequency, or ultrasound-guided foam sclerotherapy.

The exact historical point in time when saphenous vein incompetence was recognized as a source of venous hypertension is unclear; however, Trendelenburg promulgated saphenofemoral ligation in 1891.[1] In the early 20th century, stripping of the saphenous veins was added to proximal ligation. Keller[2] described an internal stripper in 1905. Hence, high ligation of the great saphenous vein (GSV) at the saphenofemoral junction (SFJ) followed by GSV stripping from groin to knee, or ankle was the standard of care and was performed in the hospital setting for about 100 years.

The two methods of thermal ablation in comprehensive vein centers at present are the VNUS ClosureFAST procedure, which uses a catheter to direct radiofrequency (RF) energy from a dedicated generator (VNUS Medical Technologies, Inc., Sunnyvale, CA), and endovenous laser (EVL) ablation, which uses a laser fiber and generator to produce focused heat (multiple manufacturers). Both RF and EVL are catheter-based endovascular interventions that use electromagnetic energy to destroy the refluxing saphenous system.

RF catheters were the first devices to become available to venous surgeons for endovenous thermal ablation of the GSV after garnering Food and Drug Administration approval in 1999. In 2002, endovascular ablation of the GSV using laser energy became available in the United States.

ETIOLOGY AND NATURAL HISTORY OF DISEASE

The majority of patients (60% to 70%) with varicose veins have an incompetent SFJ and GSV reflux.[3] It is critical to recognize that bulging varicose veins are usually associated with an underlying source of venous hypertension, and treatment of the source is as important as is treatment of the actual varicose vein.

Chronic venous disorders generally result from primary venous insufficiency or secondary processes, such as acute deep venous thrombosis (DVT) or trauma. An analysis of chronic venous disease indicated that primary valvular incompetence was present in 70% to 80% of cases; secondary valvular incompetence was due to trauma or DVT in 18% to 25%, and congenital anomaly was present in 1% to 3%.[4]

PATIENT SELECTION

Patients with chronic venous disease (CVD) will usually present to a physician with concerns referable to both medical symptoms and cosmetic appearance of their disease. Patient satisfaction results from identifying and properly treating the patient's primary concerns, which may include medical and/or cosmetic issues. Not all symptomatic patients are aware of their symptoms because the onset may be insidious. Symptoms may include leg heaviness, pain or tenderness along the course of a vein, pruritus, burning, restlessness, night cramps, edema, skin changes, and paresthesias. After treatment, patients are often surprised to realize how much discomfort they had accepted as normal. Pain caused by CVD is often improved by walking or by elevating the legs. The pain of arterial insufficiency, conversely, is worsened by ambulation and elevation. Pain and other symptoms of venous disease may intensify with the menstrual cycle, pregnancy, and in response to exogenous hormonal therapy (i.e., oral contraceptives).

As is customary for any medical condition, the physician must begin with a careful history and physical examination. The primary purpose of the clinical examination of the patient presenting with chronic venous disease (CVD) is to classify the subject using the popular CEAP system[5,6]—clinical (telangiectasias to skin damage), etiologic (primary, secondary, or congenital), anatomic (superficial, deep, or perforators), and pathophysiologic (reflux, obstruction, or both) patterns, forming the acronym CEAP. For each of these major classifications, there are subgroups. For the work described in this chapter, clinical signs emerge as the most important and are grouped as follows—C1: spider telangiectasias; C2, varicose veins (Fig. 4-1); C3, edema; C4, lipodermatosclerosis; C5, healed ulcer; and C6, active ulcer. Regarding treatment, the class (C) is the most important parameter to establish during the initial encounter. Treatment algorithms for chronic venous insufficiency (CVI) (i.e., patients with more severe disease [C4, C5, C6]) are discussed in other sections of this book. This chapter focuses on the treatment of C2 disease.

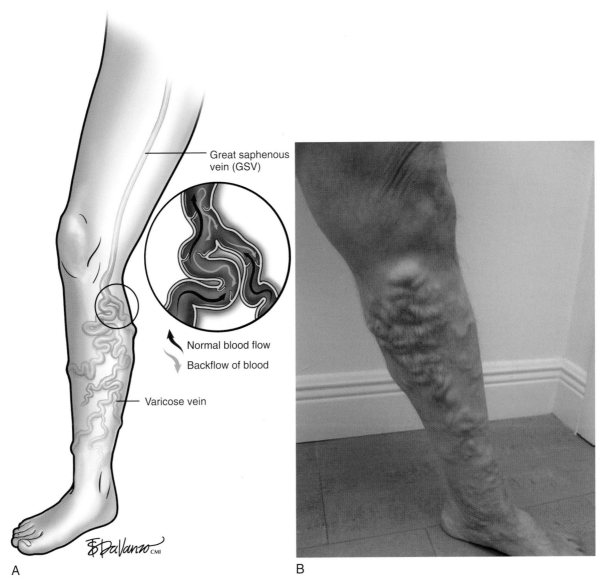

Great saphenous
vein (GSV)

Normal blood flow

Backflow of blood

Varicose vein

A

B

■ **Fig 4–1 B,** Typical varicose veins of the calf resulting from great saphenous vein (GSV) incompetence.

ENDOVASCULAR INSTRUMENTATION

Device choice is a matter of physician preference. Our center and other investigators have compared the efficacy of RF and EVL. The ablation data are slightly better for EVL.[7,8] A few years ago, we published our 3-year data showing 94% success with RF and 98% success with laser[9]; however, in current practice, the results are closer to 98% success with either technology.

Figure 4-2 depicts the general layout of an office-based venous surgery suite. An operating table with a back table is prepared in the usual sterile manner. The laptop ultrasound system is mounted on a movable cart, and the thermal ablation equipment is in close proximity to allow easy viewing of the display panels by the operator. Hemodynamic monitoring equipment (heart rate, blood pressure, oxygen saturation) is available and is used during cases offering conscious sedation. If local anesthesia without sedation is used, hemodynamic monitoring is not required in most states.

Endovascular Laser

- Diode laser: 810-, 940-, 980-, and 1470-nm wavelengths available
- Nd:YAG laser: 1319- and 1320-nm wavelengths commercially available
- A 5-Fr coaxial introducer and sheath placed over .035-inch guidewire
- Sheaths of 35-, 45-, and 65-cm lengths should be available to accommodate different length veins.
- A 600-μm-diameter laser fiber (bare tip or covered tip) is placed through sheath and deployed at the target site under ultrasound control.
- Occasionally, for ablation of short veins, the laser fiber can be placed directly through a microsheath under ultrasound control; recently, smaller, 400-μm-diameter fibers have become available.
- With EVL, one works with a long (35, 45, or 65 cm) sheath. About 2 cm of the laser fiber tip is deployed at target site by withdrawing the sheath. For GSV ablation, the fiber tip is positioned 1 cm distal to the common femoral vein (CFV).

Radiofrequency

- RF generator
- A 7-Fr coaxial introducer sheath, 7-cm length
- With RF, one works with a short (7 cm) sheath. For GSV ablation, the RF heating elements are positioned 2 cm distal to the CFV. Occasionally, the RF catheters require coaxial navigation over a .025-inch guidewire.

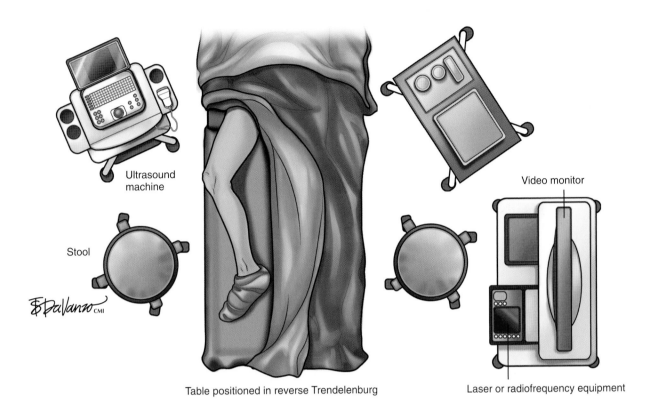

Ultrasound machine

Stool

Table positioned in reverse Trendelenburg

Video monitor

Laser or radiofrequency equipment

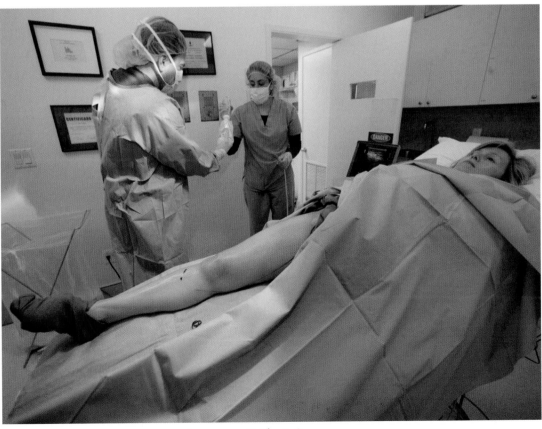

■ Fig 4-2

TUMESCENT ANESTHESIA DELIVERY

A 30-ml syringe with a 25-gauge needle is preferred if anesthesia is delivered by the operator. Extension sets with three-way stopcocks are useful if an assistant is available to push the anesthetic solution. Alternatively, tumescent anesthesia infusion pumps are commercially available.

IMAGING

- Diagnostic workup is noninvasive; physical examination followed by color flow duplex ultrasound imaging is adequate in the majority of patients presenting with lower extremity venous disease.
- One should be familiar with the anatomy of the great saphenous vein (GSV), anterior accessory saphenous vein (AASV), posterior accessory saphenous vein (PASV), thigh circumflex veins, small saphenous vein (SSV), vein of Giacomini, perforating veins of the thigh and calf, and deep venous system.
- The GSV and SSV are identified sonographically in their respective saphenous canals (Fig. 4-3). If they are determined to be incompetent on duplex imaging, they may be sources of venous hypertension and are candidates for endovenous ablation.
- Vein diameters, obtained via duplex ultrasound imaging with the patient in the standing position, must be documented to guide energy delivery.
- The ideal imaging system incorporates color flow duplex ultrasound with a 5- to 7-MHz linear array transducer. The newer "laptop" style platforms are adequate for vein work.
- A sterile bag is required to isolate the ultrasound transducer from the sterile prepped leg (see Fig. 4-2).

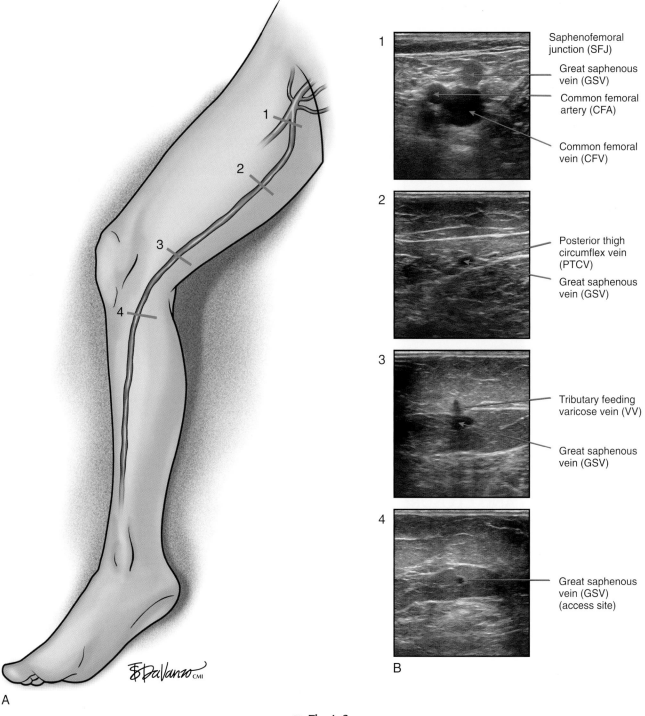

■ Fig 4–3

Continued

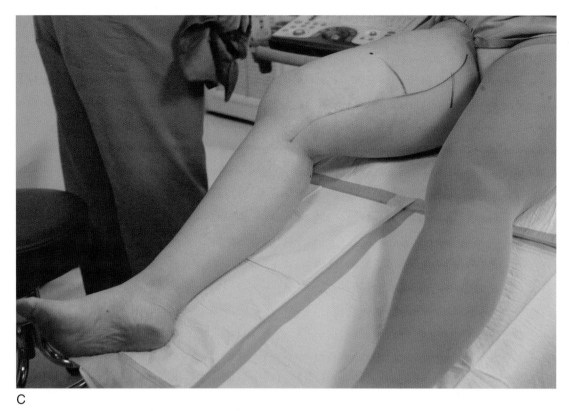

C

■ **Fig 4–3, cont'd C,** Preparing for preprocedure ultrasound scan. This is referred to as "reading" the vein. The surgeon will create an image in his or her "mind's eye" prior to beginning the procedure.

ACCESS AND CLOSURE

The surgeon begins by placing a wheal of local anesthesia on the skin access site with a syringe and small (25- to 30-gauge) needle (Fig. 4-4). The access needle is then held at an approximately 45-degree angle 1 inch from the ultrasound probe, and the target vein will be located at the tip of an imaginary triangle where the ultrasound beam and the tip of the access needle meet under the skin. For large veins (>5-mm diameter), an 18-gauge needle is used. For smaller diameter veins (<5-mm diameter), a 21-gauge needle and micropuncture assembly are preferred (Fig. 4-5).

- A 4-Fr or 5-Fr microintroducer kit contains a 21-gauge needle, .018-inch-diameter × 40-cm-length guidewire, and a microintroducer/sheath set.

- Percutaneous access is obtained with a 21-gauge needle under ultrasound control for both EVL and RF procedures

- A .035-inch-diameter, 150-cm-length, J-tipped guidewire is placed through the microintroducer sheath and navigated to the target site

- If the surgeon is unable to traverse tortuous segments, a second entry site above the tortuosity is created and the vein is treated as two separate segments. To minimize procedure costs, the use of expensive interventional wires is discouraged.

- For the GSV, access is obtained percutaneously at the most distal segment of axial vein reflux. This usually is below the knee at the level of Boyd perforating vein.

- For SSV treatment, access is obtained at the mid-calf posteriorly, where the gastrocnemius muscle becomes prominent.

- One should not introduce wires, sheaths, fibers, and/or catheters into the common femoral vein; they should be parked at the SFJ 1 cm distal to the CFV prior to treatment.

The needle tip is guided to the roof of the vein using ultrasound to visualize where the puncture will take place. Usually one will tent the roof of the vein with a gentle push, easily seen with ultrasound imaging, prior to a more forceful motion for entry. Aspiration of dark nonpulsatile blood into a connected syringe confirms venous entry (Fig. 4-6).

Text continued on p. 84

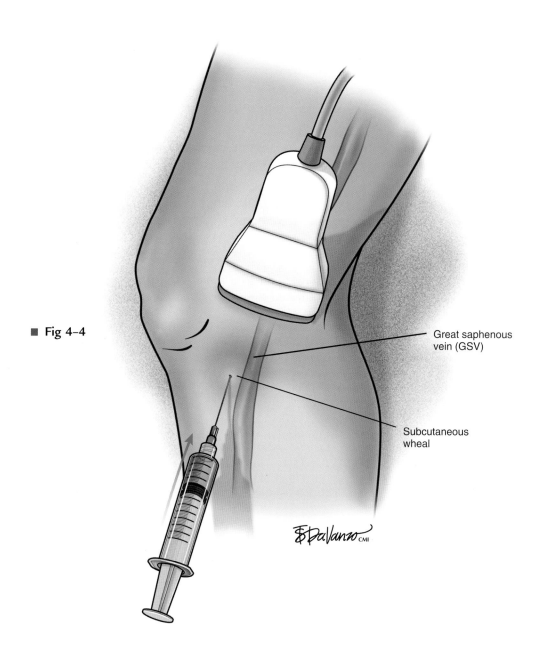

■ Fig 4–4

Great saphenous
vein (GSV)

Subcutaneous
wheal

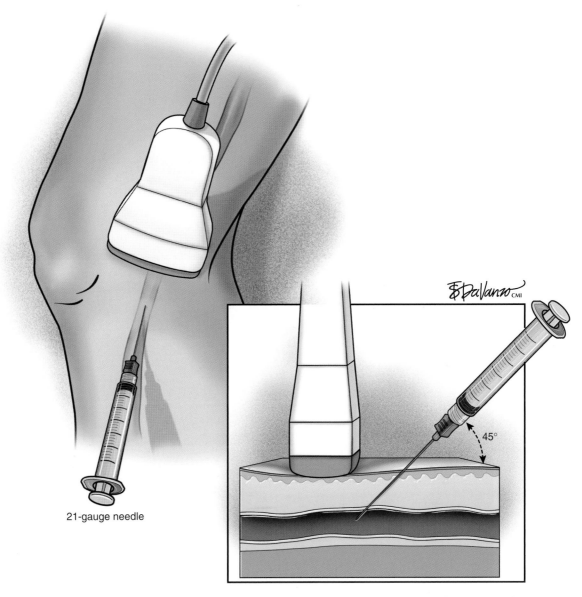

21-gauge needle

21-gauge needle positioned at 45-degree angle to ultrasound

■ **Fig 4–5**

A

Continued

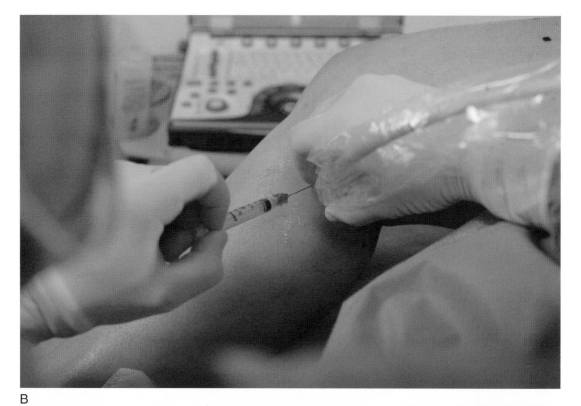

B

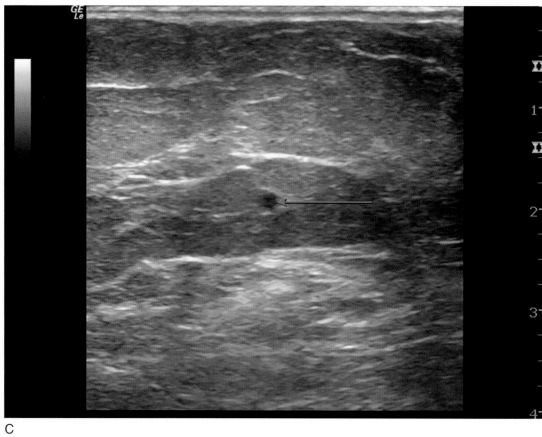

C

■ **Fig 4–5, cont'd C,** Cross-sectional ultrasound image of great saphenous vein (GSV) (the target vein) (*arrow*).

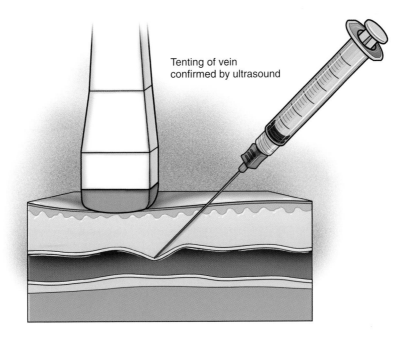

Tenting of vein confirmed by ultrasound

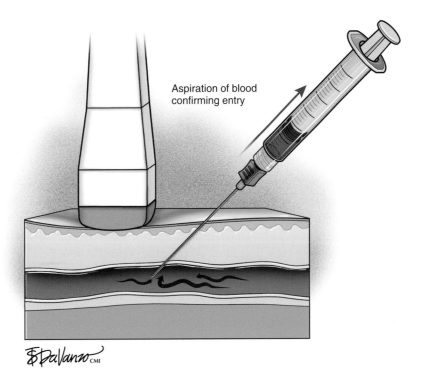

Aspiration of blood confirming entry

■ Fig 4–6

Continued

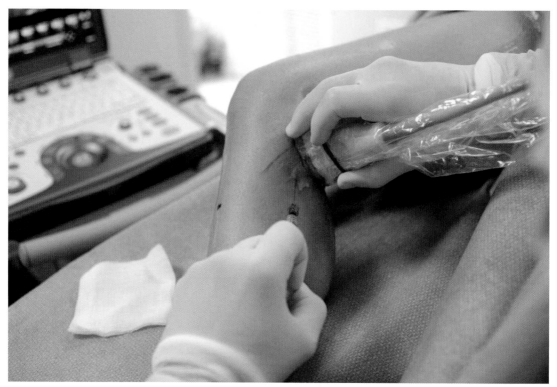

■ Fig 4–6, cont'd

HEMOSTASIS AND ANTICOAGULATION

Hemostasis at the entry site is obtained with manual pressure. As a general rule, thromboprophylaxis with anticoagulation is not required unless the patient has an underlying thrombophilia.

Patients should be stratified into mild-, moderate-, or high-risk classes to determine whether thromboprophylaxis (mechanical, pharmaceutical) is required perioperatively.

As demonstrated in Figure 4-7, we believe that on-table activation of the calf pump is very effective in preventing thromboembolic complications during thermal ablation procedures. After the ablation and before the ambulatory phlebectomy portion of the procedure (discussed in Chapter 9), we simply ask the patient to actively dorsiflex and plantarflex the foot 20 times.

OPERATIVE STEPS

Once the patient has entered the operating suite, a brief examination of the leg is performed. The skin overlying all areas of bulging varicose veins is marked with a magic marker. The patient is then placed in the supine position on the operating table. A detailed duplex ultrasound report should be readily available so the operator can review it before beginning the procedure. Our preference is to then perform a rapid scan of the medial leg with the ultrasound probe for the purpose of obtaining a high-level understanding of the venous anatomy. The operator should note areas of tortuosity, aneurysmal dilatation, and location of tributaries and perforators prior to beginning the procedure. I call this "reading" the vein; its importance is discussed later.

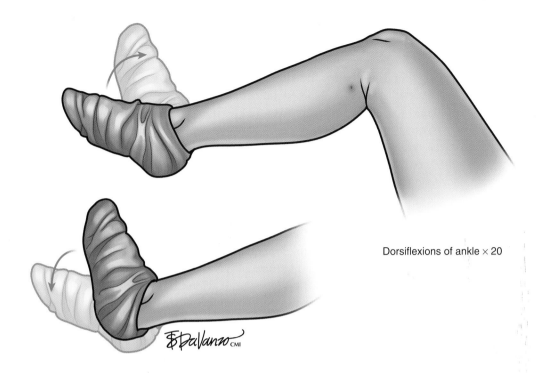

Dorsiflexions of ankle × 20

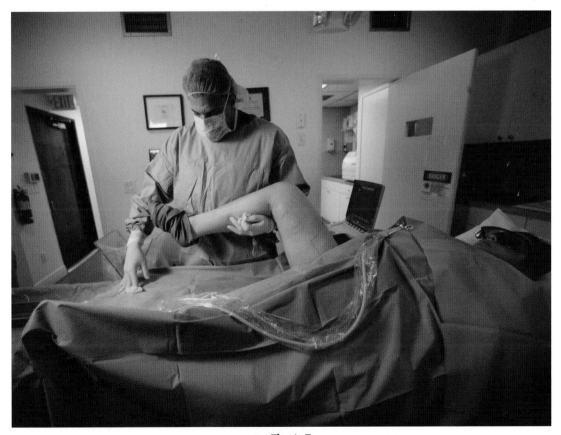

■ **Fig 4–7**

The ultrasound scan begins at the groin, and the course of the vein is followed distally until the straight segment terminates as it begins to divide and produce varicosed tributaries. These varicosed tributaries are the escape points for saphenous incompetence. This transition zone is usually found just below the knee, although many anatomic variants exist. Therefore, percutaneous access is usually obtained immediately below the knee; however, the operator must be prepared to access anywhere from below the knee to the thigh.

Once the optimal access site is chosen, preparations for entry begin. The intraluminal space of the target vein must be accessed to place a guidewire. The preferred technique is percutaneous access under ultrasound guidance. The surgeon and patient must both be comfortable. The surgeon should rest both forearms somewhere in the operative field so that his or her hands are stable.

The ultrasound probe is held perpendicular to the skin to demonstrate the target vein in either the short or long access on the ultrasound screen. Once venous entry is confirmed, a guidewire is chosen. The micropuncture needle accepts a .018-inch wire followed by a 4-Fr coaxial microsheath and its intraluminal dilator. Usually a small stab incision with a No. 11 blade scalpel is required at the wire entry site to widen the incision for the microsheath. Confirmation that the .018-inch wire is in the endoluminal space is performed with ultrasound (Fig. 4-8).

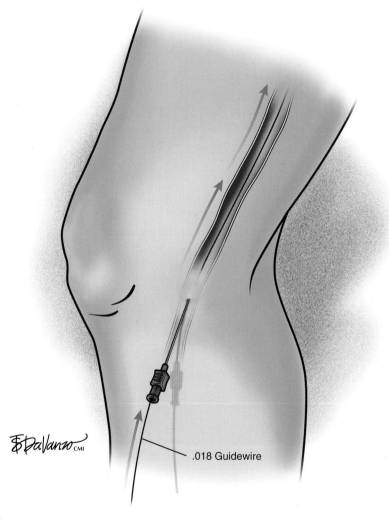

.018 Guidewire

A

■ **Fig 4-8**

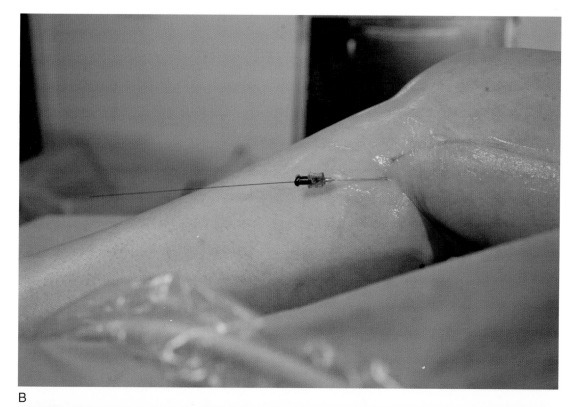

B

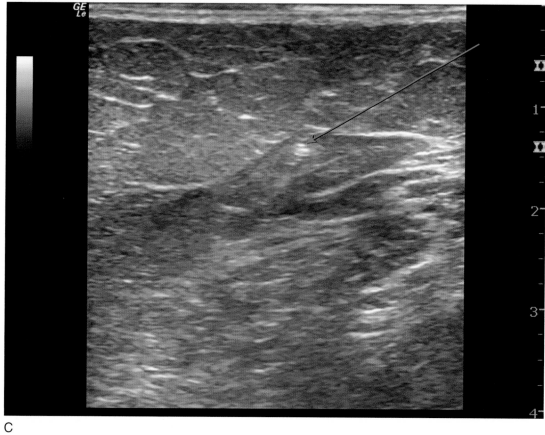

C

■ **Fig 4–8, cont'd C,** Cross-sectional ultrasound image demonstrating intraluminal placement of .018 guidewire (*arrow*).

The microsheath assembly is placed, the microdilator and .018-inch guidewire are removed, and the remaining microsheath is used to place a .035-inch guidewire (Fig. 4-9, *A*). The .035-inch guidewire is then navigated to the SFJ using ultrasound control (Fig. 4-9, *B* and *C*).

Some operators prefer to deliver the wire with the J-tip at the lead, but we prefer to send the straight end of the wire up first, especially in smaller veins. J-tipped wires may cause distention of the vein and induce friction with the inner lining of the vein wall during passage. This generally will cause pain secondary to venous distention, which activates the adrenergic sympathetic nerve fibers residing in the adventitia (Fig. 4-10).

Once the tip of the wire is positioned at the SFJ, a larger coaxial sheath is placed (Fig. 4-11).

Text continued on p. 94

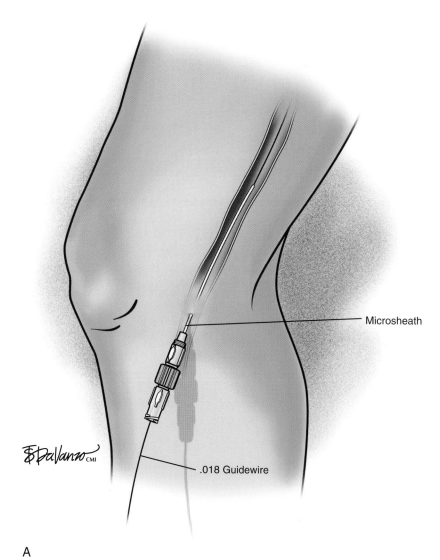

Microsheath

.018 Guidewire

A

■ **Fig 4–9 A,** A .018 guidewire and dilator will be removed, leaving microsheath in place.

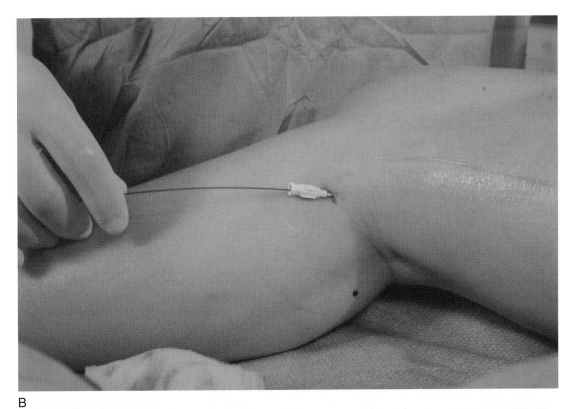

B

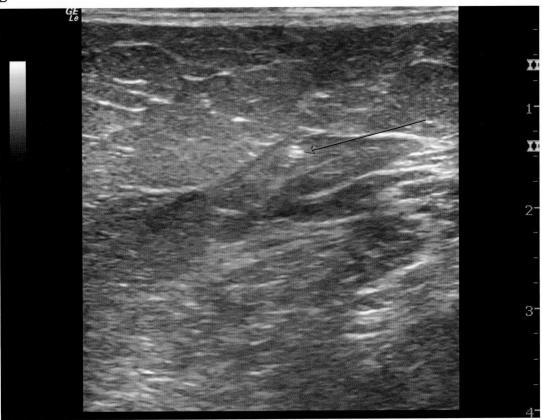

C

■ **Fig 4–9, cont'd B,** A .035 guidewire inserted into microsheath. **C,** Cross-sectional ultrasound image demonstrating intraluminal placement of .035 guidewire (*arrow*).

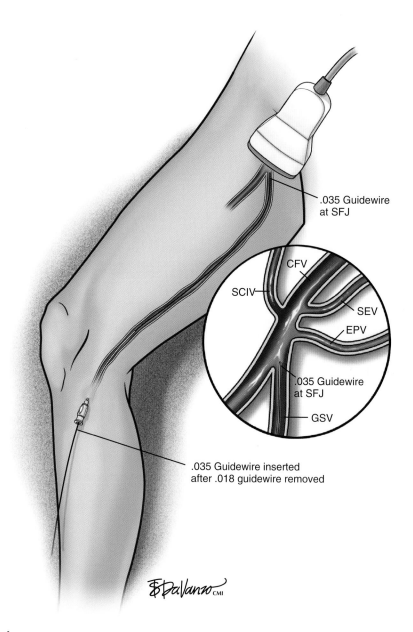

.035 Guidewire
at SFJ

CFV

SCIV

SEV

EPV

.035 Guidewire
at SFJ

GSV

.035 Guidewire inserted
after .018 guidewire removed

A

■ **Fig 4–10 A,** *CFV,* Common femoral vein; *EPV,* external pudendal vein; *GSV,* great saphenous vein; *SCIV,* superficial circumflex iliac vein; *SEV,* superficial epigastric vein; *SFJ,* saphenofemoral junction.

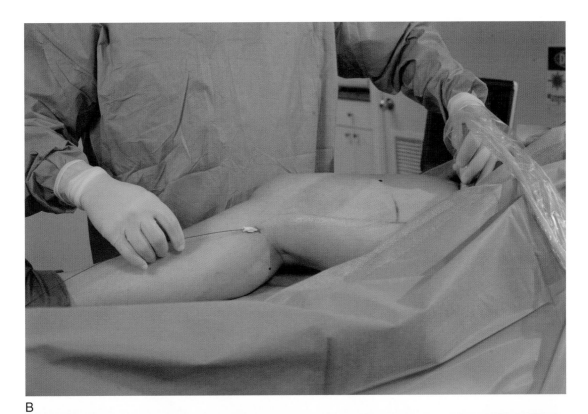

B

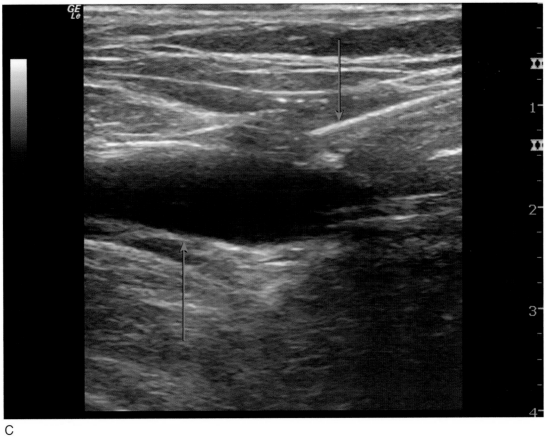

C

■ **Fig 4–10, cont'd C,** Long-access ultrasound image of saphenofemoral junction (SFJ). Top arrow points to guidewire tip at SFJ. Bottom arrow points to common femoral vein (CFV).

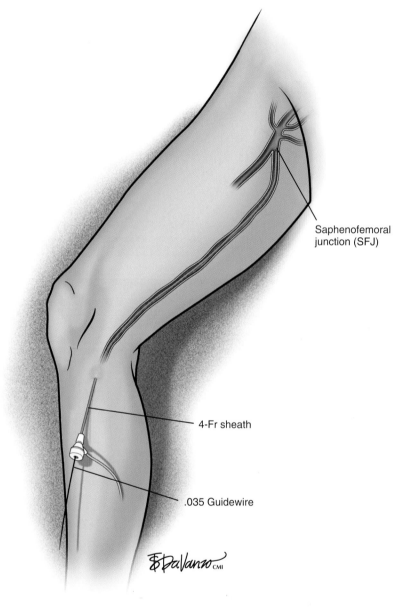

Saphenofemoral
junction (SFJ)

4-Fr sheath

.035 Guidewire

A

■ Fig 4–11

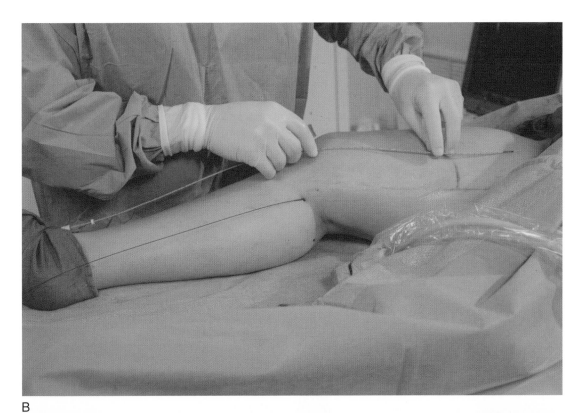

B

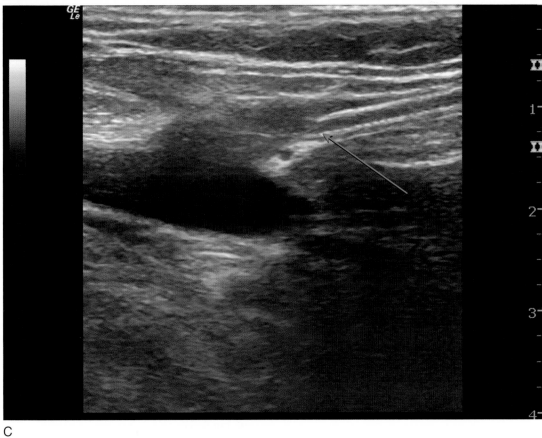

C

■ **Fig 4–11, cont'd B,** Outside of the legs, the surgeon measures the estimated sheath length. **C,** Arrow points to tip of braided sheath at saphenofemoral junction (SFJ). Black dot to the left of arrow tip is the external pudendal artery.

Placement of Perivenous Tumescent Anesthesia

The placement of a generous volume of a dilute anesthetic solution into the saphenous canal often causes these tissues to swell; therefore, one will often see this procedure referred to as tumescent anesthesia placement (Figs. 4-12 and 4-13). Most operators will use a 0.1% lidocaine solution with epinephrine. The solution is easily mixed by placing 50 mL of 1% lidocaine with 1:100,000 epinephrine in a 500-mL reservoir bag of normal saline. Bicarbonate may be added as a buffer if it is the preference of the physician. Alternatively, 50 mL of 1% lidocaine with 1:100,000 epinephrine can be mixed into 500 mL of Lactated Ringers solution, which is already buffered. Once the solution is prepared, it can be injected around the circumference of the target vein at various locations.

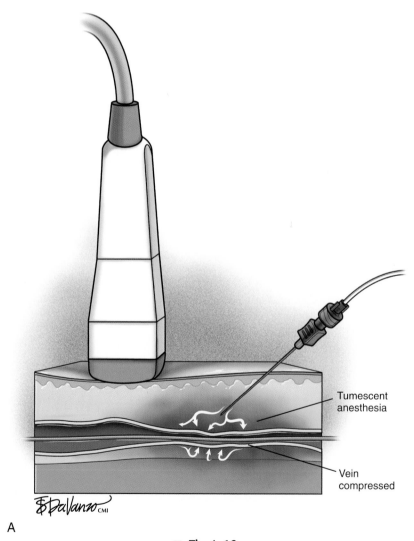

Tumescent
anesthesia

Vein
compressed

A

■ **Fig 4–12**

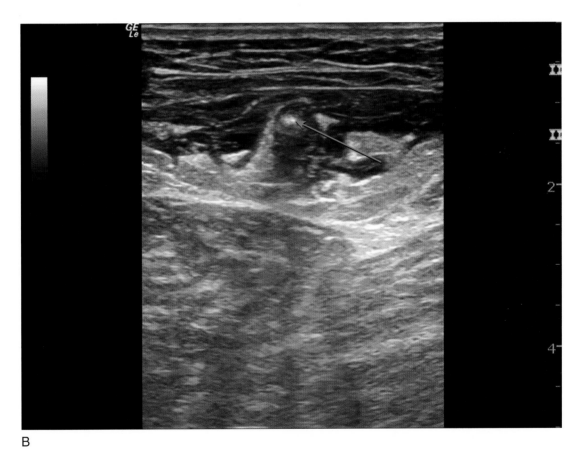

B

■ **Fig 4-12, cont'd B,** Arrow points to great saphenous vein (GSV) in cross-sectional view, catheter is seen intraluminally, there is good apposition of vein wall to catheter, and vein is completely surrounded 360 degrees with tumescent anesthesia.

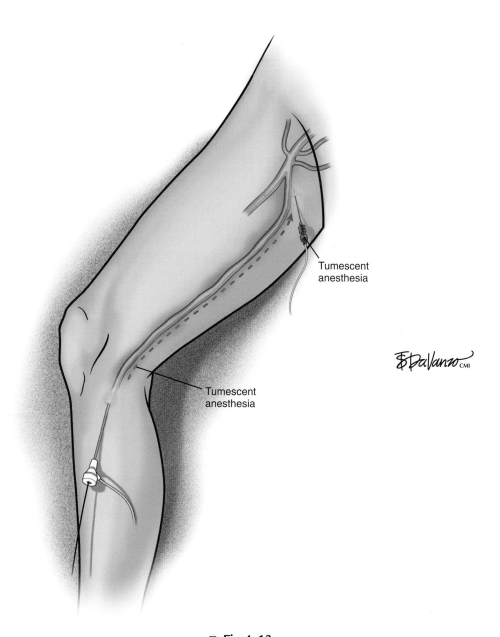

Tumescent anesthesia

Tumescent anesthesia

■ **Fig 4–13**

Perivenous tumescent anesthesia offers several benefits. First, perivenous tumescent anesthesia acts as a heat sink. By circumferentially surrounding the target vein with fluid, any heat transferred to the vein wall from the thermal ablation catheter will be effectively neutralized by the cool anesthetic fluid. Therefore, heat will not be transferred to nontarget tissues such as nerves, and damage will be localized to the vein wall. Second, perivenous tumescent anesthesia compresses the vein. The ClosureFAST radiofrequency device works by conducting heat to the vein wall. In the case of laser, heat transfer works by a combination of direct contact and convection. Regardless of the technology used, if the vein wall is brought into closer proximity with the thermal ablation catheter, the energy transfer will be more effective. As one delivers the anesthetic solution under ultrasound control, it is easy to visualize the venous diameter shrinking (by compression) as more anesthetic is injected. The goal is to see good apposition of the vein wall to the catheter shaft. Finally, perivenous tumescent anesthesia also has an analgesic effect. Patients should experience a painless procedure.

Several delivery systems are available for placement of tumescent anesthesia, ranging from an inexpensive syringe with a 25-gauge needle to specialized pumps for more rapid delivery.

Laser

In the case of EVL thermal ablation, a 4- or 5-Fr sheath is preferred. In contrast to RF ablation, the endovenous sheath for laser must be long enough to reach the SFJ. The length of the sheath chosen can be estimated by measuring on the outside of the leg from the guidewire entry site to the inguinal crease. In general, this distance is about 40 cm in length when access is obtained below the knee; therefore, a 45-cm-length sheath is most commonly used. Sheaths are commercially available in 25-, 35-, 45-, and 65-cm lengths. The sheath is then tracked over the guidewire and navigated to the SFJ. Sometimes the entry site must be widened to allow sheath entry; this is easily accomplished with a No. 11 blade scalpel. There are instances in which a patient may feel discomfort during tracking of the sheath, especially when performed in the office setting without conscious sedation. In these situations, the sheath should not be forced. The sheath tracking should be stopped momentarily to allow placement of perivenous tumescent anesthesia. With the guidewire in place, it is easy to identify and to anesthetize the vein—then tracking of the sheath may be resumed painlessly. Once the sheath has been navigated to its final position, which is about 2 cm distal to the CFV, the inner dilator and .035-inch guidewire may be removed.

The laser fiber is inserted into the sheath through the hemostatic valve and advanced to the sheath tip. The sheath is then withdrawn 1 cm, to expose the laser fiber tip at the SFJ. Some systems have a locking hub on the fiber to facilitate this process and secure the fiber-sheath components together during withdrawal. Pushing the fiber out of the sheath to expose it should be discouraged as this maneuver can inadvertently penetrate and perforate the vein wall, especially with bare-tipped fibers. Bare-tipped laser fibers are void of cladding, which renders them rather sharp. When working with covered fibers, the tips are smooth and less likely to penetrate the vein wall; therefore, "unsheathing" to expose the laser fiber tip is not as critical (Figs. 4-14 and 4-15).

Once the laser fiber tip is exposed, it should be positioned about 1 to 2 cm from the ostium of the CFV. If the superficial epigastric vein is visible, the fiber tip should be positioned distal to this entry of this vessel. There is some empirical evidence that this strategy retards the formation of thrombus extension into the CFV and that it obviates the formation of neovascular channels in the area of the groin, which may lead to recurrence.

After the vein is accessed, the device positioned, and anesthesia given, the patient is treated.

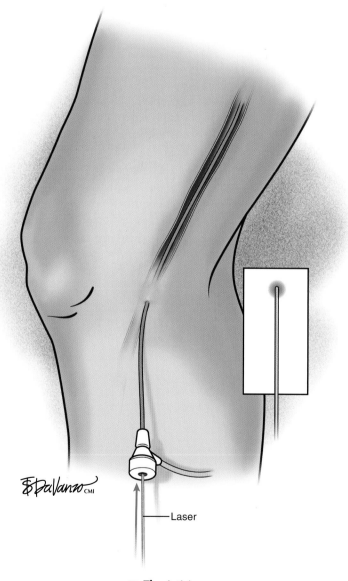

Laser

■ **Fig 4–14**

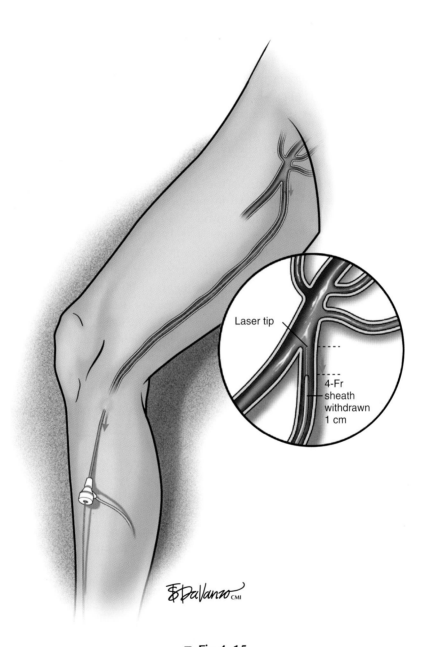

Laser tip

4-Fr
sheath
withdrawn
1 cm

■ Fig 4–15

The Pullback

Laser

The pullback protocol for endovenous laser ablation is not straightforward. Multiple wavelengths are available and no absolute energy protocols have been established. Much of the existing published work in this area is described in Chapter 6. For the three available wavelengths that target the hemoglobin molecule preferentially (810, 940, and 980 nm), the linear endovenous energy density (LEED) should range between 60 and 80 J/cm. This has produced very satisfactory results with the majority of veins and is a simple formula for the new user. As the operator gains more experience, he or she may want to tailor the therapy to the anatomy of the vein. That is, the presence of aneurysmal segments or large tributaries or perforators may sway the operator in the direction of delivering higher-energy densities than normal, whereas small-diameter veins and veins near the skin may have improved results with lower-energy densities. The pullback speed measured in millimeters per second is governed by the desired LEED.

The laser has adjustable power outputs; most laser systems, for purposes of endovenous ablation, will deliver a maximum of 15 W. One watt delivers 1 J of energy per second, and 10 W delivers 10 J/sec. With the laser set at 10 W, for most veins, the results are very satisfactory. Therefore, if one desires to treat an ordinary incompetent GSV that is 40 cm in length, the following sequence will be used. At an LEED of 60 J/cm, the total energy delivery will be 2400 J. At a power of 10 W, the total time for energy delivery will be 240 seconds. The pullback rate will therefore equal about 0.17 cm/sec, 1.7 mm/sec, or 10.2 cm/min.

If the operator does not elect a manual pullback, there is a commercially available motorized pullback device. The motor can be set to produce pullback speeds of 1 mm/sec or 2 mm/sec. The advantage of this system is that no human variability is introduced, and when looking at results, the pullback rate is a constant variable. The disadvantage is that all veins are different and a manual pullback allows for easy adjustment to treat areas of concern, such as aneurysmal segments and segments in close proximity to the skin.

By locating the aiming beam, manual application of pressure at the fiber tip (Figs. 4-16 and 4-17) facilitates the process of bringing the target vein wall in closer proximity to the energy source. Since the advent of covered fiber tips, this maneuver has become controversial. Some small pilot studies have suggested that covered tips may minimize the focal vein perforations seen with bare fiber laser ablation. The idea of external manual compression during the laser pullback is to bring the vein wall in closer proximity to the energy source. With bare fibers, this translates into areas of direct contact of the vein endothelium with the laser fiber tip (which transfers energy via conduction) and areas of vein not in direct contact with the laser fiber tip (which transfers energy via convection). Gross histologic samples suggest that the venous perforations occur at sites of direct contact. The idea of covered fibers is to not allow any areas of direct contact of the vein wall with the laser fiber, thus minimizing vein perforations.

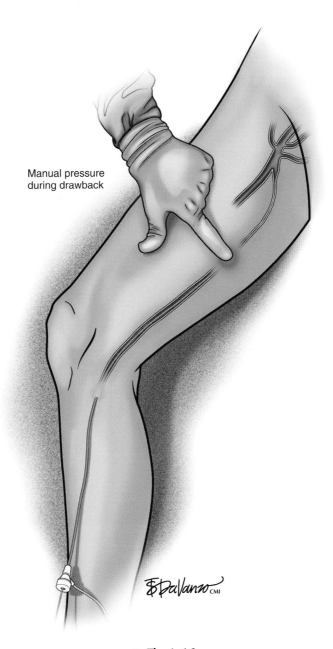

Manual pressure
during drawback

■ Fig 4–16

Continued

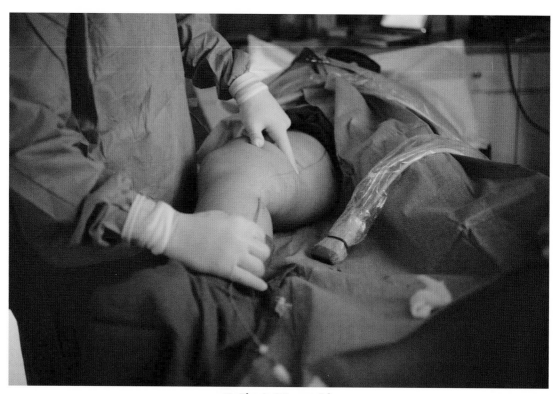

■ Fig 4–16, cont'd

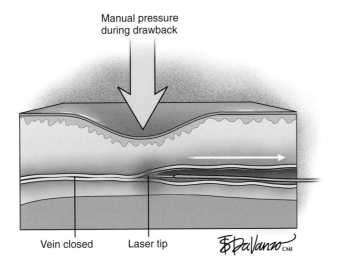

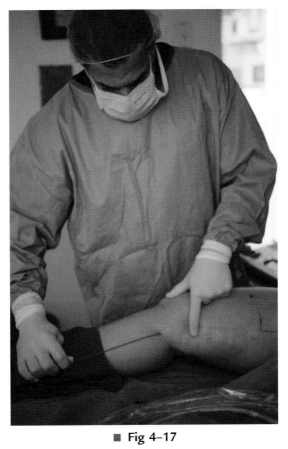

■ Fig 4–17

At termination of the laser pullback, the laser is deactivated by the surgeon's removing his or her foot from the foot pedal. The laser and the sheath are removed together in their entirety. A quick on-table duplex scan confirms vein closure. The color flow mode should demonstrate lack of flow, and the gray-scale image should demonstrate a thickened, noncompressible vein wall (Fig. 4-18).

A compression bandage is then placed by the medical assistant (Fig. 4-19). At Miami Vein Center, we prefer that the patient wear a three-layer bandage for 48 hours postprocedure. Careful application of the postoperative dressing cannot be overstated; careless dressing placement can lead to hematomas, blisters, nerve injury, ischemia, and bleeding. The limb is wrapped circumferentially from foot to groin with a compression dressing that is removed after 48 hours. The dressing should be applied with graduated pressure; the amount of pressure should decrease as one proceeds from foot to groin. During placement of the compressive bandage, it is important to pad the lateral fibular head to avoid pressure-induced injury to the deep and superficial

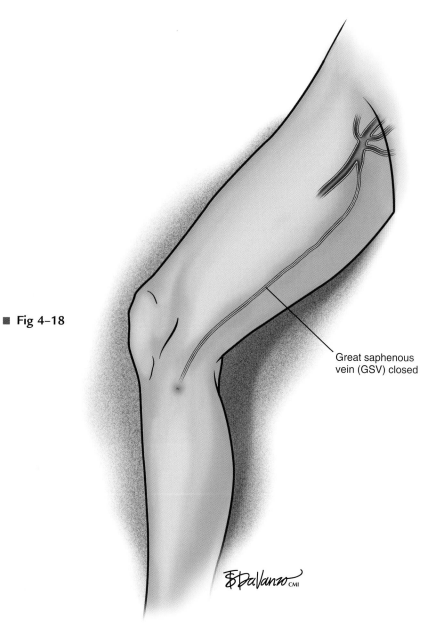

■ **Fig 4–18**

Great saphenous vein (GSV) closed

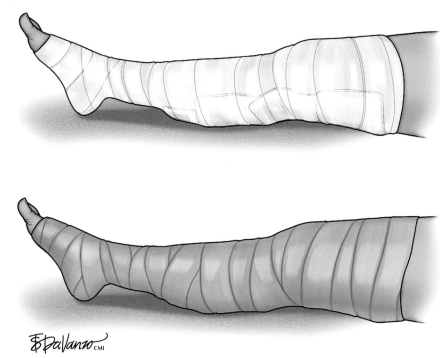

Postoperative leg bandaging

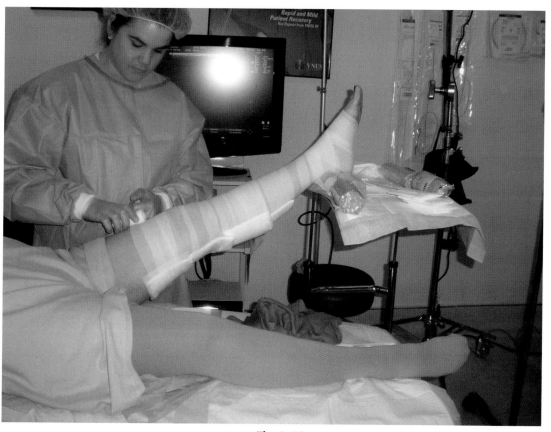

■ Fig 4–19

Continued

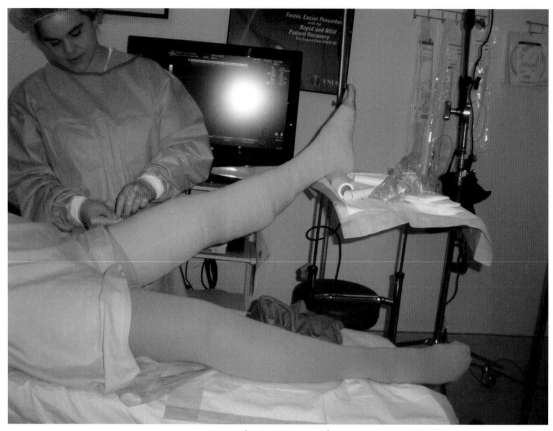

■ **Fig 4–19, cont'd**

peroneal nerves, which can lead to foot drop. Patients are encouraged to ambulate immediately after the procedure to minimize thromboembolic complications.

Application of a compressive dressing in obese patients is especially critical because the dressing has a tendency to unravel. There is a tendency to apply this dressing tightly, but this can lead to undue pressure, blistering, and/or skin necrosis.

RADIOFREQUENCY ABLATION

The VNUS Closure System includes a computer-controlled RF generator and disposable catheters (Figs. 4-20 to 4-25). RF technology has evolved from a slow continuous pullback to a rapid segmental pullback. The original device was oriented with an anode and cathode at the catheter tip. When the device was in contact with the vein wall, the vein wall acted as the resistive element of an electrical circuit analogous to a light bulb. In the case of the light bulb, an electric current passes through a thin tungsten filament, heating it until it produces light. In the case of an incompetent saphenous vein, radiofrequency current passes through the vein, heating it, causing collagen molecules to shrink. Because the heating was only 1 cm in length, a slow continuous pullback was required to adequately treat a vein. A typical 40-cm vein would take about 20 minutes to treat. Furthermore, coagulum build-up at the tip of the catheter caused an increase in the impedance, which triggered an automatic shutoff of the generator when a threshold number

Text continued on p. 116

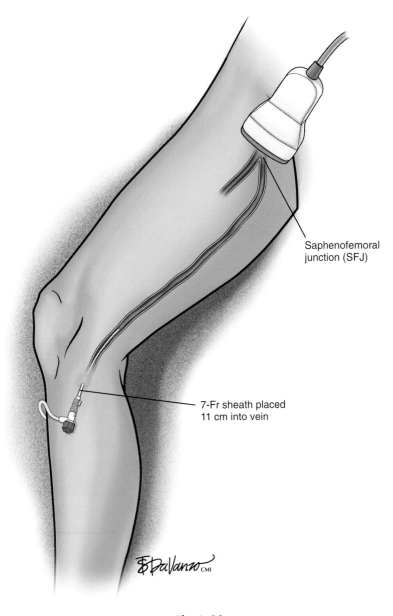

Saphenofemoral
junction (SFJ)

7-Fr sheath placed
11 cm into vein

■ **Fig 4–20**

Continued

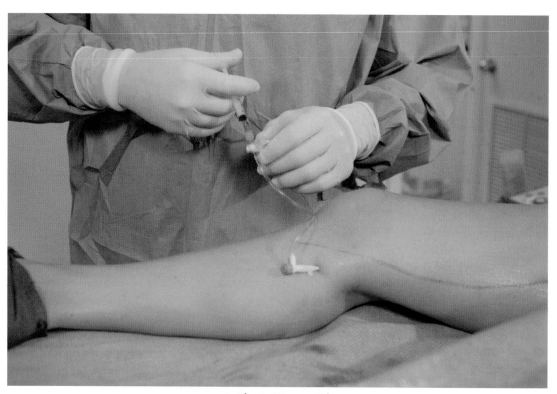

■ Fig 4–20, cont'd

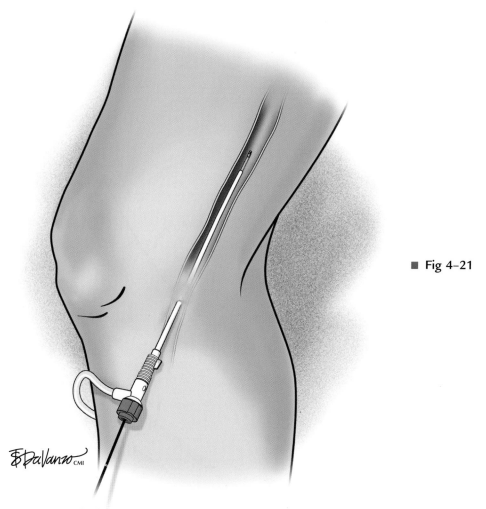

■ Fig 4–21

Radiofrequency (RF) catheter inserted into sheath

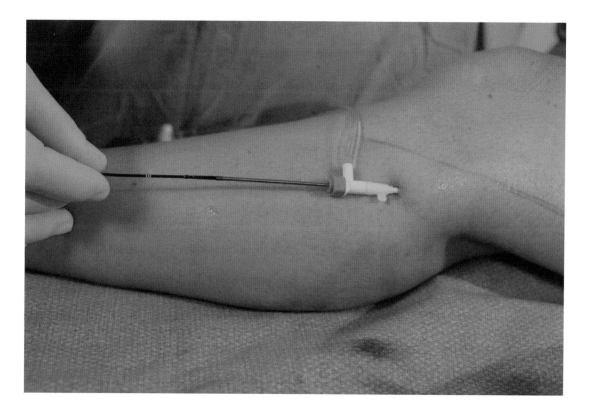

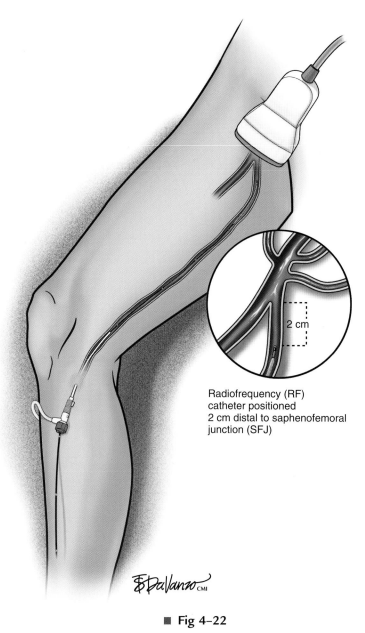

Radiofrequency (RF)
catheter positioned
2 cm distal to saphenofemoral
junction (SFJ)

■ **Fig 4–22**

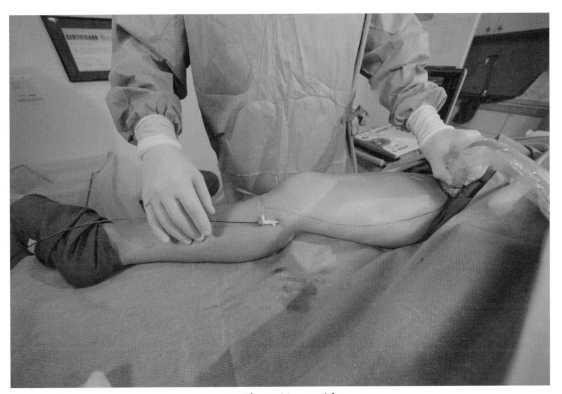

■ **Fig 4–22, cont'd**

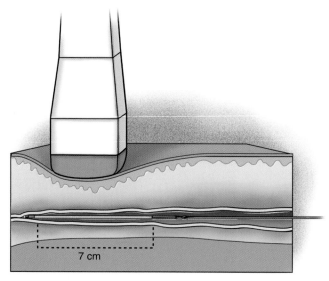

Radiofrequency (RF) catheter treating 7 cm of vein

■ **Fig 4–23**

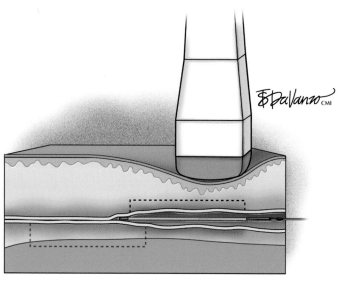

Radiofrequency (RF) catheter withdrawn 6.5 cm, treatment repeated

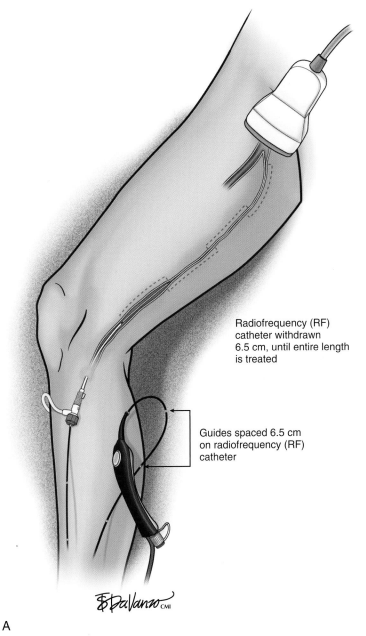

Radiofrequency (RF)
catheter withdrawn
6.5 cm, until entire length
is treated

Guides spaced 6.5 cm
on radiofrequency (RF)
catheter

A

■ **Fig 4–24**

Continued

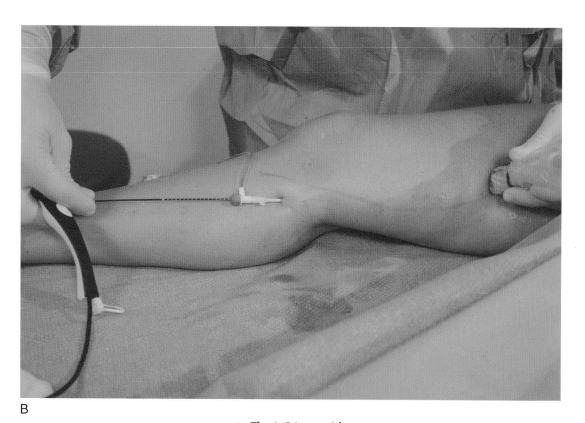

B

■ Fig 4–24, cont'd

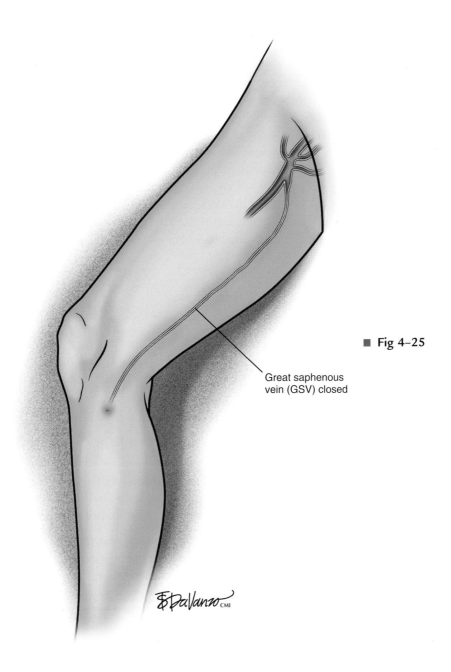

■ Fig 4–25

Great saphenous
vein (GSV) closed

was reached. In this case, catheter removal, cleaning, and reintroduction of the catheter into the vein were required. The device heated the vein wall to 85°C, and studies showed a closure rate of about 85% with 5-year follow-up.

The procedure can be performed under local anesthesia using perivenous tumescent infiltration, with or without conscious sedation. An introducer sheath is placed to allow catheter insertion into the target vein. The electrodes are deployed at the SFJ and positioned distal to the entry of the superficial epigastric vein when present or approximately 2 cm distal to the origin of the common femoral vein in cases where the superficial epigastric vein is not visualized.

The vein must be anesthetized circumferentially along the entire treatment length with a dilute lidocaine solution before treatment is begun.

Upon initiation of RF energy delivery to the electrodes, the catheter is slowly withdrawn while maintaining the treatment temperature at 85°C. The feedback mechanism of the system allows controlled energy delivery and appropriate monitoring of the procedure.

The second generation device (ClosureFAST) is fitted with a different heating element. The treatment component of the device is 7 cm in length and works with a segmental pullback protocol. That is, once the catheter is in position, activation of the generator delivers 20-second cycles of energy to the catheter tip, which heats the vein wall to 120°C. The catheter is pulled back in increments of 6.5 cm so as to overlap the treatment sites. This segmental pullback strategy with a longer length heating element translates into a treatment time of about 3 minutes for a typical saphenous vein 40 cm in length (see Fig. 4-24, *B*).

SMALL SAPHENOUS VEIN ABLATION

Gibson[10] described the anatomic differences between the SFJ and the thromboprophylaxis as well as the proximity of the sural nerve to the SSV, correctly noting that endovenous laser ablation of the SSV is slightly different than that for the GSV. The Gibson anatomic classification is depicted in Figure 4-26:

- Type A—A saphenopopliteal junction with no significant branches; 43% of limbs
- Type B—A saphenopopliteal junction with a large extension Giacomini vein; 33% of limbs
- Type C—No direct termination into a deep vein (saphenopopliteal or saphenofemoral junction), with the SSV continuing as a Giacomini vein above the popliteal fossa. The Giacomini vein was the sole termination of the SSV in 24% of limbs.

In the type A cases where the SSV enters the popliteal vein directly, the concepts remain very similar to those of GSV treatment (Fig. 4-27). The patient is taken to the office operating suite and, in the standing position, all bulging veins are marked on the skin with an indelible marker. Unlike GSV cases, where the patient is placed in the supine position, the prone position is chosen for SSV ablation. The extremity is then prepped and draped in the usual sterile manner (Fig. 4-27).

Usually, a quick preprocedure scan is performed to select the access site and determine treatment length so that the appropriate sheaths can be readied. A typical length for the SSV is about 15 cm if no cranial extension is present (Fig. 4-28). It is very important to note the anatomy of the SPJ prior to catheter placement. In the usual arrangement, best visualized with the ultrasound probe in the long axis, the SSV will deepen its course as it approaches its union with the popliteal vein. It will appear as a 45-degree bend, about 2 cm in length. We prefer to leave this 2-cm-length angled segment untreated for two reasons: (1) the gastrocnemius veins enter into this segment and are best preserved and (2) the tibial nerve comes into proximity to the SSV at this deeper level. Although it is easy to push the tibial nerve away from the vein using tumescent anesthesia, if the anesthetic diffuses onto the nerve, temporary nerve palsy may result and cause unnecessary alarm to both patient and physician.

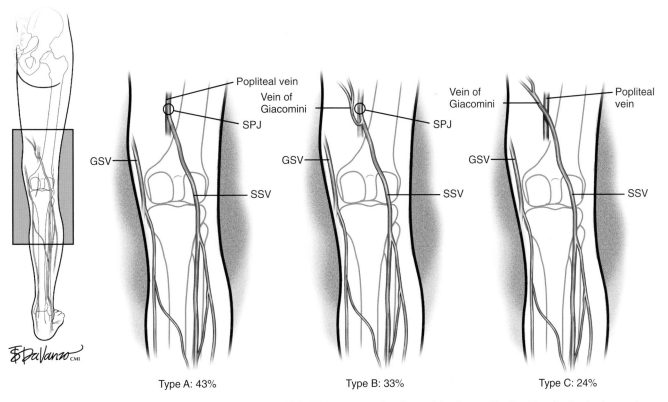

Type A: 43%   Type B: 33%   Type C: 24%

SPJ with no significant branches   SPJ with large extension Giacomini vein   No direct termination to deep vein
                                                                                    SSV continues as Giacomini vein

■ **Fig 4–26** *GSV,* Great saphenous vein; *SPJ,* saphenopopliteal junction; *SSV,* small saphenous vein.

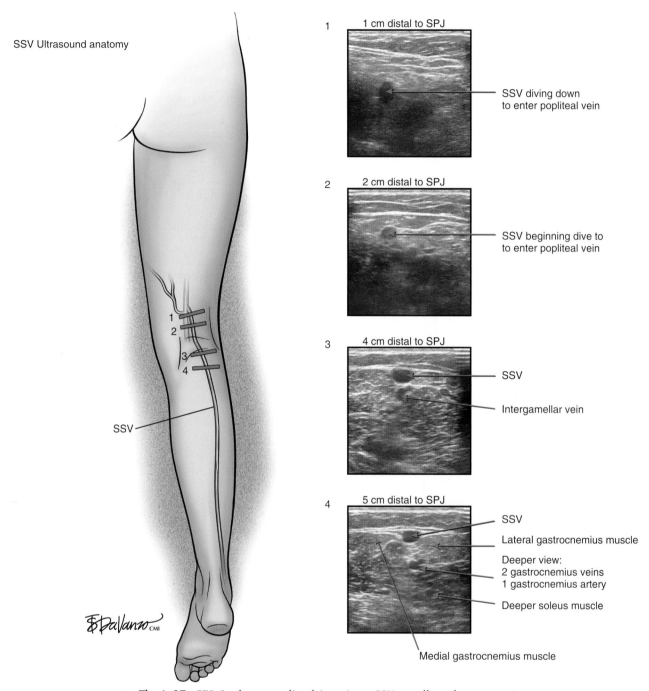

SSV Ultrasound anatomy

SSV

1 1 cm distal to SPJ

SSV diving down
to enter popliteal vein

2 2 cm distal to SPJ

SSV beginning dive to
to enter popliteal vein

3 4 cm distal to SPJ

SSV

Intergamellar vein

4 5 cm distal to SPJ

SSV
Lateral gastrocnemius muscle

Deeper view:
2 gastrocnemius veins
1 gastrocnemius artery

Deeper soleus muscle

Medial gastrocnemius muscle

■ **Fig 4–27** *SPJ,* Saphenopopliteal junction; *SSV,* small saphenous vein.

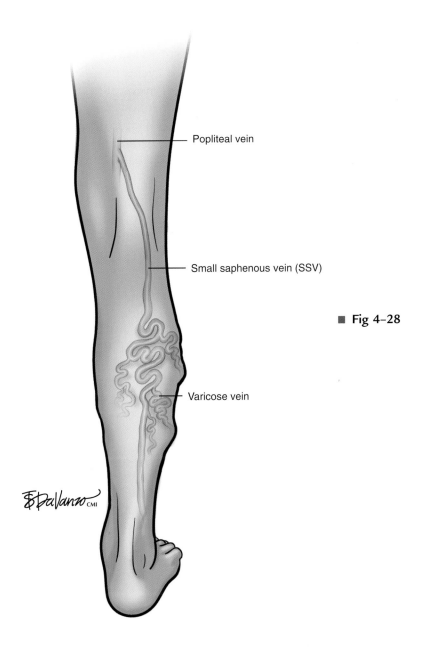

Popliteal vein

Small saphenous vein (SSV)

Varicose vein

■ **Fig 4–28**

1. ***Access*** **(FIGS. 4-29 THROUGH 4-31)**

   Percutaneous access to the SSV is achieved at mid-calf on the inferior aspect of the gastrocnemius muscles. A micropuncture kit with a 21-gauge needle and .018-inch guidewire is preferred. The .018-inch wire is advanced through the needle to the SPJ under ultrasound guidance. The microintroducer and sheath are then placed and exchanged for a .035-inch wire.

   In the case of RF, a 7-cm-length, 7-Fr sheath is placed. Keep in mind that once the RF heating element is exteriorized from the end of the sheath, the total length of the device will be about 14 cm. In the typical 15-cm-length SSV, this will translate into one double-treatment cycle at the SPJ followed by one more cycle of energy delivery after the catheter pullback—three cycles (60 seconds) total treatment.

   In the case of EVL, the laser fiber tip governs most of the decision making. Usually the vein is accessed with a 21-gauge needle followed by microintroducer placement. If using a bare-tipped 600-μm fiber, or a 400-μm fiber, the fiber will fit directly through the microintroducer sheath. However, if working with a 600-μm jacket-tip fiber, the microintroducer will need to be exchanged for a 4- or 5-Fr sheath.

2. ***Positioning*** **(FIG. 4-32)**

   The RF and laser fiber tips are positioned at the same location—about 2 cm distal to the popliteal vein opening, where the "bend" of the SSV is usually located. Because there is some forward heating with the RF ClosureFAST device, in general, I prefer laser for SSV ablations, although many operators use RF in this area with success.

3. ***Anesthesia***

   The SSV is also enveloped in a fascial compartment similar to that of the GSV, except that it is more fully developed. This fascial tissue is thicker and serves as a consistent landmark to locate the SSV. The SSV is located in the midline of the posterior calf, at the most superficial location where the medial and lateral heads of the gastrocnemius muscles meet.

   The same principles for tumescent anesthesia apply here. Using ultrasound, the solution is placed in the perivenous plane. Ideally, SSV compression and diameter shrinkage are observed.

4. ***Pullback*** **(FIG. 4-33)**

   In this area, treatment with RF can be challenging. In general, veins of shorter length require more attention from the operator because of the nature of the device with a 7-cm-length heating element. With laser, it is the same technique as for other veins, such as the GSV. First, one decides the desired LEED, the power is set, and pullback speed is determined. Vein of Giacomini ablation is demonstrated in Figure 4-34.

   Text continued on p. 128

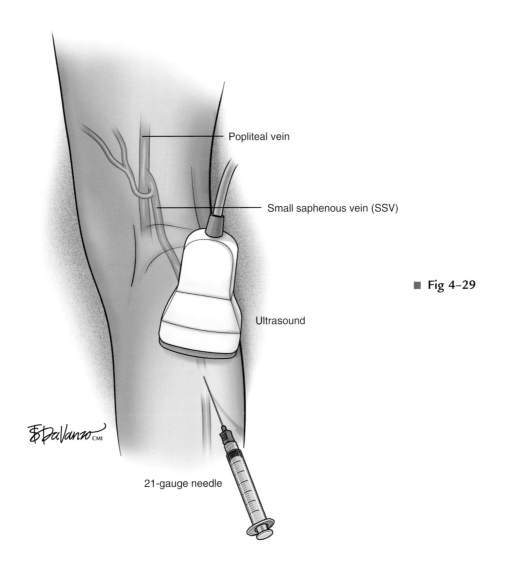

Popliteal vein

Small saphenous vein (SSV)

■ **Fig 4–29**

Ultrasound

21-gauge needle

■ Fig 4–30

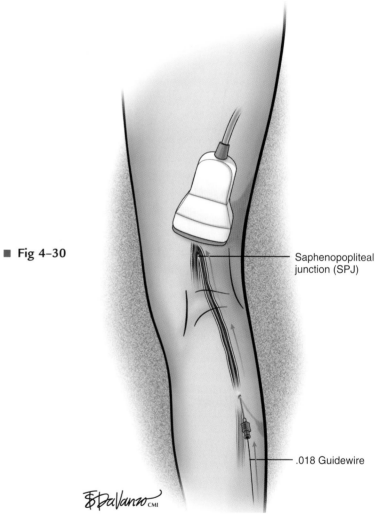

Saphenopopliteal junction (SPJ)

.018 Guidewire

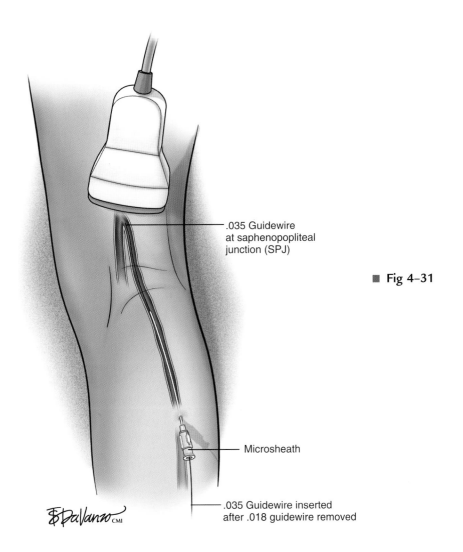

.035 Guidewire
at saphenopopliteal
junction (SPJ)

■ Fig 4–31

Microsheath

.035 Guidewire inserted
after .018 guidewire removed

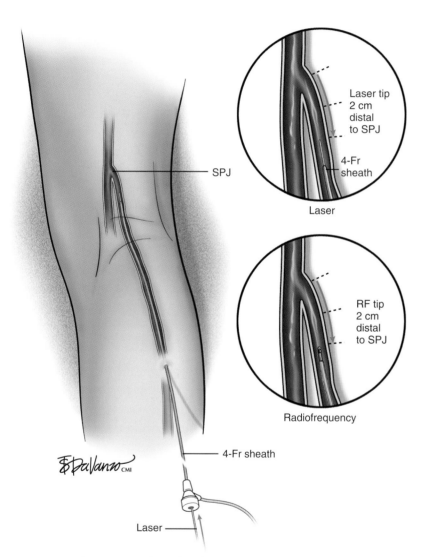

■ **Fig 4–32** Laser (*upper panel*) and radiofrequency (*RF*) (*lower panel*) catheter positioning at saphenopopliteal junction (*SPJ*).

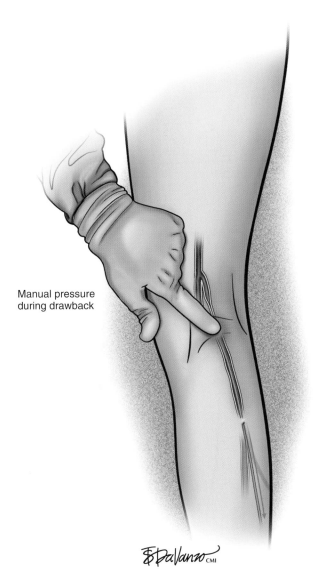

Manual pressure
during drawback

■ Fig 4–33

Continued

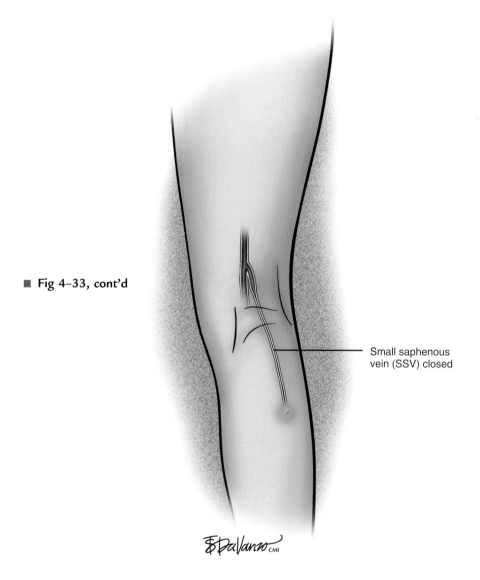

■ **Fig 4–33, cont'd**

Small saphenous vein (SSV) closed

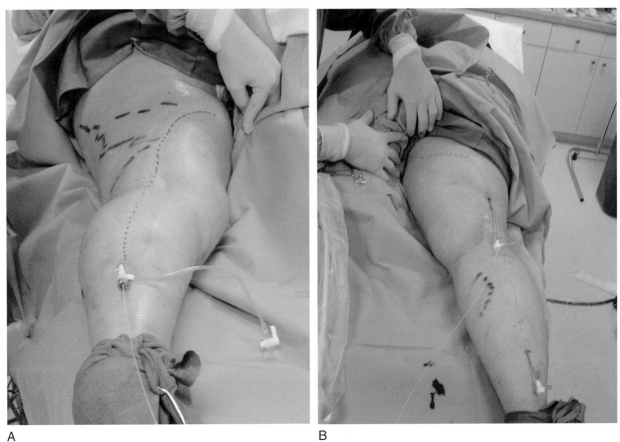

A   B

■ **Fig 4–34 A,** The vein of Giacomini can be ablated using standard principles. In this case, a single puncture allowed access to the entire vein. **B,** Sometimes two access sites are required.

TREATING ACCESSORY AND CIRCUMFLEX VEINS
(FIGS. 4-35, 4-36, and 4-37)

The aforementioned principles hold true for incompetent accessory and circumflex veins. The distalmost segment of a straight vein is chosen. For circumflex veins, these access points usually present themselves in the upper third of the thigh; thus, treatment lengths tend to be short, in the order of 5- to 10-cm lengths. Circumflex veins by definition take oblique angles, and this must be factored in during the hand-eye coordination required for access. Also, because these veins tend to have short treatment lengths, micropuncture exchanges to longer sheaths are often cumbersome. For this reason, I prefer laser for these cases. The laser fiber will fit through a micropuncture access sheath, and the energy is delivered from the tip of the laser fiber. Because the heating element for the RF catheter is 7 cm in length, it is not as versatile when treating circumflex veins.

Accessory veins are usually longer than circumflex veins but shorter than the GSV. Because they run parallel to the axis of the GSV, access resembles GSV access.

Positioning the tip of the device at the SFJ requires a little more manipulation of the ultrasound probe in order to obtain a good view of the junction.

At the groin, the anterior accessory great saphenous vein (AAGSV) is superficial to the common femoral vein and located lateral to the GSV and medial to the common femoral artery. The "alignment sign" is useful for tracking the AAGSV. The AAGSV is found directly superior to and in the same ultrasound plane as the superficial femoral artery and femoral vein. The AAGSV is found anterior and lateral to the GSV and runs parallel to the GSV; often it is confused with the anterior thigh circumflex vein (ATCV), which takes an oblique course to the GSV (Fig. 4-35, *A*).

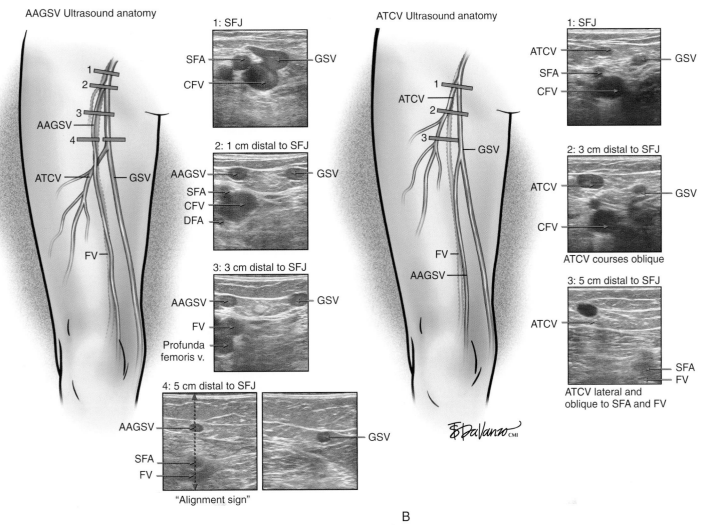

■ **Fig 4–35 A** and **B,** *AAGSV,* Anterior accessory great saphenous vein; *ATCV,* anterior thigh circumflex vein; *CFV,* common femoral vein; *DFA,* deep formal artery; *FV,* femoral vein; *GSV,* great saphenous vein; *SFA,* superficial femoral artery; *SFJ,* saphenofemoral junction.

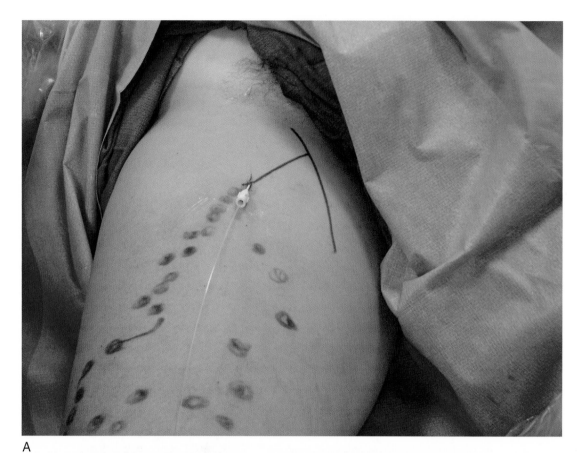

A

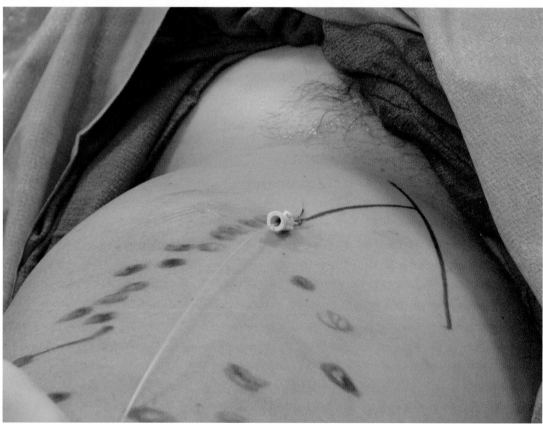

B

■ **Fig 4–36 A,** Intravenous access of anterior thigh circumflex vein (ATCV) with microsheath (bare laser fiber placed). **B,** Close-up of **A.**

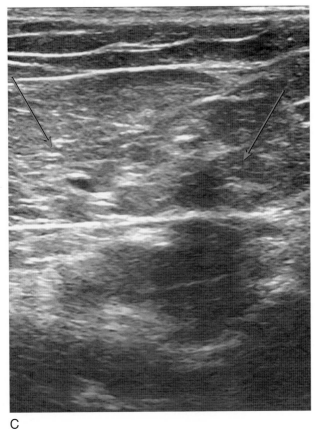

C

■ **Fig 4–36, cont'd C,** Left arrow points to anterior thigh circumflex vein (ATCV). Right arrow points to great saphenous vein (GSV).

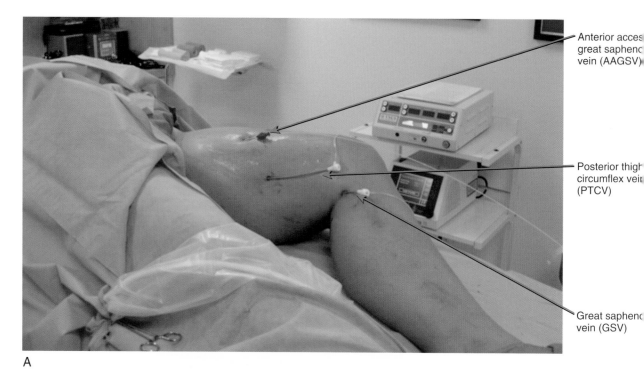

Anterior acces
great saphenc
vein (AAGSV)

Posterior thigh
circumflex vein
(PTCV)

Great saphenc
vein (GSV)

A

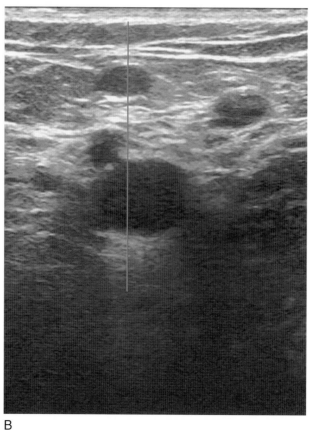

B

■ **Fig 4-37 A,** Multiple vein access. **B,** Line shows alignment of anterior accessory saphenous vein (AASV) above femoral vessels.

POPLITEAL FOSSA VEIN

Designated the popliteal fossa vein (PFV), it perforates the deep popliteal fascia and empties into the deep system (Fig. 4-38).

With a prevalence of 4.4%, the PFV presents in limbs featuring complex reflux patterns involving all three venous systems proximally and distally and high venous clinical severity scores. The PFV perforates the deep popliteal fascia terminating at the deep system (i.e., the popliteal vein in 96%) above the SSV.

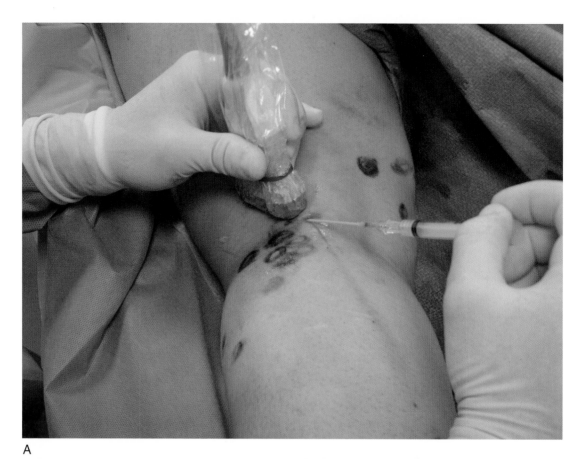

A

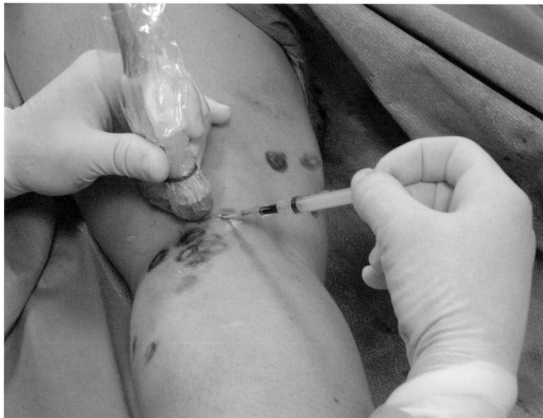

B

■ **Fig 4–38 A** and **B,** Percutaneous access of the popliteal fossa vein (PFV) under ultrasound control. Demonstrated is the use of 14-gauge angiocath through which a bare laser fiber is placed. Notice that the treatment length is only 2 cm.

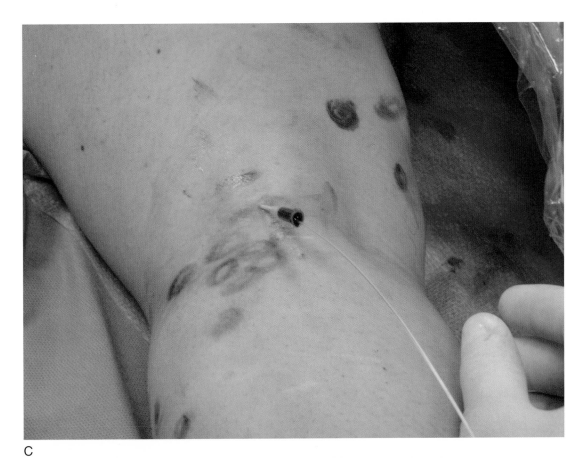

C

D

■ **Fig 4–38, cont'd C** and **D,** Percutaneous access of the popliteal fossa vein (PFV) under ultrasound control. Demonstrated is the use of 14-gauge angiocath through which a bare laser fiber is placed. Notice that the treatment length is only 2 cm.

Continued

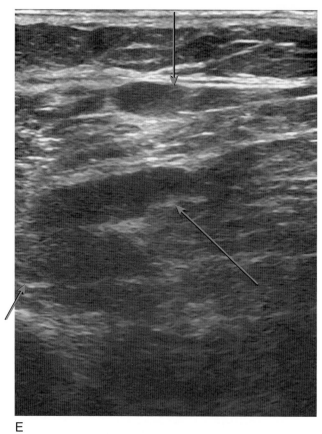

E

■ **Fig 4–38, cont'd E,** Popliteal fossa vein (PFV) ultrasound. Bottom left arrow points to the popliteal vein. Bottom right arrow points to the PFV. Top arrow points to the small saphenous vein (SSV).

LASER-ASSISTED DISTAL SAPHENECTOMY

We also developed a technique referred to as LADS (laser-assisted distal saphenectomy). This hybrid technique is useful when the GSV leaves the saphenous canal in the thigh and courses superficially under the skin down the leg (Figs. 4-39 through 4-45).

The thigh GSV is treated in the usual manner with endovenous laser, but when the superficial course of the vein is identified by the laser aiming beam, the vein is elevated via a small stab incision and exteriorized. Invagination stripping of the distal saphenous vein is performed by suturing it to the 4-Fr sheath with double-armed 2.0 Prolene suture. The sheath will serve as an invagination stripping device.

The premise behind the procedure is avoiding the discoloration associated with leaving a thermally ablated vein next to the skin. Thermal ablation causes some carbonization endoluminally, and this pigmentation transilluminates through the skin. The result is a cosmetically unpleasing "black line" where the vein courses; therefore, it is best removed to avoid this problem.

Text continued on p. 150

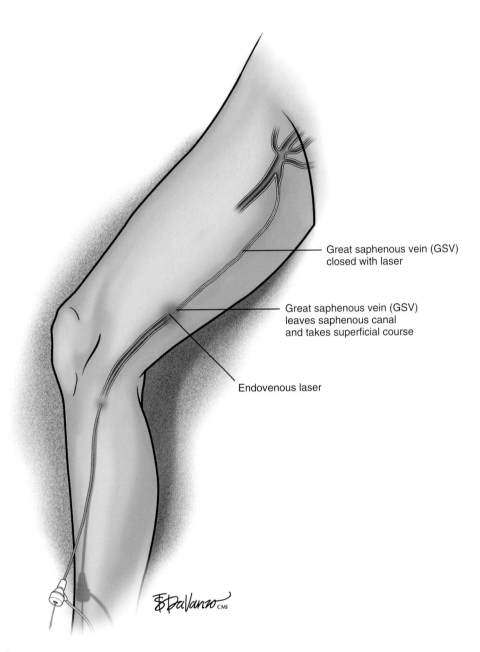

Great saphenous vein (GSV)
closed with laser

Great saphenous vein (GSV)
leaves saphenous canal
and takes superficial course

Endovenous laser

A

■ Fig 4-39

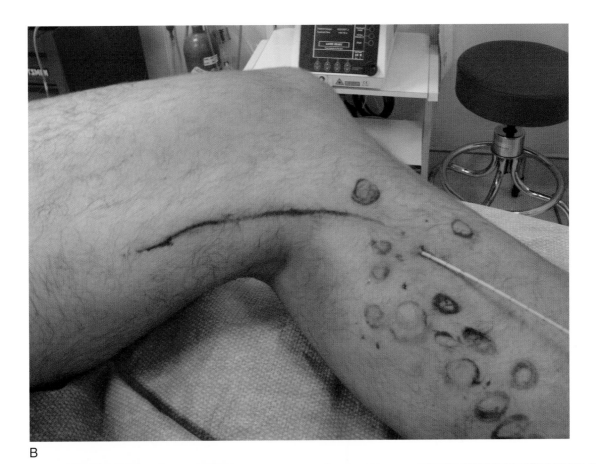

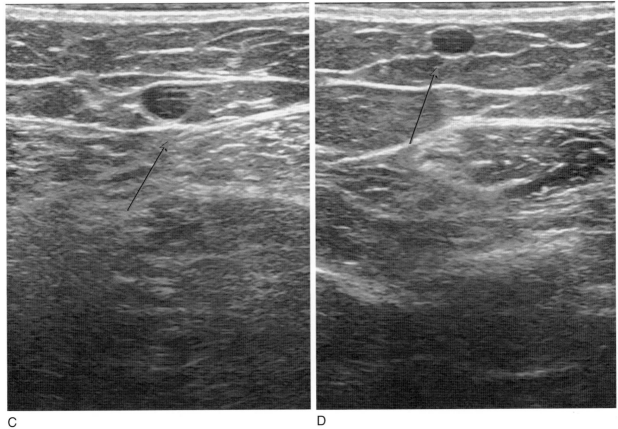

■ **Fig 4–39, cont'd C,** Great saphenous vein (GSV) in saphenous canal (*arrow*).
D, GSV close to skin; also known as superficial accessory saphenous vein (SASV)
(*arrow*).

■ **Fig 4–40**

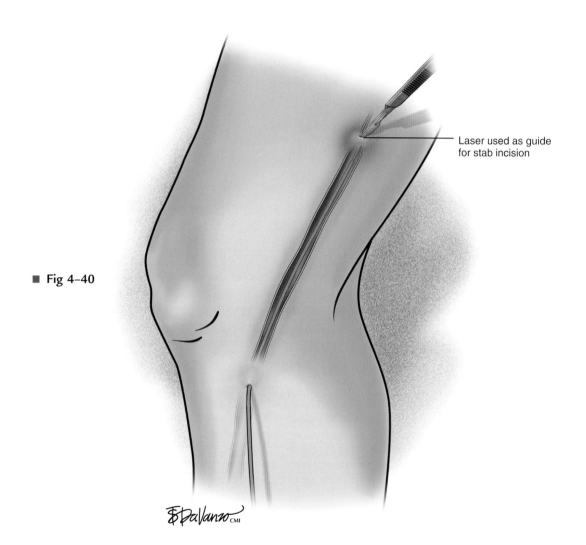

Laser used as guide
for stab incision

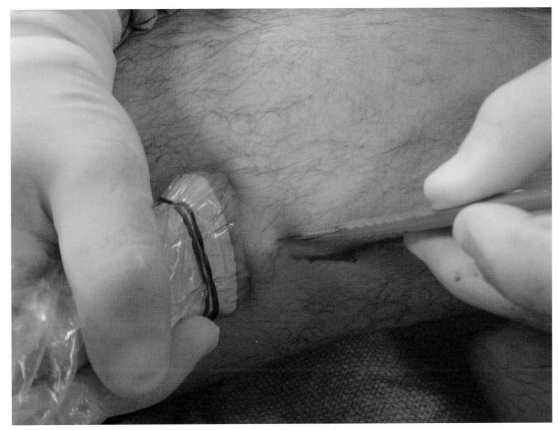

■ **Fig 4–40, cont'd**

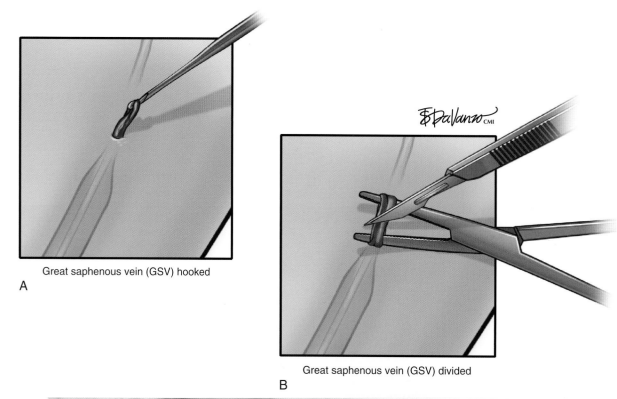

Great saphenous vein (GSV) hooked

A

Great saphenous vein (GSV) divided

B

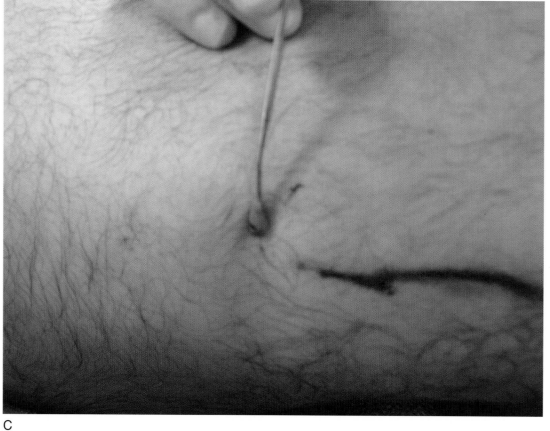

C

■ **Fig 4–41 A** through **C,** At mid-thigh, a small stab incision is made with a No. 11 blade knife. The vein is exteriorized with a crochet hook. The vein is divided, and the distal vein is carefully grasped with a hemostat.

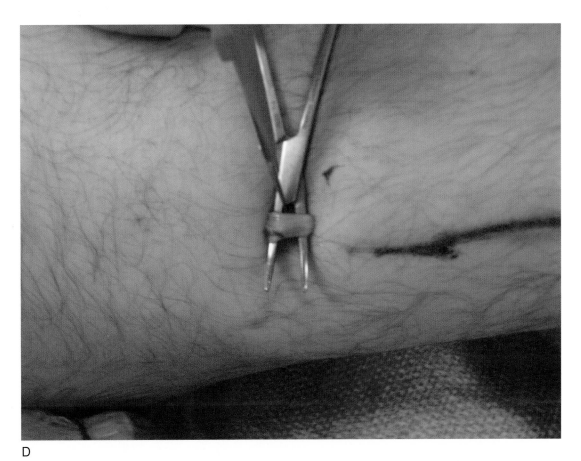

D

■ **Fig 4–41, cont'd D,** At mid-thigh, a small stab incision is made with a No. 11 blade knife. The vein is exteriorized with a crochet hook. The vein is divided, and the distal vein is carefully grasped with a hemostat.

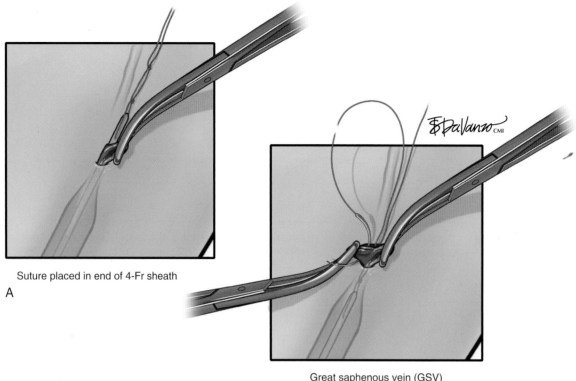

Suture placed in end of 4-Fr sheath

A

Great saphenous vein (GSV)
sutured to tip of 4-Fr sheath

B

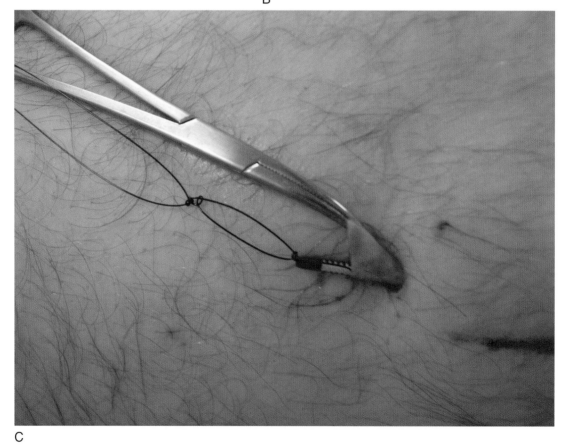

C

■ **Fig 4–42 A** through **C,** The endoluminal sheath advanced from below through
the distal vein at mid-thigh. A braided 4-Fr sheath is preferred because it
is more robust. A standard invagination saphenectomy is performed using 2.0
Prolene double-armed suture. Notice that the Prolene suture has been secured
through the open end of the 4-Fr braided sheath.

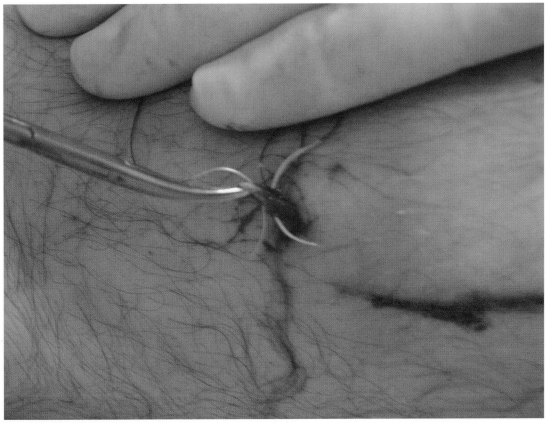

D

■ **Fig 4–42, cont'd D,** The endoluminal sheath advanced from below through the distal vein at mid-thigh. A braided 4-Fr sheath is preferred because it is more robust. A standard invagination saphenectomy is performed using 2.0 Prolene double-armed suture. Notice that the Prolene suture has been secured through the open end of the 4-Fr braided sheath.

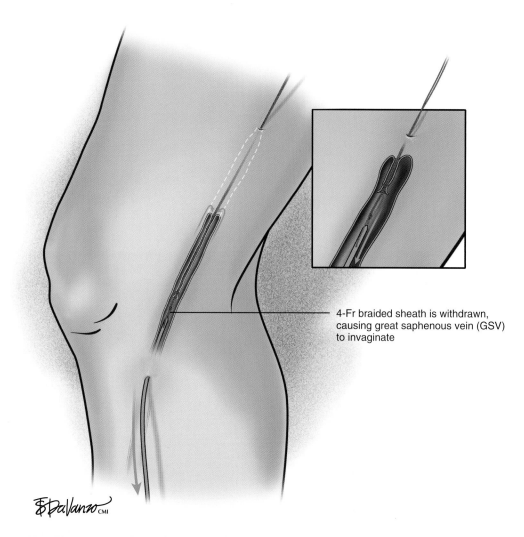

4-Fr braided sheath is withdrawn, causing great saphenous vein (GSV) to invaginate

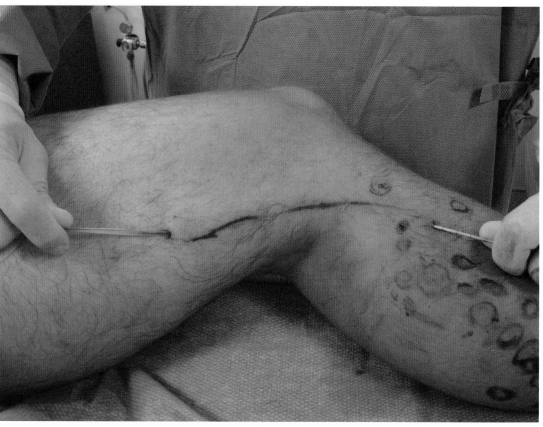

■ Fig 4–43

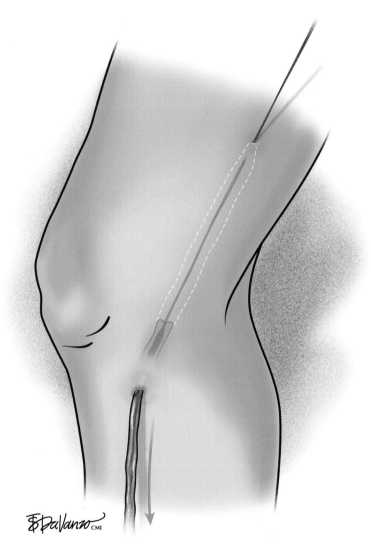

Inverted vein removed

A

■ **Fig 4-44 A,** The invaginated great saphenous vein (GSV) being harvested from the entry site at the calf. Notice how the 2.0 Prolene suture secured to the 4-Fr braided sheath has nicely invaginated the GSV.

Continued

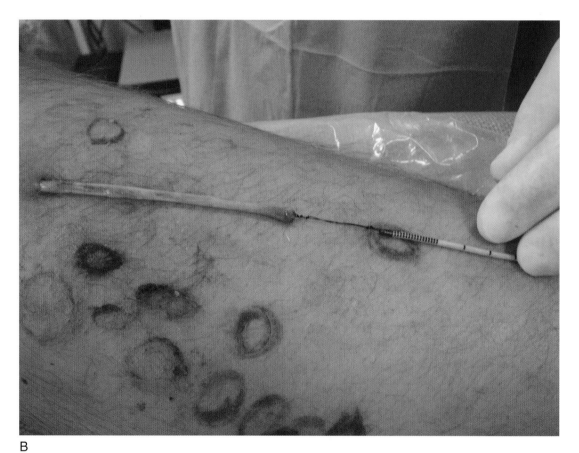

B

◾ **Fig 4–44, cont'd B,** The invaginated GSV being harvested from the entry site at the calf. Notice how the 2.0 Prolene suture secured to the 4-Fr braided sheath has nicely invaginated the GSV.

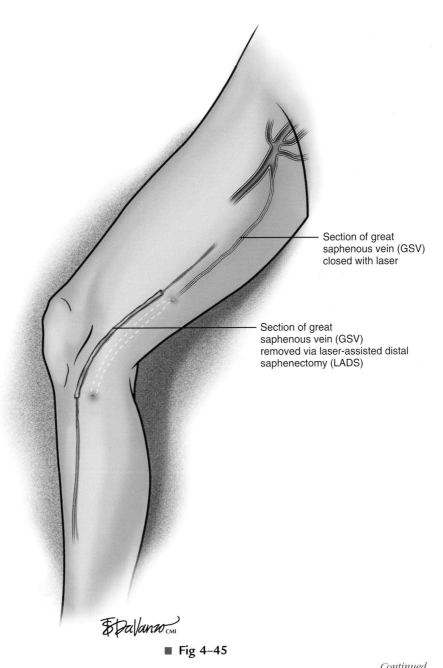

Section of great
saphenous vein (GSV)
closed with laser

Section of great
saphenous vein (GSV)
removed via laser-assisted distal
saphenectomy (LADS)

■ **Fig 4–45**

Continued

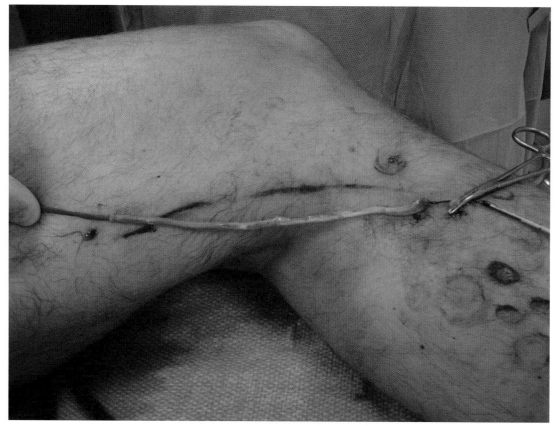

■ **Fig 4–45, cont'd**

MULTIPLE VEINS AND HYBRID PROCEDURES

At Miami Vein Center, we routinely use multiple modalities or techniques during a procedure, depending on the clinical scenario. In the case of multiple incompetent veins, each is accessed and treated individually using all of the aforementioned principles (Figs. 4-46 through 4-48). In general, to effectively deal with these cases, multimodality therapy is required—with the addition of some creativity on the part of the surgeon. If the surgeon is skilled in thermal ablation, ambulatory phlebectomy, and ultrasound-guided foam sclerotherapy, he or she can tackle 99% of the cases that present to his/her practice in the office-based surgical suite.

Text continued on p. 158

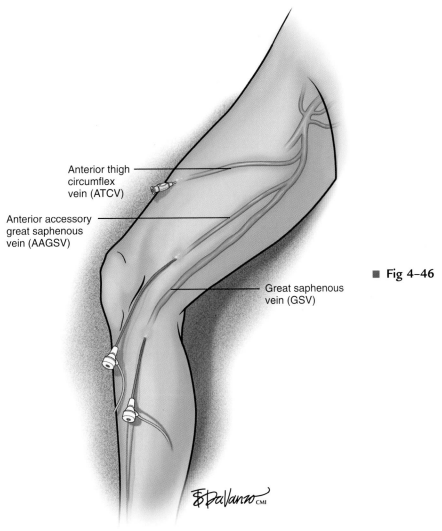

Anterior thigh circumflex vein (ATCV)

Anterior accessory great saphenous vein (AAGSV)

Great saphenous vein (GSV)

■ Fig 4–46

Multiple vein treatment

Continued

■ **Fig 4–46, cont'd**

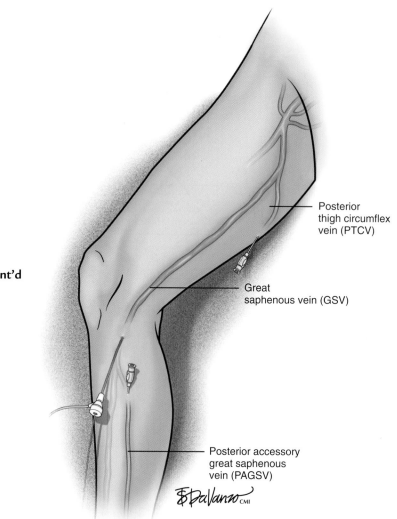

Posterior
thigh circumflex
vein (PTCV)

Great
saphenous vein (GSV)

Posterior accessory
great saphenous
vein (PAGSV)

Multiple vein treatment

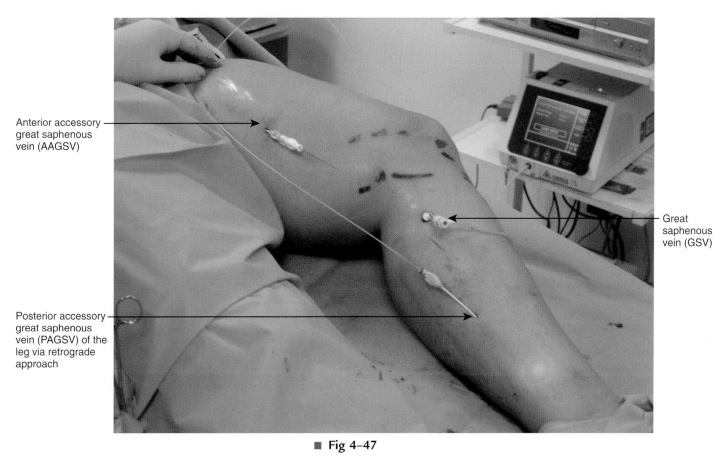

Anterior accessory
great saphenous
vein (AAGSV)

Great
saphenous
vein (GSV)

Posterior accessory
great saphenous
vein (PAGSV) of the
leg via retrograde
approach

■ Fig 4–47

Continued

Anterior thigh
circumflex vein
(ATCV)

Great saphenous
vein (GSV)

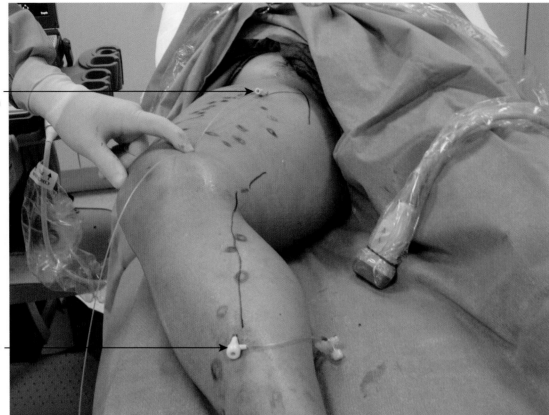

Anterior accessory
great saphenous
vein (AAGSV) of
leg via retrograde
approach

Great saphenous
vein (GSV)

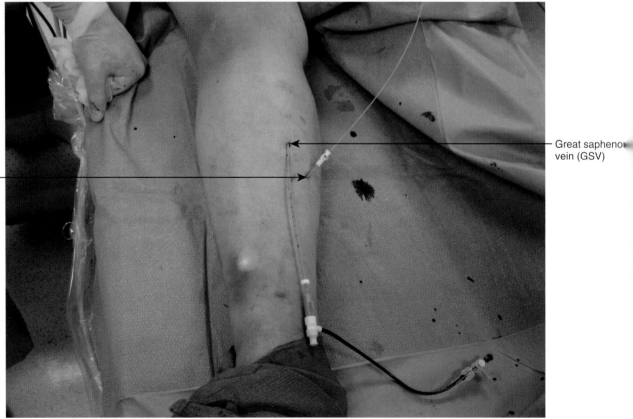

■ Fig 4-47, cont'd

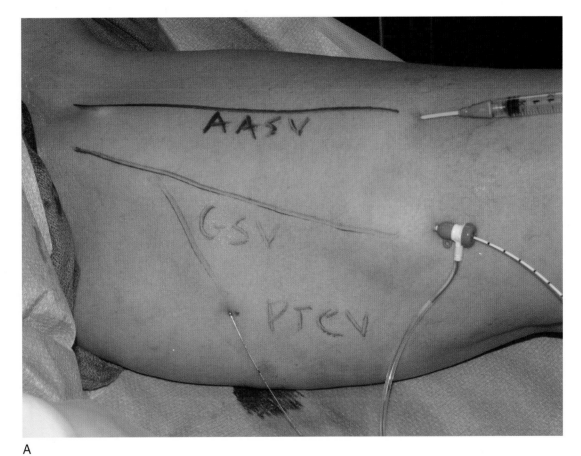

A

■ **Fig 4–48 A,** Multiple venous access using one kit. Sheath with laser fiber in the great saphenous vein (GSV). Dilator in the anterior accessory saphenous vein (AASV). Wire in the posterior thigh circumflex vein (PTCV).   *Continued*

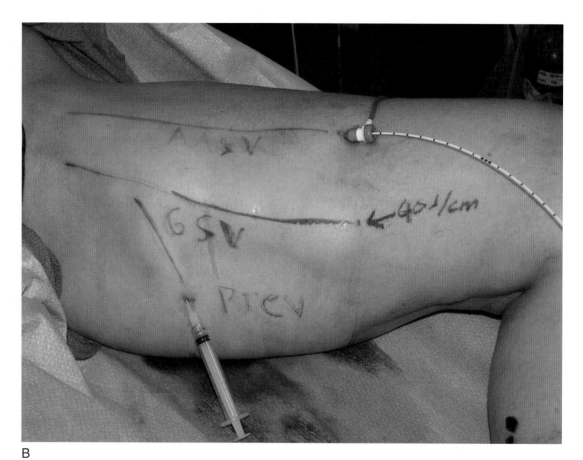

B

■ **Fig 4–48, cont'd B,** GSV treated with 40 J/cm using 1470 nm wavelength; then the sheath is transferred to the AASV. The PTCV wire was exchanged for 4-Fr microsheath in preparation for laser.

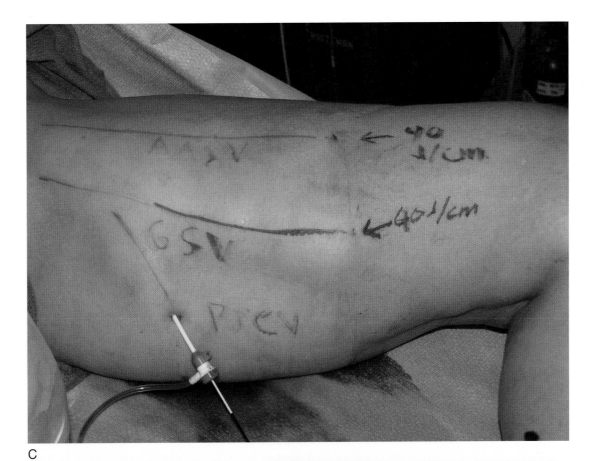

C

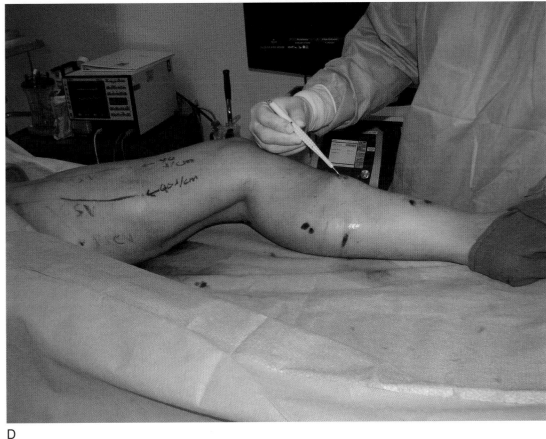

D

■ **Fig 4–48, cont'd C,** AASV treatment completed with 40 J/cm of energy, and the same sheath and laser fiber are transferred to the PTCV for treatment. **D,** After triple-truncal-vein ablation is complete, ambulatory phlebectomy is performed in the same setting of previously marked bulging varicose veins.

CONCLUSION

Endovenous thermal ablation is elegant by its mere simplicity. It is effective and safe and has acceptable cosmetic results. Ambulatory phlebectomy and ultrasound-guided foam sclerotherapy are perfect complements to endovenous thermal ablation of the saphenous veins. With this combination, virtually all patients with simple or complex superficial and perforating vein problems can be dealt with effectively, in the comfort of a physician's office. (For information on complications and for comparative effectiveness of existing treatments, see Chapters 5 and 6.)

REFERENCES

1. Trendelenberg F. Uber die Unterbindung der Vena Saphena Magna bie Unterschenkel Varicen. Beitr Z Clin Chir 1891;7:195.
2. Keller WL. A new method of extirpating the internal saphenous and similar veins in varicose conditions. N Y Med J 1905;82:385.
3. Bergan JJ, Pascarella L. Varicose vein surgery. In: Wilmore D, Souba W, Fink M, editors. ACS Surgery Online. New York: WebMD, Inc; 2003.
4. Rautio T, Ohinmaa A, Perala J, et al. Endovenous obliteration versus conventional stripping operation in the treatment of primary varicose veins: a randomized controlled trial with comparison of the costs. J Vasc Surg 2002;35:958-965.
5. Lurie F, Creton D, Eklof B, et al. Prospective randomised study of endovenous radiofrequency obliteration (closure) versus ligation and vein stripping (EVOLVeS): two-year follow-up. Eur J Vasc Endovasc Surg 2005;29:67-73.
6. Stotter L, Schaaf I, Bockelbrink A, et al. Radiofrequency obliteration, invagination or cryo stripping: which is the best tolerated treatment by the patients? Phlebologie 2005;34:19-24.
7. Hinchcliff RJ, Ubhi J, Beech A, et al. A prospective randomized controlled trial of VNUS Closure versus surgery for the treatment of recurrent long saphenous varicose veins. Eur J Vasc Edovasc Surg 2006;31:212-218.
8. Min RJ, Khilnani N, Zimmet SE. Endovenous laser treatment of saphenous vein reflux: long-term results. J Vasc Interv Radiol 2003;14:991-996.
9. Almeida JI, Raines JK. Radiofrequency ablation and laser ablation in the treatment of varicose veins. Ann Vasc Surg 2006;20:547-552.
10. Gibson KD, Ferris BL, Polissar N, et al. Endovenous laser treatment of the small saphenous vein: efficacy and complications. J Vasc Surg 2007;45:795-801.

CHAPTER 5

Radiofrequency Thermal Ablation

Jose I. Almeida

HISTORICAL BACKGROUND

Investigators in the 1960s and 1970s observed third-degree skin burns and saphenous nerve injuries after thermal ablation of the saphenous vein.[1,2] Low-wattage, bipolar current, and specific electrode designs, coupled with algorithms governed by frequent sampling of wall temperature and impedance, were expected to mitigate thermal damage to adjacent tissues. The use of bipolar electrodes, which concentrate current density along minimal impedance paths between the poles, helped resolve these problems.[3] In addition, early experiences demonstrated that procedural modifications were also needed to minimize complications and early failures.

First-Generation Device

In an industry-sponsored feasibility study: (1) the Restore catheter (VNUS Medical Technologies, Inc., Sunnyvale, CA) induced a short subvalvular constriction to improve the competence of valve leaflets and (2) the Closure catheter applied resistive heating over long vein lengths to cause maximum wall contraction for permanent obliteration.[4] Treatment with Restore catheters resulted in recurrent or persistent reflux in 81% of patients followed up for 6 to 12 months. Treatment with Closure catheters resulted in a 6% recurrent reflux rate and a 4% incidence of recurrent varicosities at a mean follow-up of 4.7 months. The authors concluded that treatment with Closure catheters was an effective, less invasive option than saphenous stripping, with complications and early failures that could be mitigated through further procedural modifications.

In 1999, VNUS Medical Technologies, Inc. (Sunnyvale, CA) received approval from the U.S. Food and Drug Administration (FDA) to market and sell a new device for closure of incompetent saphenous veins. The first-generation device, known as the Closure Procedure, used bipolar electrodes mounted on the end of a catheter to deliver radiofrequency (RF) energy to the inner vein wall. The catheter's collapsible bipolar electrodes included a temperature sensor that provided feedback to a dedicated RF generator. When deployed, the electrodes made direct contact with the endoluminal surface of the vein wall, and RF energy was delivered. The resistive effects of the vein wall tissue caused conversion of RF energy into heat. The principal mechanism of RF ablation has been demonstrated in animal studies.[5] Vein wall collagen contraction in response to thermal energy causes immediate vein wall thickening and reduction in the lumen diameter. Endothelial destruction causes an inflammatory response, which results in fibrosis and permanent vein occlusion.

The thermal effect on the vein wall is directly related to both the treatment temperature and the treatment time, the latter being a function of catheter pullback speed. The treatment protocol called for a treatment temperature of 85 °C at a pullback speed of 3 cm/min. The thermal effect produces sufficient collagen contraction to occlude the lumen while limiting heat penetration to perivenous tissue.[6,7] To assess the potential of perivenous tissue damage, the adventitial temperature was recorded in an in vitro model.[8] With the standard treatment protocol, the average peak adventitial temperature was 64.4° C and usually lasted for approximately 10 seconds at any given position along the length of the vein. Peak adventitial temperature was decreased to 51.3° C in the presence of a 2-mm perivenous saline layer.

Second-Generation Device (VNUS ClosureFAST)

With the introduction of the ClosureFAST RF ablation catheter, the elimination of the slow pullback and the implementation of stationary (segmental) treatment at 120 °C markedly improved the procedure. Controlled heating by conduction avoids vein perforations even with high dosing of thermal energy. The postprocedure inflammatory consequences often seen after endovenous laser ablation (EVL) are relatively absent with ClosureFAST.

The linear endovenous energy density (LEED) is frequently used to compare energy dosing in endovenous procedures. With the first-generation (bipolar) RF device, the catheter pullback velocity had to be slow enough to allow resistive heating of the vein wall to a target temperature of 85 °C. Measurements of the delivered energy dose to the vein were not displayed to the operator because the power delivered by the generator was subject to regulation by a feedback loop to maintain a constant temperature of 85° C. With CLF, the temperature is kept stable at 120° C during a 20-second treatment cycle. At the saphenofemoral junction (SFJ), two cycles of RF energy are delivered, averaging an LEED of 116.2 ± 11.6 J/cm for the first 7 cm of vein juxtaposed to the SFJ to ensure good vein closure at this critical site.[9] Distal to the SFJ, 68.2 ± 17.5 J/cm is delivered to each 7-cm treatment site. Thus, this aggressive "double energy cycle" at the zone of the SFJ is supported by Almeida and Raines' retrospective analysis.[10]

Proebstle reported outcomes following CLF in early 2008. The occlusion rate following segmental RFA was 99.6% at 2 years, and 70% of treated patients did not require any analgesia postprocedure.[9]

Quality-of-Life Changes

Studies of quality of life are scarce, but significant improvements in disease-specific quality-of-life following RFA were reported in the EVOLVeS study, using the CIVIQ-2 questionnaire.[11,12] Moreover, these quality-of-life statistics were improved compared to patients treated with traditional venous surgery.

ETIOLOGY AND NATURAL HISTORY OF DISEASE

Treatment Efficacy

Duplex ultrasound examination has significantly advanced our understanding of venous disease and provides both anatomic and pathophysiologic information. The morphologic and hemodynamic outcomes following RF ablation have been described in detailed ultrasound studies by Pichot et al.[13] The pathologic sequelae of a treated vein are reflected by its sonographic progression. Occluded veins were initially hypoechogenic compared with the surrounding tissue and gradually evolved into hyperechogenic and eventually isoechogenic presentations, indicating a healing process. Approximately 60% of veins were hypoechogenic and 40% were hyperechogenic at 1 week. By 6 months, they became either hyperechogenic or isoechogenic.[13] Sonographic disappearance of the saphenous vein, the desired endpoint, was observed by Weiss and Weiss in 90% of limbs at 2 years.[14]

Failures

Incomplete ablation, either segmental or total length of the vein, constitutes anatomic failure. Veins that are patent after treatment represent initial incomplete treatment or subsequent recanalization. Regardless of the presence of an anatomic failure, clinically, symptom improvement was often demonstrated in patients reported in the registry.[15]

Four types of SFJ morphologies were identified after RF ablation[15-17]: J-1, defined as complete SFJ obliteration with no SFJ flow; J-2, defined as patent SFJ tributaries draining toward the femoral vein with (J-2b) or without (J-2a) a short patent saphenous stump; and J-3, defined as terminal great saphenous vein (GSV) competence with normal antegrade flow coming from both tributaries and the saphenous vein above a limited GSV obliteration. Two years after RF ablation, the most common findings were either complete SFJ obliteration or a 5-cm or smaller patent terminal stump connecting prograde tributary flow through the SFJ, accounting for approximately 90% of the limbs treated.[15,17]

The clinical significance of a short patent SFJ stump was analyzed in a study by Merchant et al.[15] A total of 319 limbs in the Clinical Registry were followed at 1 week, 6 months, 1 year, and 2 years, with 2-year data available for 121 limbs. Comparison of symptom improvement and varicose vein absence demonstrated no statistically significant differences between patients with complete SFJ obliteration and those with a short patent SFJ stump at any follow-up time point.

While the distal trunk is occluded, SFJ competence is often restored even with a short patent stump. A patent stump can serve as a conduit and preserve the normal physiologic flow from one or more patent tributaries such as those draining blood from abdominal and perineal areas. Preservation of such physiologic flow has been considered to be an advantage of endovenous procedures over traditional vein stripping because it causes less hemodynamic disturbance. Interruption of normal tributaries in the groin is postulated to be one of the factors responsible for stimulating neovascularization following vein stripping.

Merchant and Pichot[18] categorized anatomic failure after an RF ablation procedure into three types. *Type I* failure (nonocclusion) refers to a vein that fails to occlude because of suboptimal technique, such as a rapid pullback speed resulting in an insufficient delivery of thermal dose. It has also been observed that in a very small percentage of patients, veins may be nonresponsive to thermal ablation; it has been postulated that the collagen structure might be different in these patients. Of veins that recanalized (*Type II* failure), 23% were associated with either tributary or perforator incompetence, accounting for 70% of the total anatomic failures.

The significance of tributary or thigh perforator incompetence and its relationship to the durability of endovenous ablation is not clear. Proactively addressing tributary and perforator incompetence may further improve long-term RF ablation treatment outcomes. A thorough pre-operative ultrasound study and diligent ultrasound follow-up to identify refluxing tributaries and thigh perforators can enhance a carefully designed treatment plan to address all refluxing sources. In addition to Type I and II failure, groin reflux developed in 33 limbs (18% of total failures) despite complete occlusion of the GSV trunk. The reflux often involved an accessory saphenous vein associated with or "feeding" varicosities. This type (*Type III*) of failure likely reflects disease progression associated with persistent hypertension of the venous system, but a contributing factor may also be an undiagnosed accessory vein incompetence that existed at the time of the original GSV treatment.

Risk analysis revealed that the pullback speed was a risk factor for Type I and II failures with the first-generation device. A certain level of thermal dose is required to efficiently occlude the vein, and an insufficient thermal dose may result in short-term vein occlusion, probably through formation of thrombus in the treated segment. However, thrombotic occlusions are subject to recanalization (Type II), particularly when the segment is associated with incompetent tributaries or perforators. It is important to note that anatomic failure does not necessarily result in clinical recurrence. Most patients experienced clinical improvement, and 70% to 80% were asymptomatic, regardless of anatomic failure, during a 5-year follow-up period. This suggests that the anatomic failure may not be significant enough to cause pressure-related symptoms.

On the other hand, Type II and Type III failures were risk factors for varicose vein recurrence. Type II failure patients were 3.8 times and Type III failures were 4.0 times as likely to develop varicose vein recurrence compared to patients with anatomic success. Type I failure did not reach statistical significance in this analysis. One possible explanation is lack of follow-up. Most patients had follow-up of less than 3 years. Further, some patients may have been treated with other methods and lost to follow-up. In this setting, the impact of early failure on varicose vein recurrence may not have been identified. Surveillance monitoring, early recognition of anatomic failure, and taking further corrective action that may include RF ablation retreatment may prevent or reduce varicose vein recurrence. However, it should be recognized that disease progression is likely to play a major role in Type III failure and may also account for some of Type II failure. This may contribute to an increase in varicose vein recurrence at 4 and 5 years (Fig. 5-1).

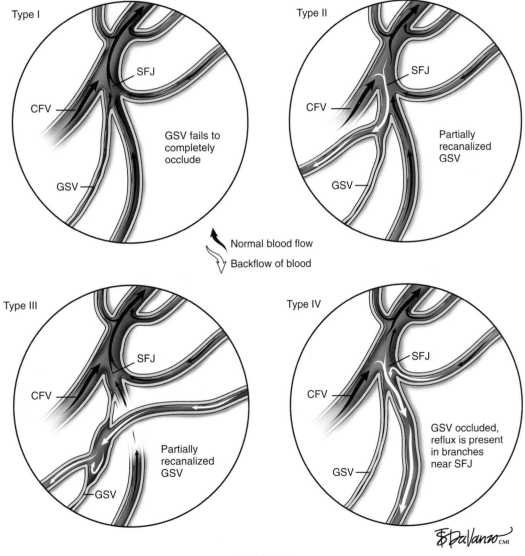

■ Fig 5-1

PEARLS AND PITFALLS

Procedural Technique

The VNUS Closure System includes a computer-controlled RF generator and disposable catheters. The catheters incorporate a central lumen for both fluid infusion and the option of using an over-the-wire approach during catheter placement. Detailed procedure techniques have been described elsewhere[14,19,20] and in Chapter 4.

Using Duplex ultrasound, a vein access site is selected, and the vein is entered either percutaneously or via a small incision. The procedure can be performed under local anesthesia using perivenous tumescent infiltration, with or without conscious sedation. An introducer sheath is placed to allow catheter insertion into the target vein. Older access kits came equipped with an 18-gauge needle, allowed for a .035-inch guidewire, and exchanged for either 6-Fr or 8-Fr. The 6-Fr catheter was paired with a 6-Fr introducer sheath, while the 8-Fr fit through an 8-Fr introducer sheath.

Currently, a 21-gauge needle with a .018-inch guidewire is manufactured to allow placement of a tapered 7-Fr sheath. The CLF catheter is placed through a 7-Fr sheath.

The catheter is navigated to the SFJ and positioned using ultrasound guidance. The catheter is usually inserted without the support of a guidewire; however, when treating tortuous veins, navigation of the catheter over a .25-inch guidewire may be required. The electrodes are deployed at the SFJ and positioned distal to the entry of the superficial epigastric vein when present, or approximately 1 cm distal to the origin of the common femoral vein in cases where the superficial epigastric vein is not visualized.

Tumescent Anesthesia

The vein must be anesthetized circumferentially along the entire treatment length with a dilute 0.1% lidocaine solution before treatment is begun. This process is facilitated by the presence of the saphenous canal. The saphenous canal is bound by superficial fascia above and muscular fascia below. The anesthetic solution is infused into the intrafascial perivenous plane with ultrasound visualization until the saphenous canal begins to swell. For this reason, most clinicians refer to this anesthetic procedure as tumescent anesthesia. Several delivery systems are available for placement of tumescent anesthesia, ranging from an inexpensive syringe with a 25-gauge needle to specialized pumps for more rapid delivery. Intrafascial perivenous tumescent anesthesia accomplishes three critical goals: (1) compression of the vein externally, causing it to shrink and thus improving contact between the RF electrodes and the vein wall; (2) development of a heat sink, obviating the inadvertent transfer of thermal energy to nontarget tissues; and (3) the provision for excellent analgesia, thereby allowing for the performance of a painless procedure.

After final positioning of the catheter tip, the electrodes are deployed. Further vein exsanguination is achieved by putting the patient in the Trendelenburg position and applying external compression. On initiation of RF energy delivery to the electrodes, the catheter is slowly withdrawn while maintaining the treatment temperature at 85° C. The feedback mechanism of the system allows controlled energy delivery and appropriate monitoring of the procedure. With the CLF system, the heating element has no electrodes and the treatment temperature is 120° C (procedure details are given in Chapter 4).

Immediate vein wall thickening and vein occlusion are expected on completion of the treatment. Incompetent tributaries, perforators, and varicosities are sometimes treated concomitantly using additional RF ablation, phlebectomy, or sclerotherapy, depending on the vein size, vein depth, and physician's preference. Patients are encouraged to ambulate immediately after the procedure. A duplex ultrasound scan should be performed within 72 hours postoperatively to confirm vein closure and rule out the presence of deep venous thrombosis (DVT).

Potential Hazards and Adverse Events

As with all endovenous interventions, RF ablation may be associated with technical difficulties in cannulation, guidewire placement, and catheter advancement. These issues are likely to resolve with increasing experience and familiarity with the equipment and technique. Complications, including DVT, skin burns, superficial thrombophlebitis, neuralgia, and bruising, have been reported, but the incidence of these problems appears low. In one study, DVT developed in 12 of 73 limbs (16%) within 30 days of RFA,[21] but the incidence of DVT in the majority of studies is in the range of 1%.

Of the 1006 patients recorded in the Closure International Registry, the reported complications were DVT (0.9%), phlebitis (2.9%), and skin burn (1.2%), although the majority of burns occurred in patients who had not received perivenous tumescent anesthesia.[18]

Minor complications such as skin burns and paresthesias were occasionally seen in the early experience with RF ablation. Contemporary data show virtual elimination of these problems since the advent of subfascial perivenous tumescent anesthesia. Tumescent anesthesia had been used for years by the dermatology and plastic surgery communities for liposuction. Since the concept was applied to veins, heat is no longer transmitted to nontarget tissues. By completely surrounding the saphenous vein with a dilute lidocaine solution, a heat sink is created. Neighboring structures such as nerves and skin are readily cooled as the intraluminal heat rises during passage of the hot catheter tips. Furthermore, the tumescent solution can act as a mechanical barrier to effectively "push" nontarget structures away from veins and other structures.

As is the case for many surgical procedures, DVT is a potential complication. In endovenous ablation, thrombosis can originate from the treated superficial vein and extend into the deep venous system. Attention is drawn to careful tip positioning to ensure treatment begins a short distance from the SFJ and to preserve the physiologic blood flow from the superficial epigastric tributary.

Massive DVT after thermal ablation is almost unheard of, but the surgeon may see a small thrombus extension on the postoperative ultrasound. Although they may look quite alarming on ultrasound imaging, they are usually about 1 cm in size. Anecdotally, these lesions are usually benign and are self-limiting. They are rarely symptomatic and they rarely propagate (Figs. 5-2 through 5-6).

Small Saphenous Vein and Other Veins

In addition to the GSV, RF ablation has also been used to treat small saphenous vein (SSV) and anterior accessory saphenous vein (AASV) incompetence in clinical practice. In this series, 4.3% veins treated were SSVs and 1.3% were AASVs. Although there were not enough samples and follow-up to demonstrate their long-term efficacy, one would not expect a dramatic difference between these treatments and GSV treatment. In this series, no serious adverse event such as motor nerve damage was reported with SSV treatment. The paresthesia rate in the SSV group was 8.9% at 1 week and 9.5% at 6 months; this is similar to the results of GSV treatment. The technical aspects of perivenous tumescent infiltration, catheter tip placement, and patient response monitoring during the procedure demand special attention with SSV treatment to protect the sural nerve and other surrounding nerves. When these elements were applied to SSV procedures, the

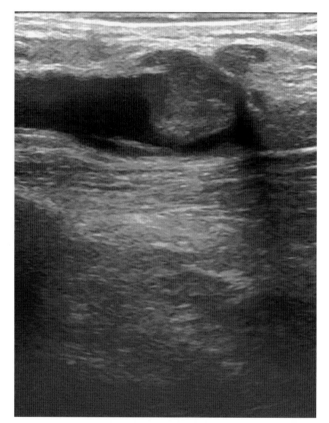

■ Fig 5–2

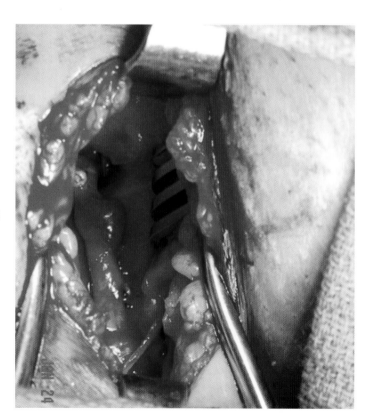

■ Fig 5–3

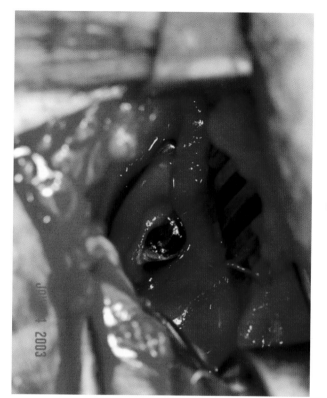

■ Fig 5–4

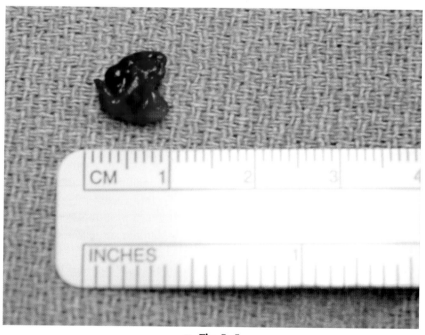

■ Fig 5–5

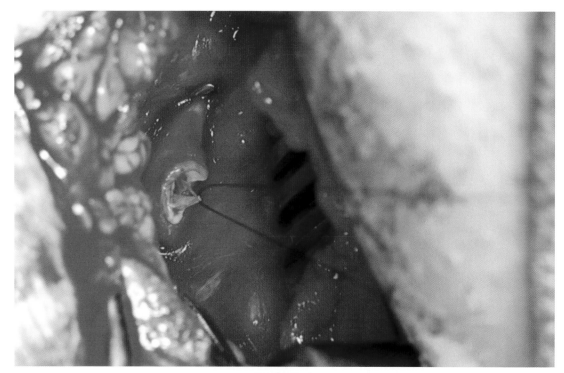

■ **Fig 5-6**

paresthesia incidence dropped to as low as 0.3% (1 of 30) in one center.[11] As has already been emphasized, tumescent infiltration can significantly decrease complications of this procedure.

Treatment efficacy of RF ablation on large veins was also analyzed by Merchant et al.[22] There were 39 veins with a diameter greater than 12 mm (maximum, 24 mm) in the registry. Vein occlusion rates were 97.4% within 1 week and 96.2% at 6 months and 1 year.

COMPARATIVE EFFECTIVENESS OF EXISTING TREATMENTS

First-generation RF devices had marginally higher recanalization rates than EVL, but the new ClosureFAST catheter results rival those of EVL at about 98% primary closure. The literature database is populated mostly with first-generation device studies. Reported vein closure rates vary between 67% and 100%* (Table 5-1). In a recent meta-analysis, the early technical success following RF ablation was found to be 89% (3 months), reducing to 80% after 5 years.[24] These values compared favorably to those for traditional surgery and foam sclerotherapy but were lower than those for EVL ablation. By far, the largest patient series treated by RF ablation was published in 2005 and reported 5-year clinical and anatomic outcomes following RF ablation in 1006 patients (1222 limbs).[18] Data were collected from a prospective international registry and occlusion rates of 87.2% were seen at 5 years. Significant improvements in pain, fatigue, and edema were seen up to 5 years; interestingly, these improvements were present despite recurrent truncal reflux. Recurrent varicosities were seen in 27% of patients at 5 years, and anatomic failure of RF ablation was an independent risk factor for varicosity recurrence.[18] In randomized studies, recurrent varicosities were seen in 48 of 217 (22%) of patients at 4 years.[23]

*References 4, 9, 11, 12, 14, 15, 17, 18, 20, 21, 23-35.

TABLE 5–1 Published Prospective Clinical Studies of Radiofrequency Ablation

Author	Year	Study Design	Limbs	Follow-up, mo	Occlusion Rate, %	DVT	Skin Burn
Luebke and Brunkwall[23]	2008	Meta-analysis	315	36	81	N/A	N/A
van den Bos et al.[24]	2008	Meta-analysis	N/A	60	80	N/A	N/A
Rautio et al.[25]	2002	RCT	15	36	67	0	0
Perala et al.[26]	2005	RCT	15	36	67	0	0
Lurie et al.[11]	2003	RCT	65	24	86	0	N/A
Lurie et al.[12]	2005	RCT	65	24	86	0	N/A
Hingorani et al.[27]	2006	RCT	16	1	81	0	N/A
Chandler et al.[20]	2000	Prospective	120	12	90	0	N/A
Manfrini et al.[4]	2000	Prospective	151	6	96	0	N/A
Goldman and Amiry[28]	2002	Prospective	50	24	68	0	N/A
Merchant et al.[15]	2002	Prospective	1222	60	87	11	15
Merchant and Pichot[18]	2005	Prospective	1222	60	87	11	15
Sybrandy and Wittens[29]	2002	Prospective	26	12	88	N/A	1
Weiss and Weiss[14]	2002	Prospective	140	24	90	0	0
Fassiadis et al.[30]	2003	Prospective	59	12	98	N/A	N/A
Hingorani et al.[21]	2004	Prospective	73	1	96	12	N/A
Pichot et al.[17]	2004	Prospective	63	25	90	N/A	N/A
Ogawa et al.[31]	2005	Prospective	25	1	100	0	N/A
Nicolini[32]	2005	Prospective	330	36	75	0	N/A
Kianifard et al.[33]	2006	Prospective	51	12	100	N/A	N/A
Dunn et al.[34]	2006	Prospective	85	6	90	0	0
Zan et al.[35]	2007	Prospective	24	24	96	N/A	N/A
Proebstle et al.[9]	2008	Prospective	252	6	99.6	0	0

RCT, Randomized controlled trial; N/A, not applicable.

A direct comparison of postoperative recovery endpoints between RF ablation and EVL was conducted in the RECOVERY trial. Results showed reduced pain and ecchymosis scores after CLF.[36]

Four randomized controlled trials have compared endovenous RF ablation to surgical vein stripping. In the first, Rautio et al. randomized 28 patients to either RF ablation or vein stripping and reported significantly less postoperative pain, fewer postoperative analgesia requirements, and faster recovery in the RF group.[37] The second trial, called the EVOLVeS study, was a multi-center, prospective, randomized study comparing quality-of-life factors between RF ablation and vein stripping. In all outcome variables, RF ablation demonstrated superior results compared to vein stripping: faster recovery, less postoperative pain, fewer adverse events, and superior quality-of-life scores.[11] EVOLVeS patients seen at 2 years' follow-up demonstrated virtually identical treatment results between RF ablation and vein stripping, with 91% versus 92% of limbs free of reflux, respectively. In addition, quality-of-life and pain scores were significantly better ($p < .05$) at 2 years for RF ablation over vein stripping, demonstrating a lasting benefit for patients.[12] A third trial compared RF ablation to invaginated stripping and to cryostripping in a single-center trial with 20 patients in each treatment arm. RF ablation showed significantly better quality-of-life score improvement, less pain, and superiority in patient return to normal activity and work.[38] The fourth comparative trial involved patients with recurrent GSV reflux after a previous vein stripping. RF ablation treatment resulted in better scores related to bruising and procedure times.[27]

Vein clinical severity scores have been previously reported with endovenous RF ablation. In the EVOLVeS trial of RF versus vein stripping, mean Venous Clinical Severity Scores were reduced from an average pretreatment score of 4.8 to 2.5 at 3 weeks after treatment.[29]

Meta-analysis

This meta-analysis of randomized controlled trials reviews the current evidence base, comparing open and endovascular treatment of varicose veins. Systematic review of studies reporting duplex scan follow-up after open surgical, laser (endovenous laser therapy [EVLT]), or radiofrequency (VNUS Closure device; VNUS Medical Technologies Inc.) treatment of refluxing GSVs was completed. Primary outcome measures were occlusion and complication rates and time to resume work. No significant difference were found in recurrence rates at 3 months between open surgery and EVLT (risk ratio [RR] 2.19; 95% confidence interval [CI] 0.99-4.85, $p = .05$) or VNUS device (RR 7.57; 95% CI 0.42-136.02). Return to work is significantly faster after VNUS device (by 8.24 days; 95% CI 10.50-5.97) or EVLT (by 5.02 days; 95% CI 6.52-3.52). Endovascular treatment of varicose veins is safe and effective and offers the significant advantage of rapid recovery.[39]

REFERENCES

1. Politowski M, Zelazny T. Complications and difficulties in electrocoagulation of varices of the lower extremities. Surgery 1966;59:932-934.
2. Watts GT. Endovenous diathermy destruction of internal saphenous. Br Med J 1972;4:53.
3. Pearce JA. Electrosurgery. New York: John Wiley & Sons; 1986:62-65.
4. Manfrini S, Gasbarro V, Danielsson G, et al. Endovenous management of saphenous vein reflux. J Vasc Surg 2000;32:330-342.
5. Weiss RA. RF-mediated endovenous occlusion. In: Weiss RA, Feied CF, Weiss MA, eds. Vein Diagnosis and Treatment: A Comprehensive Approach. New York: McGraw-Hill Medical Publishing Division; 2001:211-221.
6. Weiss RA. Comparison of endovenous radiofrequency versus 810 nm diode laser occlusion of large veins in an animal model. Dermatol Surg 2002;28:56-61.
7. Goldman MP, Mauricio M, Rao J. Intravascular 1320-nm laser closure of the great saphenous vein: a 6- to 12-month follow-up study. Dermatol Surg 2004;30:1380-1385.
8. Zikorus AW, Mirizzi MS. Evaluation of setpoint temperature and pullback speed on vein adventitial temperature during endovenous radiofrequency energy delivery in an in-vitro model. Vasc Endovascular Surg 2004;38:167-174.
9. Proebstle TM, Vago B, Alm J, et al. Treatment of the incompetent great saphenous vein by endovenous radiofrequency powered segmental thermal ablation: first clinical experience. J Vasc Surg 2008;47:151-156.
10. Almeida JI, Raines JK. Radiofrequency ablation and laser ablation in the treatment of varicose veins. Ann Vasc Surg 2006;20:547-552.
11. Lurie F, Creton D, Eklof B, et al. Prospective randomized study of endovenous radiofrequency obliteration (Closure) versus ligation and stripping in a selected patient population (EVOLVeS study). J Vasc Surg 2003;38:207-214.
12. Lurie F, Creton D, Eklof B, et al. Prospective randomised study of endovenous radiofrequency obliteration (Closure) versus ligation and vein stripping (EVOLVeS): two-year follow-up. Eur J Vasc Endovasc Surg 2005;29:67-73.

13. Pichot O, Sessa C, Chandler JG, et al. Role of duplex imaging in endovenous obliteration for primary venous insufficiency. J Endovasc Ther 2000;7:451-459.

14. Weiss RA, Weiss MA. Controlled radiofrequency endovenous occlusion using a unique radiofrequency catheter under duplex guidance to eliminate saphenous varicose vein reflux: a 2-year follow-up. Dermatol Surg 2002;28:38-42.

15. Merchant RF, DePalma RG, Kabnick LS. Endovascular obliteration of saphenous reflux: a multicenter study. J Vasc Surg 2002;35:1190-1196.

16. Pichot O, Sessa C, Chandler JG, et al. Role of duplex imaging in endovenous obliteration for primary venous insufficiency. J Endovasc Ther 2000;7:451-459.

17. Pichot O, Kabnick LS, Creton D, et al. Duplex ultrasound scan findings two years after great saphenous vein radiofrequency endovenous obliteration. J Vasc Surg 2004;39: 189-195.

18. Merchant RF, Pichot O, for the Closure Study Group. Long-term outcomes of endovenous radiofrequency obliteration of saphenous reflux as a treatment for superficial venous insufficiency. J Vasc Surg 2005;42:502-509.

19. Goldman MP, Weiss RA, Bergan JJ. Varicose veins and telangiectasias. Circulation 1999;12: 219-223.

20. Chandler JG, Pichot O, Sessa C, et al. Defining the role of extended saphenofemoral junction ligation: a prospective comparative study. J Vasc Surg 2000;32:941-953.

21. Hingorani AP, Ascher E, Markevich N, et al. Deep venous thrombosis after radiofrequency ablation of greater saphenous vein: a word of caution. J Vasc Surg 2004;40:500-504.

22. Merchant RF, Pichot O, Mayers KA. Four-year follow-up on endovascular radiofrequency obliteration of great saphenous reflux. Dermatol Surg 2005;31:129-134.

23. Luebke T, Brunkwall J. Systematic review and meta-analysis of endovenous radiofrequency obliteration, endovenous laser therapy, and foam sclerotherapy for primary varicosis. J Cardiovasc Surg (Torino) 2008;49:213-233.

24. van den Bos R, Arends L, Kockaert M, et al. Endovenous therapies of lower extremity varicosities: a meta-analysis. J Vasc Surg 2009;49:230-239.

25. Rautio T, Ohinmaa A, Perala J, et al. Endovenous obliteration versus conventional stripping operation in the treatment of primary varicose veins: a randomized controlled trial with comparison of the costs. J Vasc Surg 2002;35:958-965.

26. Perala J, Rautio T, Biancari F, et al. Radiofrequency endovenous obliteration versus stripping of the long saphenous vein in the management of primary varicose veins: 3-year outcome of a randomized study. Ann Vasc Surg 2005;19:669-672.

27. Hinchcliffe RJ, Ubhi J, Beech A, et al. A prospective randomised controlled trial of VNUS closure versus surgery for the treatment of recurrent long saphenous varicose veins. Eur J Vasc Endovasc Surg 2006;31:212-218.

28. Goldman MP, Amiry S. Closure of the greater saphenous vein with endoluminal radiofrequency thermal heating of the vein wall in combination with ambulatory phlebectomy: 50 patients with more than 6-month follow-up. Dermatol Surg 2002;28:29-31.

29. Sybrandy JEM, Wittens CHA. Initial experiences in endovenous treatment of saphenous vein reflux. J Vasc Surg 2002;36:1207-1212.

30. Fassiadis N, Holdstock J, Whiteley MS. Endoluminal radiofrequency ablation of the long saphenous vein (VNUS Closure): a minimally invasive management of varicose veins. Minim Invasive Ther Allied Technol 2003;12:91-94.

31. Ogawa T, Hoshino S, Midorikawa H, et al. Clinical results of radiofrequency endovenous obliteration for varicose veins. Surg Today 2005;35:47-51.

32. Nicolini P. Treatment of primary varicose veins by endovenous obliteration with the VNUS closure system: results of a prospective multicentre study. Eur J Vasc Endovasc Surg 2005;29:433-439.

33. Kianifard B, Holdstock JM, Whiteley MS. Radiofrequency ablation (VNUS Closure) does not cause neovascularisation at the groin at one year: results of a case controlled study. Surgeon 2006;4:71-74.

34. Dunn CW, Kabnick LS, Merchant RF, et al. Endovascular radiofrequency obliteration using 90 degrees C for treatment of great saphenous vein. Ann Vasc Surg 2006;20:625-629.

35. Zan S, Contessa L, Varetto G, et al. Radiofrequency minimally invasive endovascular treatment of lower limbs varicose veins: clinical experience and literature review. Minerva Cardioangiol 2007;55:443-458.

36. Almeida J, Kaufman J, Göckeritz O, et al. Radiofrequency endovenous ClosureFAST versus laser ablation for the treatment of great saphenous reflux: a multicenter, single-blinded, randomized study (RECOVERY study). J Vasc Interv Radiol 2009;20:752-759.

37. Rautio T, Ohinmaa A, Perälä J, et al. Endovenous obliteration versus conventional stripping operation in the treatment of primary varicose veins: a randomized controlled trial with comparison of costs. J Vasc Surg 2002;35:958-965.

38. Stötter L, Schaaf I, Bockelbrink A, et al. Radiowellenobliteration, invaginierendes oder Kryo-stripping. Welches Verfahren belastet den Patienten am wenigsten? Phlebologie (German) 2005;34:19-24.

39. Brar R, Nordon IM, Hinchliffe RJ, et al. Surgical management of varicose veins: meta-analysis. Vascular 2010;18:205-220.

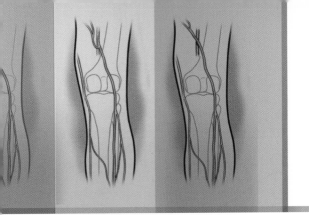

CHAPTER 6

Laser Thermal Ablation

Jose I. Almeida

HISTORICAL BACKGROUND

Bruising, transient pain, and induration of the thigh are common adverse events after endovenous laser (EVL) therapy and are most likely caused by laser-induced perforation of the vein wall with extravasation of blood into surrounding tissue.[1-3] It is known that conversion of an incompetent vein into a fibrous cord, with subsequent sonographic disappearance, will guarantee permanent occlusion. At the onset of EVL therapy, little was known about the mechanism of action and durability of treatment after intervention with these devices. Studies have indicated that heat-related damage to the inner vein wall leads to thrombotic occlusion of the treated vein.[4,5]

EVL can be classified into hemoglobin-specific laser wavelengths (HSLWs) and water-specific laser wavelengths (WSLWs) (Fig. 6-1). Wavelengths of 808, 810, 940, 980, 1064, 1319, and 1320 nm have been successfully used for great saphenous vein (GSV) ablation[4,6-10] and for other superficial axial and perforating veins.[11] Hemoglobin and, to a lesser extent, myoglobin in venous smooth muscle cells are the dominant chromophores at the lower end of this range, while at the 1320-nm wavelength range, water dominates as the energy-absorbing molecule.[4,7]

Published reports suggest that delivery of higher energy is required to effect secure vein closure; however, with increased energy delivery, pain and bruising after treatment are encountered more frequently. After EVL, studies have demonstrated 70% of limbs experience some degree of pain, and 50% require analgesics for pain management.[12] Kabnick[13] reported an average pain score of 2.6 on a scale of 0 to 5 after EVL. There is increasing focus on reducing perioperative pain and bruising in the field of EVL saphenous ablation. The most recent WSLW to become available is the 1470 nm, which requires less energy delivery for closure, and reports of less pain and bruising postprocedure are beginning to populate the literature.

The WSLWs were developed to target the interstitial water in the vein wall and minimize perforations.[7] Two WSLW (1319 and 1320 nm) lasers are in widespread clinical use, and trends in the literature suggest that these longer wavelength lasers may produce fewer side effects than HSLW lasers at comparable linear endovenous energy density (LEED). Two comparisons of different wavelengths with similar delivered laser energy have been performed. One study compared 940-nm and 1320-nm wavelengths in a retrospective analysis, and another compared 810-nm and 980-nm wavelengths in a randomized prospective study.[13,14] The two studies demonstrated

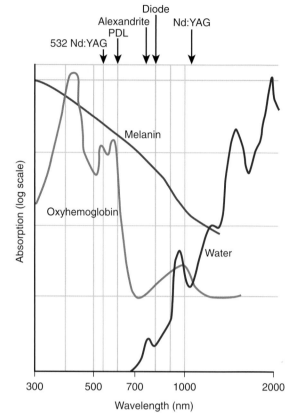

■ **Fig 6-1** Light absorption curve.

equivalent safety and efficacy at similar energy dosing. However, EVL performed at comparable LEED with either the 940-nm (HSLW) or the 1320-nm (WSLW) lasers showed a reduction in postoperative pain and bruising with the 1320-nm device. Also, use of less power (5 W) demonstrated a lower rate of side effects than did 8 W with a laser operating at a wavelength of 1320 nm.[14] A low rate of pain and bruising was reported after GSV treatment for GSV reflux with the 1470-nm wavelength at 5 W, 30 J/cm.[15]

ETIOLOGY AND NATURAL HISTORY OF DISEASE

There remains controversy over the mechanism of action of EVL and most of the investigations were performed with HSLWs. Proebstle found in vitro with an HSLW that the extensive heat damage of the endothelium and the intima came from steam bubble formation and induced full-length thrombotic occlusion of the vein.[4] Bush et al.,[16] in a histologic study, found that the mechanism of injury with HSLWs is secondary to steam bubbles caused by water evaporation of the blood followed by transmitted heat injury to the tissue. Acutely, there is complete loss of the endothelium and early thrombus formation, followed by the injury response with inflammatory cellular infiltration into the subintimal layers. Eventually, fibroblasts deposit collagen and represent the predominant histologic finding at 4 months postoperatively.

Opposed to the steam bubble theory, Fan and Rox-Anderson[17] studied existing histologic reports from studies with excellent closure rates using tumescent anesthesia and found that HSLWs produce a transmural vein wall injury, typically associated with perforations and carbonization. The pattern of injury was eccentrically distributed, with maximum injury occurring along the path of laser contact. The authors concluded that steam production during EVL accounted for only 2% of applied energy dose (i.e., EVL causes permanent vein closure through a high-temperature photothermolytic process at the point of contact between the vein and the laser). Precise mechanism-of-action studies with ample histologic information are lacking with WSLWs.

Although it is not known exactly how much damage to the individual layers of the vein wall is required, it seems that at a minimum, intimal and medial coagulation are necessary for long-term closure. Technically, the depth of penetration of a 940-nm laser beam into blood is limited to approximately 0.3 mm.[18] Qualitative analysis with optical coherence tomography in an ex vivo model matched with histologic cross sections showed a symmetric, complete, circular disintegration of intima and media structures, without any transmural tissue defects after radiofrequency ablation (RFA).[19] However, with an HSLW laser, pronounced semicircular tissue ablations and complete vessel wall perforations were detected at 35 J/cm LEED. The quantitative analysis demonstrated a significant ($p < .0001$) increase in intima-media thickness after RF ablation (38% to 67%) and EVL (11% to 46%) and a significant ($p < .0001$) reduction in vessel lumen diameter (36% to 42%) after RF ablation. No linear correlation could be identified between laser energy level and effects on tissue such as ablation/perforation, media thickening, or vein lumen diameter.[22]

Weiss[20] examined the gross tissue effects and tissue temperatures generated during EVL with an 810-nm diode laser in an in vivo goat model. Using thermal sensors mounted adjacent to the laser optical fiber, they determined the mean temperature at the firing tip was 729° C (peak 1334° C). The intense thermal heating zone appeared to be focally situated around the laser tip; the mean temperature decreased to 231° C and 307° C, 2 mm proximal and distal to the fiber tip, respectively. At 4 mm distal from the fiber tip, the mean temperature decreased further to 93° C. Recently, Disselhoff et al,[10] with intravascular temperature measurements in an in vitro system, found that despite the intense heat at the laser tip, the thermal heating zone is predominantly contained within the venous lumen. Zimmet and Min[21] demonstrated in a swine model that during EVL with an 810-nm diode laser, ear vein outer wall temperatures ranged from 40° to 49° C. In hind extremity veins, these investigators showed that with tumescent anesthesia, the external vein wall temperatures never exceeded 40° C.

These findings were corroborated in humans by Beale et al.[22] when he inserted thermocouples percutaneously, positioned at 3, 5, and 10 mm from a small saphenous vein (SSV), after administration of tumescent anesthesia. He recorded temperatures during EVL with an 810-nm diode laser, using 1-second pulse application at 12 W, and found peak temperatures of 43°, 42°, and 36° C at 3, 5, and 10 mm, respectively, in perivenous tissues.

PEARLS AND PITFALLS

Dosing

Data on the dose-response relationship between laser energy and durability of vein occlusion began to be published in 2004, when parameters describing the LEED and endovenous fluence equivalent (EFE) were introduced.[23] LEED is a linear energy density quantity measured in joules per centimeter, and EFE is an energy parameter that uses a cylindric approximation of the inner vein surface area expressed in joules per centimeter squared.

In a retrospective study,[24] recanalization was reported in 20% of cases treated with administration of less than 80 J/cm and was significantly reduced if laser energy exceeded 80 J/cm at a wavelength of 980 nm. However, in a follow-up prospective study by the same author, 9% of veins treated with LEEDs exceeding 80 J/cm unexpectedly recanalized at 6-month follow-up.[25]

Multiple regression analysis determined that EFE was the most significant predictor of recanalization events and, when exceeding 20 J/cm^2, was associated with durable GSV occlusion after 1-year follow-up.[26] Another study reported on 129 GSVs and found that 52 J/cm^2 EFE was ideal to produce long-term occlusion; this author cautioned that recanalization can occur in patients treated with higher fluence.[27]

A sliding scale approach has been used at Miami Vein Center since 2002 and has yielded excellent results.[11] High rates of vein occlusion and ultimate sonographic disappearance were noted when the thermal dose in each segment of the GSV was tailored to the diameter in that segment. The ranges of energies used fell between 50 J/cm for veins 5 mm in diameter and 120 J/cm for veins 10 mm in diameter at the saphenofemoral junction (SFJ). No increase in complications were seen with any of the higher energy strategies.[28]

Reports from John Hopkins University on "low-energy" EVL treatment of 34 consecutive GSVs with a 980-nm diode laser at 11 W in continuous mode (mean GSV diameter 12 mm) using mean LEED of 35 J/cm resulted in zero recanalization (100% success) at a mean follow-up of 1 year.[29] Interestingly, the same author reported later in the same year that 60 consecutive GSVs demonstrated a reduced treatment success of 95%; the mean follow-up for this series was 6.8 months and mean LEED for successful and failed treatments was 33 J/cm. The mean maximum diameter of successfully treated GSVs was 11 mm, and that for failed treatments was 21 mm (p = .008). The investigators concluded that there were no significant differences in mean unit energy applied for successful, failed, and repeat treatments (p > .05); however, larger GSV diameter was associated with early treatment failures.[30]

A recent clinical trial indicated that energy density may not be the most important determinant of recanalization. In 471 segments, 11 failures were encountered, including 4 in a group treated with less than 60 J/cm (4%), 2 in a 60 to 80 J/cm group (3%), 4 in an 81 to 100 J/cm group (3%), and 1 in a group treated with more than 100 J/cm (1%). There were no statistically significant differences in failure rates among energy density ranges. The authors concluded that EVL has a low failure rate and that failure rate is not a function of energy density.[31]

Complications

Significant adverse events reported following EVL include skin burns, sensory nerve injuries, and deep vein thrombosis (DVT). Early experience[32] reported skin burn rates as high as 4%; this decreased to almost zero as the use of tumescent anesthesia became the standard of practice. The overall rate for these complications has been shown to be higher in low-volume centers compared to high-volume centers; the rate of skin burns in one series using RFA was 1.7% before and 0.5% after the initiation of the tumescent technique.[33] The nerves at highest risk include the saphenous nerve, located adjacent to the GSV below the midcalf perforating vein, and the sural nerve, adjacent to the SSV in the midcalf and lower calf. The most common manifestations of a nerve injury are paresthesias, which are usually transient. The nerve injuries can occur during venous access, the delivery of tumescent anesthesia, or lasering by transfer of thermal energy to perivenous tissues.

Patients treated with EVL, using extraordinarily high rates of energy delivery without tumescent anesthetic infiltrations, demonstrated a high rate of nerve injuries and skin burns.[34] However, in a series using RF ablation, delivery of perivenous fluid was thought to be responsible for the low rate of cutaneous and neurologic thermal injuries, where the 1-week paresthesia rate was shown to decrease from 15% to 9% after the introduction of tumescent anesthesia.[35] The addition of tumescent anesthesia has been demonstrated to reduce outer vein wall temperatures during EVL and RFA in animal models.[36,37]

Fortunately, thromboembolic events are uncommon after endovenous thermal ablation, probably because tumescent anesthesia has allowed for speedy procedures, which promotes ambulation immediately after surgery.[11] The thrombus extensions at the SFJ seen occasionally after thermal ablation were discussed in Chapter 5.

Small Saphenous Vein

Ablation of the SSV with either laser or radiofrequency is a very attractive alternative to SSV ligation and stripping because open dissection of the popliteal fossa is not required. The popliteal space has traditionally been referred to as "tiger country" in many vascular surgery circles because of the anatomy. While the usual reason for surgery in this area is for popliteal artery treatment, those who begin an open dissection in this area can injure the popliteal vein and tibial nerve if great care is not taken. Fewer reports of endovenous laser treatment of the SSV than of the GSV have been published.

In a 2003 report[38] on the treatment of SSV in 41 limbs using a 940-nm diode laser, 39 SSVs (95%) were successfully treated with EVL. During a median follow-up interval of 6 months, no recanalization was observed. Apart from one thrombosis of the popliteal vein in a patient with polycythemia vera, four transient sural nerve paresthesias were reported.

Almeida and Raines[11] reported on 987 treated veins in 2006, 115 of which were SSVs. Most recanalizations occurred in the first 12 months and developed in the SSV proximal to May's perforator. Five of 115 treated SSVs recanalized partially (4%), most likely as a result of cooler blood (37 °C) entering the treatment site from a midcalf perforating vein. No thrombus extensions into the popliteal vein or other thrombotic complications of the deep system were identified. Ravi et al.[39] then reported the series in 2006, which consisted of 981 patients and included 101 SSV procedures. There were 9 (9.0%) failures among the 101 SSVs treated with EVL.

Gibson et al.[40] published their series of 210 SSVs treated with EVL. Their data demonstrated that EVL of the SSV is feasible and safe and has excellent clinical outcomes in combination with concomitant therapies where indicated. All procedures were technically successful; 96% of SSVs remained closed at a mean follow-up of 4 months. The incidence of nerve injury is acceptably low and not clinically significant. Three patients (1.6%) had numbness at the lateral malleolus at the 6-week follow-up. Only three patients (1.6%) complained of numbness at the 6-week follow-up. In only one of these patients could EVL alone be implicated in causing numbness, because two of the patients also had microphlebectomy of large varicose vein branches at the lateral malleolus. None of the patients found the numbness to be a significant concern. The incidence of DVT, defined as a tail of thrombus protruding into the popliteal vein, was noted in 12 limbs (5.7%) at the 1-week follow-up examination. The incidence of DVT after treatment of the SSV was 5.7%, higher than in the other reported series. The reason for this difference is unclear; DVT was present in 11.4% of type A anatomy compared with 2.9% of limbs with type B anatomy and 0% of limbs with type C anatomy.

In an effort to understand the reason for the high rate of DVT, the authors incorrectly describe the Giacomini vein as analogous to the inferior epigastric vein in EVL of the GSV in the case of type A and type B anatomy. That EVL ablation the of the GSV should commence with the tip of the laser distal to the superficial epigastric vein (not the inferior epigastric vein) has become dogma in the endovenous community and is based purely on empirical data. Theoretically, this preserves flow at the SFJ, which in turn may prevent extension of thrombus into the common femoral vein. There is an analogous arrangement at the SFJ; however, the similarity exists with drainage of the gastrocnemius veins into the most proximal aspect of the SFJ and not the Giacomini vein as the authors stated. It is correct that patients with type C anatomy may have a reduced risk of DVT because of the absence of communication between the SSV and the popliteal vein. That type B anatomy has the benefit of flow from the Giacomini vein into the SFJ to maintain patency remains to be proved.

In a multicenter prospective study[41] on 229 limbs, the feasibility, safety, and efficacy of endovenous laser ablation to treat SSVs were evaluated. Duplex ultrasound imaging showed immediate occlusion of the SSV with no thrombosis in the proximal veins. No complications occurred intraoperatively. All patients had postoperative ecchymosis, but it was minimal. Complete occlusion with absence of flow at less than 2 months of follow-up was detected in 226 SSVs (98.7%). It occurred in 22 patients with large SSV diameters. Recanalization was found in one patient at 12 months and in two patients at 24 months. After 1 year, eight limbs developed reflux in new locations and four underwent treatment. Symptoms resolved in most patients soon after the operation. The mean follow-up was 16 months. After 8 to 12 months postprocedurally, the laser-treated veins were fibrotic and almost indistinguishable from the surrounding tissues on duplex ultrasound imaging. In five patients (2.25%), postoperative paresthesia occurred more than 2 to 3 days postoperatively and persisted in the follow-up period.

It is important to be able to identify true SSV incompetence. The SSV is an important reentry site for refluxing blood from the GSV. There are usually several intersaphenous connections present on the anteromedial calf that directly connect the GSV to the SSV. With the use of color flow duplex imaging, one can easily discern true SSV incompetence from retrograde flow in the SSV as a result of reentry from the GSV. In the case of true SSV incompetence, the reflux and dilatation are present throughout the entire length of the vein, whereas in the case of reentry, the proximal SSV has antegrade flow without dilatation. At the point of reentry, a large tributary is seen entering the SSV, and flow below this site is retrograde. In cases of reentry, once the retrograde flow in the GSV is corrected with thermal ablation, the SSV physiology corrects automatically.

In the case of true SSV incompetence, the vein map generated from the diagnostic ultrasound examination should include the presence or absence of a cranial extension of the SSV and its termination. Significant tributaries and perforators and their locations should be documented in the planning stages.

COMPARATIVE EFFECTIVENESS OF EXISTING TREATMENTS

Nonrandomized Studies*

There have been several large case series describing outcomes for endovenous laser ablation. Most report GSV ablation rates of over 90% with associated improvement in symptoms and minimal complications (Table 6-1).

Summary of Randomized Controlled Trials

These randomized studies suggest that abolition of GSV reflux, improvements in quality of life, patient satisfaction, and cosmesis are similar for surgery and EVL[51-55] (Table 6-2). Three studies also show that posttreatment discomfort was no different for either technique.

---

*References 2, 3, 6, 7, 9, 11, 13, 14, 23-25, 28, 30, 38-40, and 42-50.

TABLE 6–1 Published Observational Series of Endovenous Laser for Saphenous Reflux

Study Author, Year	Limbs, n	Vein	Anatomic Success, %	DUS Follow-up, mo	Major Complication Rate, %
Navarro et al., 2001[42]	40	GSV	100	4.2	0
Min et al., 2001[3]	90	GSV	97	9	0
Proebstle, 2003[2]	104	GSV	90	12	0
Oh et al., 2003[9]	15	GSV	100	3	0
Min et al., 2003[6]	499	GSV	98	17	0
Proebstle et al., 2003[38]	39	SSV	100	6	2
Perkowski et al., 2004[43]	154	GSV	97	12	0
	37	SSV	97	12	0
Sadick and Waser, 2004[44]	31	GSV	97	24	0
Timperman et al., 2004[24]	111	GSV	78	7	0
Proebstle et al., 2004[23]	106	GSV	90	3	0
Goldman et al., 2004[7]	24	GSV	100	9	0
Proebstle et al., 2005[14]	282	GSV	95	3	0
Timperman, 2005[25]	100	GSV	91	9	1
Puggioni et al., 2005[45]	77	GSV/SSV	94	1	2
Kabnick, 2006[13]	60	GSV	92	12	0
Almeida and Raines, 2006[11]	578	GSV	98	24	0
	115	SSV	96	24	0
Yang et al., 2006[46]	71	GSV	94	13	–
Kim and Paxton, 2006[30]	60	GSV	95	3	–
Kavaturu et al., 2006[47]	66	GSV	97	12	0
Myers et al., 2006[48]	404	GSV/SSV	80	36	0
Sadick and Wasser, 2007[49]	94	GSV	96	48	0
Theivacumar et al., 2007[50]	68	SSV	100	6	4
Gibson et al., 2007[40]	210	SSV	100	1.5	6
Ravi et al., 2006[39]	990	GSV	97	36	0
	101	SSV	90	36	0
Desmyttere et al., 2007[28]	511	GSV	97	48	0

DUS, duplex ultrasound; *GSV*, great saphenous vein; *SSV*, small saphenous vein.

TABLE 6–2 Summary of Outcomes for Randomized Trials of Surgery Versus Endovenous Laser Ablation

	de Medeiros and Luccas[51]	Ying et al.[52]	Rasmussen et al.[53]	Kalteis et al.[54]	Darwood et al.[55]
No. of limbs (surgery vs. EVLA)	20 vs. 20	80 patients	68 vs. 69	48 vs. 47	35 vs. 79 (1:2 randomization)
Anesthesia for EVLA	Regional		Tumescent and LA sedation	General or regional	Tumescent and LA sedation
Surgical treatment	SFJ ligation, GSV stripping, and phlebectomy		SFJ ligation, GSV stripping, and phlebectomy	SFJ ligation, GSV stripping, and phlebectomy	SFJ ligation, GSV stripping, and phlebectomy
Addition therapy for EVLA patients	SFJ ligation and phlebectomy		Concomitant phlebectomy	SFJ ligation and phlebectomy	Delayed sclerotherapy (6 weeks)
Outcome measures	Bruising, abolition of reflux and pain	Pain, blood loss, hospital stay	Bruising, QOL, normal activity, abolition of reflux, and pain	Bruising, QOL, normal activity, abolition of reflux and pain, and patient satisfaction	QOL, normal activity, abolition of reflux and pain, and patient satisfaction
Results	EVLA: less bruising; patients preferred EVLA; EVLA: 95% ablation; pain: equivalent	All reduced by EVLA	EVLA: less bruising; QOL: equivalent; NA: equivalent; ablation: 96% vs. 94%; and pain: less with EVLA	EVLA: less bruising; QOL: equivalent; EVLA: delayed NA; ablation: 100% both; pain: equivalent; and cosmesis: equivalent	QOL: equivalent; NA: earlier with EVLA; Ablation: 88% vs. 94%; Pain: equivalent, and satisfaction: equivalent
Duration of follow-up	60 days		6 months	16 weeks	3 months (limited 12-month data)

EVLA, endovenous laser ablation; *GSV*, great saphenous vein; *LA*, local anesthesia; *NA*, not applicable; *QOL*, quality of life; *SFJ*, saphenofemoral junction.

Although this may be surprising, it is likely to reflect GSV and adjacent soft tissue inflammation ("phlebitis") following the thermal injury inflicted by EVL. Although pain levels appear similar for surgery and EVL, return to normal activity or work is variously reported as occurring earlier after EVL[56] at the same time following either modality[53] or delayed after laser therapy.[54]

It is evident from these trials that there is no consensus as to the optimum treatment protocol for EVL. Given the results reported by Rasmussen et al.[53] and Darwood et al.,[55] it seems that concomitant saphenofemoral ligation is unnecessary, thus allowing EVL to be performed without general or regional anaesthesia in an outpatient or office setting. The question of adjuvant treatment for the varicosities has not been answered by these studies. Only Darwood et al.[55] used delayed sclerotherapy for persisting varicose veins after EVL. Provided that truncal vein ablation is commenced at the lowest point of reflux, it is still not known how many patients require additional treatment—thus, many operators support a policy of delayed sclerotherapy, while others prefer synchronous phlebectomy with EVL.

Meta-analysis

This meta-analysis of randomized controlled trials reviews the current evidence base, comparing open and endovascular treatment of varicose veins.[56] Systematic review of studies reporting duplex scan follow-up after open surgical, laser (endovenous laser therapy [EVLT]), or radiofrequency (VNUS Closure device, VNUS Medical Technologies, San Jose, CA) treatment of refluxing great saphenous veins was completed. Primary outcome measures were occlusion and complication rates and time taken to resume work. Meta-analysis finds no significant difference in recurrence rates at 3 months between open surgery and endovenous laser ablation (EVLA) (relative risk [RR] 2.19, 95% confidence internal [CI] 0.99 to 4.85, p = .05) or VNUS (RR 7.57; 95% CI 0.42 to 136.02). Return to work is significantly faster following VNUS (by 8.24 days, 95% CI 10.50 to 5.97) or EVLA (by 5.02 days, 95% CI. 6.52 to 3.52). Endovascular treatment of varicose veins is safe and effective and offers the significant advantage of rapid recovery.

REFERENCES

1. Mundy L, Merlin TL, Fitridge RA, et al. Systematic review of endovenous laser treatment for varicose veins. Br J Surg 2005;92:1189-1194.
2. Proebstle TM, Gul D, Lehr HA, et al. Infrequent early recanalization of greater saphenous vein after endovenous laser treatment. J Vasc Surg 2003;38:511-516.
3. Min RJ, Zimmet SE, Isaacs MN, et al. Endovenous laser treatment of the incompetent greater saphenous vein. J Vasc Interv Radiol 2001;12:1167-1171.
4. Proebstle TM, Lehr HA, Kargl A, et al. Endovenous treatment of the greater saphenous vein with a 940 nm diode laser: thrombotic occlusion after endoluminal thermal damage by laser generated steam bubbles. J Vasc Surg 2002;35:729-736.
5. Proebstle TM, Sandhofer M, Kargl A, et al. Thermal damage of the inner vein wall during endovenous treatment: key role of energy absorption by intravascular blood. Dermatol Surg 2002;28:596-600.
6. Min RJ, Khilnani N, Zimmet S. Endovenous laser treatment of saphenous vein reflux: long-term results. J Vasc Interv Radiol 2003;14:991-996.
7. Goldman MP, Mauricio M, Rao J. Intravascular 1320-nm laser closure of the great saphenous vein: a 6- to 12-month follow-up study. Dermatol Surg 2004;30:1380-1385.
8. Goldman MP. Intravascular lasers in the treatment of varicose veins. J Cosmetic Dermatol 2004;3:162-166.
9. Oh CK, Jung DS, Jang HS, et al. Endovenous laser surgery of the incompetent greater saphenous vein with a 980-nm diode laser. Dermatol Surg 2003;29:1135-1140.

10. Disselhoff B, Rem AI, Verdaasdonk R, et al. Endovenous laser ablation: an experimental study on the mechanism of action. Phlebology 2008;23:69-76.

11. Almeida JI, Raines JK. Radiofrequency ablation and laser ablation in the treatment of varicose veins. Ann Vasc Surg 2006;20:547-552.

12. Lurie F, Creton D, Eklof B, et al. Prospective randomised study of endovenous radiofrequency obliteration (closure) versus ligation and vein stripping (EVOLVeS): two-year follow-up. Eur J Vasc Endovasc Surg 2005;29:67-73.

13. Kabnick LS. Outcome of different endovenous laser wavelengths for great saphenous vein ablation. J Vasc Surg 2006 Jan;43:88-93.

14. Proebstle TM, Moehler T, Gul D, et al. Endovenous treatment of the great saphenous vein using a1,320 nm Nd:YAG laser causes fewer side effects than using a 940 nm diode laser. Dermatol Surg 2005;31:1678-1683.

15. Almeida JI, Mackay EG, Javier JJ, et al. Saphenous laser ablation at 1470 nm targets the vein wall, not blood. Vasc Endovascular Surg 2009;43:467-472.

16. Bush RG, Shamma HN, Hammond K. Histological changes occurring after endoluminal ablation with two diode lasers (940 and 1319 nm) from acute changes to 4 months. Lasers Surg Med 2008;40:676-679.

17. Fan CM, Rox-Anderson R. Endovenous laser ablation: mechanism of action. Phlebology 2008;23:206-213.

18. Roggan A, Friebel M, Dorschel K, et al. Optical properties of circulating human blood in the wavelength range 400-2500 nm. J Biomed Opt 1999;4:36-46.

19. Schmedt CG, Meissner OA, Hunger K, et al. Evaluation of endovenous radiofrequency ablation and laser therapy with endoluminal optical coherence tomography in an ex vivo model. J Vasc Surg 2007;45:1047-1058.

20. Weiss RA. Comparison of endovenous radiofrequency versus 810 nm diode laser occlusion of the large veins in an animal model. Dermatol Surg 2002;28:56-61.

21. Zimmet SE, Min RJ. Temperature changes in perivenous tissue during endovenous laser treatment in a swine model. J Vasc Interv Radiol 2003;14:911-915.

22. Beale RJ, Mavor AID, Gough MJ. Heat dissipation during endovenous laser treatment of varicose veins—is there a risk of nerve injury? Phlebology 2006;21:32-35.

23. Proebstle TM, Krummenauer F, Gül D, et al. Non-occlusion and early reopening of the great saphenous vein after endovenous laser treatment is fluence dependent. Dermatol Surg 2004;30(2 Pt 1):174-178.

24. Timperman PE, Sichlau M, Ryu RK. Greater energy delivery improves treatment success of endovenous laser treatment of incompetent saphenous veins. J Vasc Interv Radiol 2004;15: 1061-1063.

25. Timperman PE. Prospective evaluation of higher energy great saphenous vein endovenous laser treatment. J Vasc Interv Radiol 2005;16:791-794.

26. Proebstle TM, Moehler T, Herdemann S. Reduced recanalization rates of the great saphenous vein after endovenous laser treatment with increased energy dosing: definition of a threshold for the endovenous fluence equivalent. J Vasc Surg 2006;44:834-839.

27. Vuylsteke M, Liekens K, Moons P, et al. Endovenous laser treatment of saphenous vein reflux: how much energy do we need to prevent recanalizations. Vasc Endovasc Surg 2008;42: 141-149.

28. Desmyttere J, Grard C, Wassmer B, et al. Endovenous 980-nm laser treatment of saphenous veins in a series of 500 patients. J Vasc Surg 2007;46:1242-1247.

29. Kim HS, Nwankwo IJ, Hong K, et al. Lower energy endovenous laser ablation of the great saphenous vein with 980 nm diode laser in continuous mode. Cardiovasc Intervent Radiol 2006;29:64-69.

30. Kim HS, Paxton BE. Endovenous laser ablation of the great saphenous vein with a 980-nm diode laser in continuous mode: early treatment failures and successful repeat treatments. J Vasc Interv Radiol 2006;17:1449-1455.

31. Prince EA, Ahn SH, Dubel GJ, et al. An investigation of the relationship between energy density and endovenous laser ablation success: does energy density matter? J Vasc Interv Radiol 2008;19:1449-1453.

32. Merchant RF, dePalma RG, Kabnick LS. Endovascular obliteration of saphenous reflux: a muticenter study. J Vasc Surg 2002;35:1180-1186.

33. Merchant RF, Pichot O, Meyers KA. Four-year follow-up on endovascular radiofrequency obliteration of great saphenous reflux. Dermatol Surg 2005;31:129-134.

34. Chang C, Chua J. Endovenous laser photocoagulation (EVLP) for varicose veins. Lasers Surg Med 2002;31:257-262.

35. Merchant RF, Pichot O, for the Closure Study Group. Long-term outcomes of endovenous radiofrequency obliteration of saphenous reflux as a treatment of superficial venous insufficiency. J Vasc Surg 2005;42:502-509.

36. Zikorus AW, Mirizzi MS. Evaluation of setpoint temperature and pullback speed on vein adventitial temperature during endovenous radiofrequency energy delivery in an in-vitro model. Vasc Endovascular Surg 2004;38:167-174.

37. Dunn CW, Kabnick LS, Merchant RF, et al. Endovascular radiofrequency obliteration using 90°C for treatment of great saphenous vein. Ann Vasc Surg 2006;20:625-629.

38. Proebstle TM, Gul D, Kargl A, et al. Endovenous laser treatment of the lesser saphenous vein with a 940-nm diode laser: early results. Dermatol Surg 2003;29:357-361.

39. Ravi R, Rodriguez-Lopez JA, Traylor EA, et al. Endovenous ablation of incompetent saphenous veins: a large single-center experience. J Endovasc Ther 2006;13:244-248.

40. Gibson KD, Ferris BL, Polissar N, et al. Endovenous laser treatment of the small saphenous vein: efficacy and complications. J Vasc Surg 2007;45:795-801.

41. Kontothanassis D, Di Mitri R, Ferrari Ruffino S, et al. Endovenous laser treatment of the small saphenous vein. J Vasc Surg 2009;49:973-979.

42. Navarro L, Min RJ, Bone C. Endovenous laser: a new minimally invasive method of treatment of varicose veins—preliminary observations using an 810 nm diode laser. Dermatol Surg 2001;27:117-122.

43. Perkowski P, Ravi R, Gowda RCN, et al. Endovenous laser ablation of the saphenous vein for treatment of venous insufficiency and varicose veins: early results from a large single-center experience. J Endovasc Ther 2004;11:132-138.

44. Sadick NS, Waser S. Combined endovascular laser with ambulatory phlebectomy for the treatment of superficial venous incompetence: a 2-year perspective. J Cosmet Laser Ther 2004;24:149-153.

45. Puggioni A, Kalra M, Carmo M, et al. Endovenous laser therapy and radiofrequency ablation of the great saphenous vein: analysis of early efficacy and complications. J Vasc Surg 2005;42:488-493.

46. Yang CH, Chou HS, Lo YF. Incompetent great saphenous veins treated with endovenous 1,320-nm laser: results for 71 legs and morphologic evolvement study. Dermatol Surg 2006;32:1453-1457.

47. Kavuturu S, Girishkumar H, Ehrlich F. Endovenous laser ablation of saphenous veins is an effective treatment modality for lower extremity varicose veins. Am Surg 2006;72:672-675.

48. Myers K, Fris R, Jolley D. Treatment of varicose veins by endovenous laser therapy: assessment of results by ultrasound surveillance. Med J Austral 2006;185:199-202.

49. Sadick NS, Wasser S. Combined endovascular laser plus ambulatory phlebectomy for the treatment of superficial venous incompetence: a 4-year perspective. J Cosmet Laser Ther 2007;9:9-13.

50. Theivacumar NS, Beale RJ, Mavor AI, et al. Initial experience in endovenous laser ablation (EVLA) of varicose veins due to small saphenous vein reflux. Eur J Vasc Endovasc Surg 2007;33:614-618.

51. de Medeiros C, Luccas G. Comparison of endovenous treatment with an 810 nm laser versus conventional stripping of the great saphenous vein in patients with primary varicose veins. Dermatol Surg 2005;31:1685-1694.

52. Ying L, Sheng Y, Ling H, et al. Random, comparative study on endovenous laser therapy and saphenous veins stripping for the treatment of great saphenous vein incompetence. Zhonghua-Yi-Xue-Za-Zhi 2007;87:3043-3046.

53. Rasmussen LH, Bjoern L, Lawaetz M, et al. Trial comparing endovenous laser ablation of the great saphenous vein with high ligation and stripping in patients with varicose veins: short term results. J Vasc Surg 2007;46:308-315.

54. Kalteis M, Berger I, Messie-Werndl S, et al. High ligation combined with stripping and endovenous laser ablation of the great saphenous vein: early results of a randomised controlled study. J Vasc Surg 2008;47:822-829.

55. Darwood R, Theivacumar N, Dellagrammaticus D, et al. Randomised clinical trial comparing endovenous laser ablation with surgery for the treatment of primary great saphenous varicose veins. Br J Surg 2008;95:294-301.

56. Brar R, Nordon IM, Hinchliffe RJ, et al. Management of varicose veins: meta-analysis. Vascular 2010;18:205-220.

Chemical Ablation

Jose I. Almeida

HISTORICAL BACKGROUND

Historical data suggest that chemical ablation of the great saphenous vein (GSV) using liquid sclerosant delivered percutaneously via syringe and needle will fail (recanalize) in over 50% of cases at 1 year. Sclerotherapy in Europe became less frequently performed in the latter part of the 20th century, at least in part, because of the work of Hobbs.[1] His 10-year randomized controlled study showed the clinical recurrence of varices was common in patients with truncal saphenous reflux managed with sclerotherapy.[2] Hobbs found that after 10 years, 71% of patients treated with traditional surgery for saphenous incompetence had a good outcome; this compared with only 6% of patients treated by sclerotherapy. Recent scientific evidence has shown that liquid sclerotherapy is not very effective at eliminating truncal saphenous incompetence and failure to eliminate reflux leads to early recurrence of varices. Scientific evidence is limited when comparing sclerotherapy and surgery due to the fact that many of the trials had methodologic flaws such as lack of evaluation by independent observers, high dropout rates, poorly defined outcomes, and the lack of intention-to-treat analyses.[3,4] However, despite these defects, most of the studies clearly demonstrated very high recurrence rates of varicose veins after sclerotherapy, ranging from 20% to 70%.

Investigators have shown that if endothelial damage is not extensive, thrombi will form and layer endoluminally. Some thrombus is expected because of platelet deposition and initiation of the intrinsic coagulation pathway once collagen is exposed; however, excessive thrombosis is undesirable because it can lead to recanalization of the vessel. Furthermore, excessive thrombus can lead to perivenous inflammation resulting in patient discomfort on an acute basis and unwanted pigmentation of the surrounding skin thereafter.

ETIOLOGY AND NATURAL HISTORY OF DISEASE

Sclerotherapy refers to the introduction of a drug into the vein lumen for the specific purpose of producing endoluminal fibrosis and subsequent vein closure. Clinically, the reason vein closure is desired is to mitigate the effects of venous hypertension caused by retrograde venous flow; however, other reasons are also present in clinical practice. The mechanism of action of sclerosing solutions is directed toward complete destruction of the endothelial cells lining the venous lumen, exposure of subendothelial collagen fibers, and, ultimately, the formation of a fibrous cord. In accomplishing this process, sclerosing agents must significantly alter the endothelium and to a lesser extent the media of the vein wall. The most important qualities that a sclerosant should possess are safety, efficacy, and lack of untoward side effects. Other important features should be the ability to produce durable and repeatable results, painless treatments, accurate placement with ultrasound guidance, ease of availability, and low cost.

The efficacy of sclerosing agents is a function of concentration and vein diameter.[5] If the target vein diameter is greater than 3 mm, liquid sclerosants do not properly reach the vein wall secondary to dilution. Sclerosant in the form of foam has clearly improved the results of sclerotherapy. Foam is more efficacious than liquid[6-8] and is more readily monitored with ultrasound imaging. Foam is the reason chemical ablation has made a resurgence. Foam will expand and fill a vein of less than 12-mm diameter, offering better contact with the vein wall. Cabrera and colleagues[9] published a clinical series of 500 lower limbs treated with foam sclerotherapy and reported that after 3 or more years, 81% of treated great saphenous trunks remained occluded and 97% of superficial varices had disappeared. This required one session of sclerotherapy in 86% of patients, two sessions in 11% of patients, and three sessions in 3% of patients.

Sclerosants

Sclerosing solutions are categorized as either detergent, chemical, or osmotic; in the United States, although many are used, only one drug is approved by the U.S. Food and Drug Administration (FDA). Sodium tetradecyl sulfate (STS) was originally approved by the FDA for manufacture by Elkins Sinn in 1946. Under the Elkins Sinn trade name Sotradecol, STS became the preferred agent for sclerotherapy. In Europe, the popular sclerosants are STS 1% to 3% (Fibrovein; STD Pharmaceuticals, Hereford, UK) and polidocanol (POL) 0.5% to 3% (Sclerovein; Resinag AG, Zurich, Switzerland). The sclerotherapy community is therefore limited in its choices of drug, and currently investigators are focused on two methods of enhancing sclerotherapy—one method changes the biologic behavior of the drug, and the other method alters the drug delivery system.

When Elkins Sinn discontinued production of Sotradecol in the United States in 2000, a nationwide shortage ensued. Since no other manufacturer had FDA approval to produce STS, compounding pharmacies were the only source from which physicians could obtain this agent. The shortage of STS and the stopgap role of compounding pharmacies ended in November 2004 when the FDA granted approval to Bioniche Pharma USA, Inc. (Belleville, Ontario, Canada) to manufacture STS in 1% and 3% strengths. Today, FDA-approved Sotradecol is manufactured by Bioniche Pharma in an FDA-approved facility and sold exclusively by AngioDynamics, Inc. (Queensbury, NY). In a study of compounded STS versus pharmaceutical-grade STS, several findings were reported.[10] Compounded STS was found to contain measured levels of impurities, the most important of which was carbitol. Analysis of pharmaceutical-grade STS revealed no detectable levels of impurities. Although the level of STS impurity necessary to precipitate a clinical event is unknown, impurities in other drugs have been linked to significant unexpected adverse events. Concentrations of different compounded STS formulations showed significant variation when measured by an independent laboratory. In one sample, the concentration was 20% below the desired 3% concentration level.

Regarding efficacy, in the compounded STS group 45.7% of treated great saphenous veins demonstrated segments of incomplete ablation some time during follow-up. In the pharmaceutical-grade STS group, incomplete ablation occurred in only 12.5% of veins ($p = .02$).

PATIENT SELECTION

Sclerotherapy is a good choice for the treatment of nonsaphenous varicose veins, residual veins after surgical correction of axial vein reflux, and recurrent varicose veins secondary to neovascularization or incompetent perforating veins. Sclerotherapy is also the treatment of choice in spider telangiectasias, venectasias, and isolated reticular veins.[11] The mode of action is induction of irritation of the vein wall followed by inflammation and fibrosis. Different agents are used such as hypertonic glucose that act by dehydrating the endothelium and substances like ethanolamine oleate[8] that have a detergent effect in the endothelial layer.

OPERATIVE STEPS

The three different methods of injecting large veins are:

1. ***Fegan's method***: In this method the distal perforators are injected first followed by the proximal veins.[12] The saphenous trunk and the junctions are not injected. This is followed by prolonged strong compression with bandaging from bottom to top in order to minimize thrombophlebitis and induce fibrosis.

2. ***Tournay's method***: In this method the proximal points of reflux are injected, including the saphenofemoral and saphenopopliteal junctions (SFJs and SPJs, respectively). The final step is distal injection. Short periods of local compression are used.[13]

3. ***Sigg's method***: In this method, the most distal varicose vein is injected first, followed by proximal stepwise injection until the most proximal reflux point is reached. Following the procedure, prolonged compression is used[14] (Figs. 7-1 through 7-5).

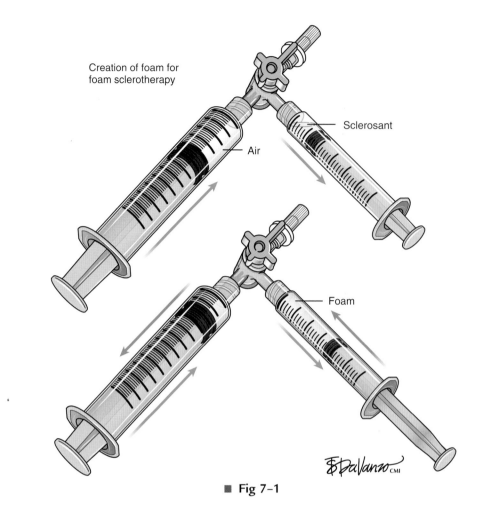

Creation of foam for
foam sclerotherapy

Air

Sclerosant

Foam

■ Fig 7–1

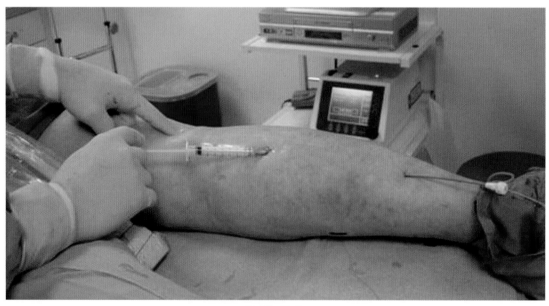

■ Fig 7–2

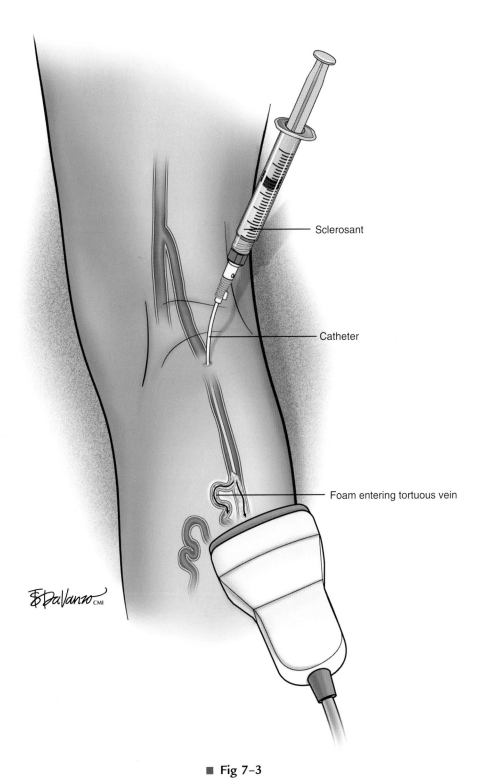

Sclerosant

Catheter

Foam entering tortuous vein

■ **Fig 7–3**

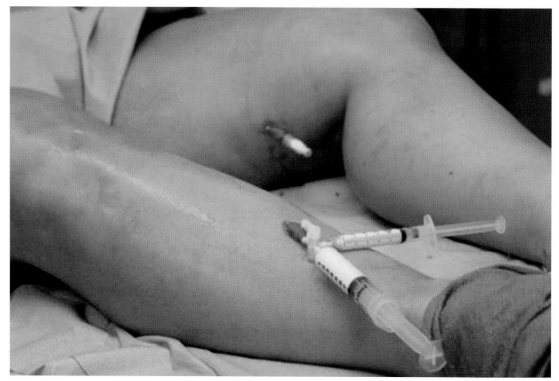

■ Fig 7–4

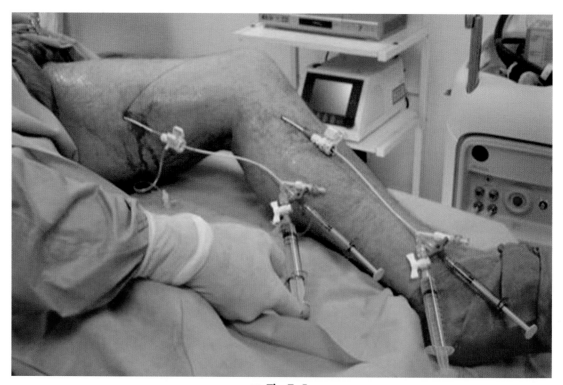

■ Fig 7–5

IMAGING

Recent trends have demonstrated a growing use of duplex-guided sclerotherapy, which was first described in 1989.[15] It not only minimizes the chances of intraarterial injection and extravasation but also allows the estimation of the degree of spasm, length of vein treated, and position of the deep veins (Figs. 7-6 and 7-7).

Foam Sclerotherapy

A recent revolution in the treatment of venous disease has been the emergence of foam sclerotherapy. Egmont James Orbach in 1944 first proposed the use of foam generated by a simple process of shaking a sclerosant with air. However, interest faded because it could only be used for small veins owing to large bubbles and a high air-to-liquid ratio.[16] The renaissance of foam sclerotherapy is credited largely to the work of Cabrera et al.[17] and Monfreux et al.[18] in the 1990s.

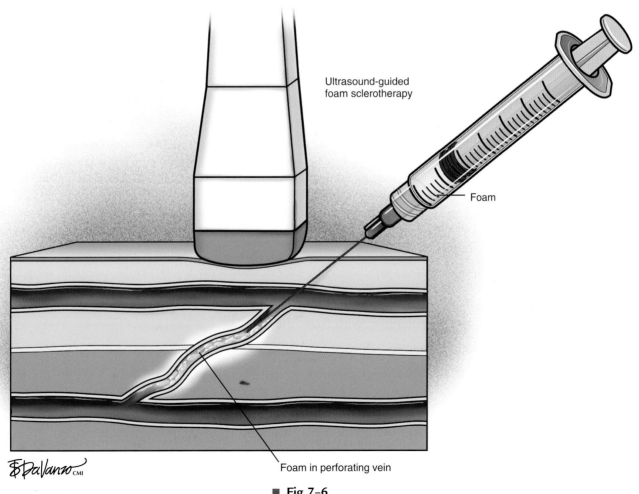

Ultrasound-guided
foam sclerotherapy

Foam

Foam in perforating vein

■ **Fig 7-6**

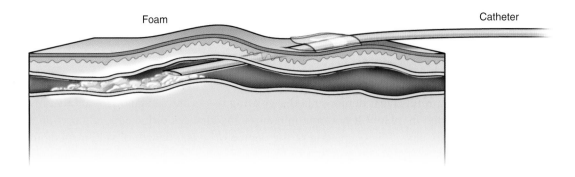

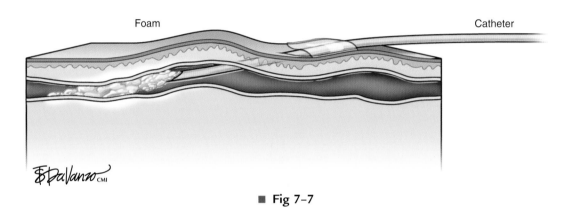

■ **Fig 7–7**

Foam for the purpose of vein wall destruction is a nonequilibrated dispersion of gas bubbles in a sclerosing solution in which the gas fraction is 0.5221 or greater. The foam is composed of tiny bubbles of gas covered by a tensioactive liquid.[19] Small bubbles make the foam highly interactive, whereas large bubbles produce ineffective foam. The foam mechanically displaces the blood and comes into contact with the endothelium. Therefore, the same concentration of the sclerosant is suitable for large and small veins. There is sufficient clinical evidence to demonstrate several advantages of foam preparations over conventional liquid sclerotherapy[6,20]:

1. Liquid sclerosants are diluted by blood, thus reducing delivered concentration to the vein wall. Foam, on the other hand, displaces the blood and allows direct contact with the endothelium. It follows that the efficacy of a given concentration of a sclerosant can be enhanced with foam therapy.

2. There is increased safety with foam preparations as lower concentrations of sclerosants are used.

3. Extravasated foam is much better tolerated than liquid extravasation.

4. The air contained in the foam is echogenic and thus increases the visibility and accuracy of placement when performing duplex-guided sclerotherapy.[21]

Variables like type and concentration of the sclerosing agent, gas, gas-to-liquid ratio, bubble size, and time between preparation and use determine the efficacy of the agent.[21] An ideal foam should be durable enough to allow injection before separating into gas and liquid components.[22]

It is accepted that microfoams with bubble diameters less than 250 μm are commonly used and the ideal effective choice (macrofoams have bubbles larger than 500 μm and minifoams have bubbles ranging from 250 to 500 μm). There are various techniques in the literature that describe effective ways to produce microfoam.

In reference to the biologic behavior of STS, Schneider and Fischer[23] showed that endothelial damage is concentration dependent and occurs immediately after injection, with resulting rapid thrombus formation leading to vascular sclerosis. Importantly, 3% STS foam has not yielded 100% GSV closure when injected with a standard needle and syringe; therefore, catheters that can enhance the interaction of drug to vein wall are under investigation.

Foam is an option for controlling saphenous reflux in veins of less than 12 mm and has been shown to be a viable treatment for sclerosis of perforators. Foam is of value in the treatment of varicosed tributaries, tortuous vessels, and venous malformations. Foam also has limitations and carries liability concerns. In veins larger than 12 mm, the sclerosant–blood interface compromises treatment.[24] It has been recommended that a 10-mL limit be placed with regard to total foam volume injected because of possible paradoxical embolization via the patent foramen ovale.[19] For this reason there has been some interest in maximizing sclerosant contact time with the vein wall through the use of catheters. Future studies will likely focus on maximizing results of liquid or foamed sclerosants through innovations in catheter technology. The known methods of producing foam sclerotherapy include the following:

Cabrera method: Juan Cabrera in 1997 published his 7-year experience of excellent results with special foam that is prepared with a sclerosing agent, CO_2, and an unknown tensioactive agent.[17]

Monfreux method: In this method, foam is produced in a glass syringe with the tip closed by a sterile plug; tension is applied by compressing the piston. While the foam is long lasting, the larger bubbles formed by this method can reduce the effectiveness of the therapy.[18]

Tessari method: Described in 1999 by Lorenzo Tessari, high-quality foam is produced with two disposable syringes and a three-way tap.[24] STS was initially described with this method. The advantages of this method are use of disposable materials, compact foam with small bubble diameter, and the ability to reconstitute the foam if the treatment session takes more time.

Frullini method: Described by Frullini and Cavezzi in 2000, the foam generation uses the same turbulence effect as the Tessari method.[18] Foam is generated by a vial and syringe joined by a connector.

COMPARATIVE EFFECTIVENESS OF EXISTING TREATMENTS

Results of Clinical Trials

A prospective randomized control trial involving more than 800 patients over 10 years compared six treatment options: liquid sclerotherapy, high-dose liquid sclerotherapy, multiple ligations, stab avulsions, foam sclerotherapy, and ligation followed by sclerotherapy. The conclusion was that the results of foam sclerotherapy were superior to those of liquid sclerotherapy and comparable with those of surgery.[25]

The listed complications ranged from phlebitis, skin necrosis, transient visual disturbance, and, on rare occasions, deep venous thrombosis (DVT). There have been suggestions that foam sclerotherapy may have a slightly higher rate of pigmentation, inflammation, and minimal necrosis when used in small reticular veins and telangiectasias.[18] There have been uncertainties regarding the safety of foam preparations as animal studies demonstrated increased pulmonary hypertension. The stress on the human respiratory system is still unclear. The volume used per session depends on the size of the veins. No cases of DVT were reported in a prospective study of large volume foam sclerotherapy for varicose veins.[26]

Two randomized controlled trials (RCTs) compared foam sclerotherapy with high ligation and stripping (HL/S). The first RCT showed that HL/S is superior to foam sclerotherapy using Varisolve (BTG plc, London, UK) for occlusion and elimination of reflux (86% versus 63%) but that foam sclerotherapy was superior to conventional sclerotherapy (90% versus 76%).[26] The second RCT showed that foam sclerotherapy combined with high ligation was less expensive, involved shorter treatment time, and resulted in more rapid recovery compared with HL/S.[27]

Although foam sclerotherapy is used universally and has become the standard of care, foamed sclerosants can embolize to the arterial circulation via patent foramen ovale. Only three permanent adverse events from paradoxical embolization of foam have been published[28,29]; however, several transient neurologic events have been reported anecdotally, and therefore foam remains controversial.

Outcomes Using Foam

A detailed review of the outcomes of ultrasound-guided foam sclerotherapy was published in 2007.[30] Some important publications and more recent data are discussed here. Cabrera et al.[17] published a clinical series of 500 legs treated with foam sclerotherapy. They reported that after 3 or more years, 81% of treated great saphenous trunks remained occluded and 97% of superficial varices had disappeared. This required one session of sclerotherapy in 86% of patients, two sessions in 11% of patients, and three sessions in 3% of patients. No DVT or pulmonary embolism was encountered in this series.

Subsequently, a number of authors have published clinical series based on this technique including Frullini and Cavezzi,[18] who reported a series of 453 patients, and Barrett et al.,[31] who reported a series of 100 limbs. Cavezzi et al.[32] subsequently published a detailed analysis of the efficacy of foam sclerotherapy in 194 patients, reporting a good outcome in 93% of patients. In fact, this technique has become widely used in southern Europe, Australia, New Zealand, South America, and the United States.[33] However, few surgeons in the United Kingdom use this method, perhaps because of limited evidence of efficacy. One series has been reported from the United Kingdom involving 60 patients in comparing surgical treatment with foam sclerotherapy combined with saphenofemoral ligation.[34]

One randomized study of foam sclerotherapy in comparison with surgery has been published. This was a multicenter European study.[26] This randomized controlled trial included two separate studies: a surgical part undertaken by surgeons who randomized patients to saphenous stripping or ultrasound-guided foam sclerotherapy. In addition, sclerotherapists randomized patients to ultrasound-guided sclerotherapy conducted using either foam or liquid sclerosant. In all, 654 patients were treated during this study. Up to four sessions of ultrasound-guided foam sclerotherapy were allowed over 3 months to obliterate the saphenous trunks. After 12 months, the surgeons had eliminated truncal saphenous reflux in 130 of 176 patients (74%) by foam sclerotherapy and in 84 of 94 patients (88%) by surgery. In comparison, sclerotherapists had eliminated reflux in 239 of 254 patients (91%) by foam and 104 of 125 patients (83%) by liquid sclerotherapy. Posttreatment pain was assessed by a visual analog scale, which showed that surgery was much more painful during the first week. Normal activities were resumed after a median of 13 days in the surgery group and 2 days in the foam group. DVT was seen in 10 patients treated by foam and one patient treated by liquid sclerotherapy.

The relative efficacy of foam and liquid sclerotherapy has been investigated in a detailed study.[35] Patients with truncal saphenous incompetence were injected with either 2 to 2.5 mL of 3% POL liquid or foam into the GSV under ultrasound guidance on only one occasion. Obliteration of saphenous incompetence was obtained in 35% of liquid-treated patients and 85% of foam-treated patients after 3 weeks. At 2 years, 53% of foam-treated and 12% of liquid-treated patients had successful obliteration of the GSV. A further study was performed to assess the relative efficacy of 1% and 3% sclerosant foam.[36] Patients with truncal saphenous reflux were randomized to treatment with either 1% or 3% POL foam in a single session. An average of 4.5 mL of foam was injected in both groups. Immediate occlusion rates were 96% (3% concentration) and 86% (1% concentration). After 2 years, saphenous occlusion was seen in 69% of the 3% group and 68% of the 1% group.

In both of these studies, a rather small volume of foam was used; it was well below the maximum of 10 mL recommended in the Tegernsee document[37] and the 20 mL suggested earlier in this text. This probably prejudiced the outcome but allowed the authors to demonstrate clearly the advantages of foam and lack of increased efficacy with 3% POL.

A number of papers have addressed particular problems in the management of varicose veins. Recurrent varices managed surgically have a poor outcome, with further recurrence from neovascularization as a common feature.[38] The clinical series mentioned found similar outcomes in primary and recurrent varices managed by foam sclerotherapy, with 88% of SFJs and saphenous trunks remaining obliterated at 11-month follow-up.[39] Creton and Uhl[40] have reported a combined surgical and foam sclerotherapy technique (in one session) for patients with recurrent varices, with obliteration of 93% of varices and saphenous trunks at 40-day follow-up. Perrin and Gillet[41] reviewed the available literature on recurrent varices of the popliteal fossa and concluded that unless a grossly incompetent SPJ stump is present, ultrasound-guided foam sclerotherapy is the most appropriate treatment. They acknowledge that this conclusion is supported by reports of clinical series and not randomized clinical trials.

A number of papers have discussed the outcome of foam sclerotherapy in patients with venous ulceration and severe venous disease. One hundred eighty-five truncal veins were treated in 165 patients. A high proportion of veins were complicated (109 CEAP classes 4-6, 76 CEAP 1-3). There was no significant difference in occlusion rates between primary (45/60-75%) and recurrent (23/32-72%) veins; CEAP 2-3 (22/30-73%) and CEAP 4-6 (46/62-74%) veins; and veins with a diameter less than 7 mm (29/38-76%) and veins with a diameter more than or equal to 7 mm (13/23-57%). The authors concluded that foam sclerotherapy was equally effective for complicated and uncomplicated varicose veins.[42] The clinical outcome of treatment has been reported in a number of papers.[43-45] In general, rapid healing of ulcers is reported following foam sclerotherapy, confirming that this treatment can probably achieve the same outcomes that result from saphenous obliteration in leg ulcer patients.

PEARLS AND PITFALLS

The major contraindication to the use of sclerotherapy is known allergy to the agent. The minor side effects seen are hyperpigmentation, pruritus, and neovascularization. Other reported side effects include night cramps, swollen foot, thrombophlebitis, and blisters.[46,47] Sclerotherapy must be performed with caution in patients with arterial insufficiency, recent or recurrent DVT, hypercoagulability syndromes, and severe systemic diseases. Dangerous complications like intraarterial injection and thromboembolism can be avoided by following a meticulous protocol.

COMPLICATIONS

Systemic complications of foam sclerotherapy have been examined in some detail in view of occasional visual disturbance reported by some patients following both foam and liquid sclerotherapy.[48] Visual disturbance has been reported following the injection of a range of liquid sclerosants, although it is clear that it is far more common following foam sclerotherapy. Some serious neurologic adverse events, from which recovery was eventually complete, have also been reported.[31] This has led to attention focusing on the effects of a patent foramen ovale. This was the subject of a study by Morrison et al.,[49] in which 20 patients with visual or respiratory symptoms following foam sclerotherapy were studied by transthoracic echocardiography during treatment. In this study, 65% of patients were found to have echoes in the left atrium after the injection of foam sclerosant. Five of nine patients who then underwent transcranial Doppler investigation during foam sclerotherapy were found to have high-intensity events in the middle cerebral artery during treatment.

Clearly, gas bubbles injected in the lower limb may reach the cerebral circulation, but the relationship to this phenomenon and the visual disturbances reported in some patients is yet to be established. Morrison et al. also reported the outcome of treating patients with foam made with CO_2 in comparison with air foam. This resulted in a substantial reduction in visual and other adverse events following treatment. It seems logical to consider moving to CO_2 foams to minimize these side effects, even if they are usually benign and resolve swiftly. In general, the number of serious adverse events is very small compared with the number of treatments performed. However, this reminds us that even minimally invasive treatments may have significant side effects and that we should take all reasonable precautions.

One study has examined the relative efficacy of minimally invasive means of treating incompetent saphenous trunks in comparison with surgical management.[50] A meta-analysis of 119 studies including 12,320 limbs was undertaken. The main outcome measure was obliteration of the saphenous trunk assessed by duplex ultrasonography at an average of 30 months following treatment.

A small advantage in favor of endovenous laser ablation was found, but the authors concluded that surgery and endovenous laser ablation, endovenous radiofrequency ablation, and ultrasound-guided foam sclerotherapy are equally effective.

MIAMI VEIN CENTER EXPERIENCE

At Miami Vein Center we have worked with two different chemical ablation catheter systems, each quite different in design, which enhance drug interaction with venous endothelium. At the 2006 American Venous Forum, we presented the results of 75 saphenous veins treated with an endovenous catheter with an occlusive balloon at the SFJ (VeinRx, Miami, FL). The idea was to isolate a column of 3% STS *foamed* sclerosant at the desired target site with a controlled dwell time of 4 minutes. The amount of drug delivered by the catheter was calculated based on vein volume of the target saphenous vein.[51] Primary closure was 87% and primary assisted closure was 96% at 6-month follow-up. Three limbs (4%) were treated for asymptomatic DVT. Interestingly, in our series thrombus formed only at sites of decreased flow in duplicated femoral veins. In all three cases of DVT, the foam was forced into the femoral vein via a thigh perforator from the GSV because the balloon blocked the outflow to the common femoral vein.[52] Also of interest in this trial was the difference that drug quality played in the role of effective ablation. Pharmaceutical-grade drug was profoundly more effective than drug prepared by a compounding pharmacy.[10] In the compounded STS group, 45.7% of veins demonstrated segments of incomplete ablation (SIAs) at some time during follow-up. In the pharmaceutical-grade STS group, SIAs were observed in only in 12.5% of veins. This difference was statistically significant at $p = .02$.

The second catheter device, presented at the 2008 American Venous Forum, attempts to maximize the effectiveness of 3% *liquid* STS sclerosant by delivery under pressure, in a pulsed fashion (AngioDynamics, Inc., Queensbury, NY), to the GSV endoluminally. In a pilot study of

10 limbs followed for 1 year, we reported 80% primary occlusion.[53] Sixty percent of treated veins demonstrated SIAs at some point during the 1-year follow-up. This catheter does not occlude the SFJ, and one thrombus extension into the common femoral vein was observed postprocedure. The thrombus extension resolved spontaneously without anticoagulation. All treated GSVs were limited to a size of less than 10 mm in diameter.

Catheter-directed sclerotherapy (CDS) is attractive because it requires no power source. Lasers and radiofrequency generators cost about $25,000, in addition to the disposables required per case. CDS requires no delivery of time-consuming and often uncomfortable perivenous anesthesia to the extremity. Although we commonly see SIAs in follow-up after CDS, these areas are easily closed with needle injection of additional sclerosant to the affected area (assisted-closure). On balance, sclerotherapy still has a cosmetic connotation and is not reimbursed by many third party payers. Primary occlusion rates are lower than with thermal ablation of the GSV, but with adjunctive ultrasound-guided sclerotherapy, failing veins can be rescued. Thrombus identified in the deep system has been seen more frequently in our experience, as compared with thermal ablation.

SCLEROTHERAPY FOR SUPERFICIAL VARICES AND TELANGIECTASES

Conventional liquid sclerotherapy is useful in the management of isolated small superficial varices not associated with truncal saphenous incompetence. Foam treatment has little advantage here and ultrasound guidance is unnecessary. A frequent presentation involves patients with reticular varices and telangiectases. Reticular varices can be managed surgically, but better outcomes are usually obtained with sclerotherapy. All patients should be carefully evaluated for the presence of saphenous truncal incompetence or other possible sources of varices by duplex ultrasonography. This commonly reveals an underlying problem that may lead to an unsatisfactory outcome if it is ignored.

Most saphenous trunks and varices can be managed by foam sclerotherapy where they play a significant part in the development of reticular varices and telangiectases. Small veins are probably best managed by liquid, rather than foam, sclerotherapy. Foam sclerosants tend to be very strong and can cause even more telangiectases to develop if injected overenthusiastically. After preparation of the area with 70% alcohol, small needles (25 to 33 gauge) are used to inject the veins. Treatment intervals depend on physician preference; in general, patients are seen for follow-up every 2 weeks.

Most publications mention the injection of 0.25% to 0.5% POL as being the most appropriate. STS 0.2% may also be used with similar outcomes.[54] In Europe, chromated-glycerine is commonly used, and a randomized trial has been published comparing this to POL and POL foam.[55] A good result can only be expected when the methods used by European phlebologists are followed.[56] The essence is to treat the "feeding veins" as well as the telangiectases. The feeding veins comprise the reticular veins that drain the telangiectases plus any incompetent saphenous veins. A region of telangiectases is selected and reticular veins in this area are injected with 0.5% POL liquid, injecting 0.25 to 0.5 mL at each location. Sclerosant will often enter telangiectases, demonstrating that the valves in the reticular veins are incompetent. Then, all telangiectases in the affected area should be injected with small amounts of 0.5% POL using 0.1 to 0.2 mL at each site.

If the reticular varices are not treated, a reasonable outcome will be obtained in about half of patients but may not be sustained. The other half of patients may obtain a disappointing outcome or more telangiectases may develop. The use of compression following sclerotherapy for small veins varies widely. A recent randomized trial showed that it is of value,[57] and it is advised that patients wear Class 2 compression stockings for at least 3 days after telangiectases and reticular varices have been injected. Postsclerotherapy compression can be used, although it was shown that the degree and duration of compression made no difference in recurrence rates, symptom improvement, or cosmesis.[58]

In the United States, the aforementioned techniques are useful; however, STS is preferred for liability reasons.

SYSTEMIC COMPLICATIONS

Visual disturbance occurs in about 2% of patients and is probably dose related. This occurs following both liquid and foam sclerotherapy but is more frequent after the use of foam. It often occurs in patients who have a previous history of migraine but may occur in anyone. A scotoma develops associated with other visual phenomena such as ground-glass appearance in part of the visual field and irregular colored patterns. This normally resolves within 30 minutes in most patients. It is highly likely to return in subsequent sessions of treatment; it is suggested that affected patients lie supine for up to 30 minutes following injection of foam to attempt to prevent this complication.

Some patients may develop tightness in the chest or coughing after foam. This is probably a direct effect of the foam on the lungs and can also occur following injections of liquid sclerosant. This also resolves in about 30 minutes. Again, lying supine for 30 minutes after treatment may be useful. The incidence of visual disturbances and chest symptoms has been reported to be reduced by using CO_2 foams.[59] Severe allergic reactions may follow injection of either of the sclerosants mentioned in this text. Appropriate drugs and equipment must be available to manage these potential complications.

REFERENCES

1. Hobbs JT. Surgery or sclerotherapy for varicose veins: 10-year results of a random trial. In: Tesi M, Dormandy JA, eds. Superficial and Deep Venous Diseases of the Lower Limbs. Turin, Italy: Panminerva Medica; 1984:243-248.
2. Fegan WG. Injection with compression as a treatment for varicose veins. Proc R Soc Med 1965;58:874-876.
3. Einarsson E, Eklof B, Neglen P. Sclerotherapy or surgery as treatment for varicose veins: a prospective randomized study. Phlebology 1993;8:22-26.
4. Neglen P, Einarsson E, Eklof B. The functional long-term value of different types of treatment for saphenous vein incompetence. J Cardiovasc Surg 1993;34:295-301.
5. Guex JJ. Indications for the sclerosing agent polidocanol. J Dermatol Surg Oncol 1993;19: 959-961.
6. Hamel-Desnos C, Desnos P, Wollmann JC, et al. Evaluation of the efficacy of polidocanol in the form of foam compared with liquid form in sclerotherapy of the greater saphenous vein: initial results. Dermatol Surg 2003;29:1170-1175.
7. Goldman MP. Sodium tetradecyl sulfate for sclerotherapy treatment of veins: is compounding pharmacy solution safe? Dermatol Surg 2004;30:1454-1456.
8. Rao J, Wildemore JK, Goldman MP. Double-blind prospective comparative trial between foamed and liquid polidocanol and sodium tetradecyl sulfate in the treatment of varicose and telangiectatic leg veins. Dermatol Surg 2005;31:631-635.
9. Cabrera J, Cabrera J Jr, Garcia-Olmedo MA. Sclerosants in microfoam: a new approach in angiology. Int Angiol 2001;20:322-329.
10. Almeida JI, Raines JK. FDA-Approved sodium tetradecyl sulfate (STS) versus compounded STS for venous sclerotherapy. Dermatol Surg 2007;33:1037-1044.

11. Guex JJ. Foam sclerotherapy—an overview: use for primary venous insufficiency. Semin Vasc Surg 2005;18:25-29.
12. Fegan WG. Continuous compression technique for injecting varicose veins. Lancet 1963;2: 109.
13. Anonymous. Consensus conference on sclerotherapy of varicose veins of the lower limbs. Phlebology 1997;12:2-160.
14. Sigg K. Treatment of Varicose Veins by Injection Sclerotherapy as Practised in Basle. Treatment of Venous Disorders of the Lower Limb. Lancaster, UK: MTP Press; 1976.
15. Kanter A, Thibault P. Saphenofemoral incompetence treated by ultrasound-guided sclerotherapy. Dermatol Surg 1996;22:648-652.
16. Orbach EJ. Sclerotherapy of varicose veins: utilization of intravenous airblock. Am J Surg 1944;66:362-366.
17. Cabrera J Jr, Garcia-Olmedo MA. Treatment of varicose long saphenous veins with sclerosant in microfoam: long term outcomes. Phlebology 2000;15:19-23.
18. Frullini A, Cavezzi AM. Sclerosing foam in the treatment of varicose veins and telangiectases: history and analysis of safety and complications. Dermatol Surg 2002;28:11-15.
19. Breu FX, Guggenbichler S. European consensus meeting on foam sclerotherapy, April, 4Đ6, 2003, Tegernsee, Germany. Dermatol Surg 2004;30:709-717.
20. Yamaki T, Nozaki M, Iwasaka S. Comparative study of duplex-guided foam sclerotherapy and duplex-guided liquid sclerotherapy for the treatment of superficial venous insufficiency. Dermatol Surg 2004;30:718-722.
21. Barrett JM, Allen B, Ockelford A, Goldman MP. Microfoam ultrasound-guided sclerotherapy of varicose veins in 100 legs. Dermatol Surg 2004;30:6-12.
22. Hsu T-SM, Weiss R. Foam sclerotherapy: a new era. Arch Dermatol 2003;139:1494-1496.
23. Schneider W, Fischer H. Fixierung and bindegewebige organization artefizieller thrombin bei der varizenuerodung. Dtsch Med Wochenschr 1964;89:2410.
24. Tessari LM. Preliminary experience with a new sclerosing foam in the treatment of varicose veins. Dermatol Surg 2001;27:58-60.
25. Belcaro G. Foam-sclerotherapy, surgery, sclerotherapy, and combined treatment for varicose veins: a 10-year, prospective, randomized, controlled, trial (VEDICO* Trial). Angiology 2003; 54:307-315.
26. Wright D, Gobin JP, Bradbury AV, et al. Varisolve polidocanol microfoam compared with surgery or sclerotherapy in the management of varicose veins in the presence of trunk vein incompetence: European randomized controlled trial. Phlebology 2006;21:180-190.
27. Bountouroglou DG, Azzam M, Kakkos SK, et al. Ultrasound guided foam sclerotherapy combined with saphenofemoral ligation compared to surgical treatment of varicose veins: early results of a randomized controlled trial. Eur J Vasc Endovasc Surg 2006;31:93-100.
28. Forlee MV, Grouden M, Moore DJ, et al. Stroke after varicose vein foam injection sclerotherapy. J Vasc Surg 2006;43:162-164.
29. Bush RG, Derrick M, Manjoney D. Major neurological events following foam sclerotherapy. Phlebology 2008;23:189-192.
30. Jia X, Mowatt G, Burr JM, et al. Systematic review of foam sclerotherapy for varicose veins. Br J Surg 2007;94:925-936.
31. Barrett JM, Allen B, Ockelford A, et al. Microfoam ultrasound-guided sclerotherapy of varicose veins in 100 legs. Dermatol Surg 2004;30:6-12.
32. Cavezzi A, Frullini A, Ricci S, et al. Treatment of varicose veins by foam sclerotherapy: two clinical series. Phlebology 2002;17:13-18.
33. Breu FX, Guggenbichler S, Wollmann JC. 2nd European Consensus Meeting on Foam Sclerotherapy, 2006. Tegernsee, Germany. VASA 2008;3(suppl 1):1-29.
34. Bountouroglou DG, Azzam M, Kakkos SK, et al. Ultrasound-guided foam sclerotherapy combined with sapheno-femoral ligation compared to surgical treatment of varicose veins: early results of a randomised controlled trial. Eur J Vasc Endovasc Surg 2006;31: 93-100.
35. Ouvry P, Allaert FA, Desnos P, et al. Efficacy of polidocanol foam versus liquid in sclerotherapy of the therapy. Phlebology 2007;22:34-39.

36. Hamel-Desnos C, Ouvry P, Benigni JP, et al. Comparison of 1% and 3% polidocanol foam in ultrasound guided sclerotherapy of the great saphenous vein: a randomised, double-blind trial with 2 year-follow-up. "The 3/1 Study". Eur J Vasc Endovasc Surg 2007;34:723-729.

37. Breu FX, Guggenbichler S, Wollmann JC. Second European Consensus Meeting on Foam Sclerotherapy. Duplex ultrasound and efficacy criteria in foam sclerotherapy from the Second European Consensus Meeting on Foam Sclerotherapy 2006, Tegernsee, Germany. VASA 2008;37:90-95.

38. Winterborn RJ, Foy C, Heather BP, et al. Randomised trial of flush saphenofemoral ligation for primary great saphenous varicose veins. Eur J Vasc Endovasc Surg 2008;36:477-484.

39. Coleridge Smith P. Chronic venous disease treated by ultrasound guided foam sclerotherapy. Eur J Vasc Endovasc Surg 2006;32:577-583.

40. Creton D, Uhl JF. Foam sclerotherapy combined with surgical treatment for recurrent varicose veins: short term results. Eur J Vasc Endovasc Surg 2007;33:619-624.

41. Perrin M, Gillet JL. Management of recurrent varices at the popliteal fossa after surgical treatment. Phlebology 2008;23:64-68.

42. O'Hare JL, Parkin D, Vandenbroeck CP, et al. Mid term results of ultrasound guided foam sclerotherapy for complicated and uncomplicated varicose veins. Eur J Vasc Endovasc Surg 2008;36:109-113.

43. Hertzman PA, Owens R. Rapid healing of chronic venous ulcers following ultrasound-guided foam sclerotherapy. Phlebology 2007;22:34-39.

44. Ergan J, Pascarella L, Mekenas L. Venous disorders: treatment with sclerosant foam. J Cardiovasc Surg (Torino) 2006;47:9-18.

45. Pascarella L, Bergan JJ, Mekenas LV. Severe chronic venous insufficiency treated by foamed sclerosant. Ann Vasc Surg 2006;20:83-91.

46. Norris MJ, Carlin MC, Ratz JL. Treatment of essential telangiectasia: effects of increasing concentrations of polidocanol. J Am Acad Dermatol 1989;20:643-649.

47. Scurr JH, Coleridge-Smith P, Cutting P. Varicose veins: optimum compression following sclerotherapy. Ann R Coll Surg Engl 1985;67:109-111.

48. Guex JJ, Allaert FA, Gillet JL, et al. Immediate and midterm complications of sclerotherapy: report of a prospective multicenter registry of 12,173 sclerotherapy sessions. Dermatol Surg 2005;31:123-128.

49. Morrison N, Rogers C, Neuhardt D, et al. Large volume, ultrasound guided polidocanol foam sclerotherapy: a prospective study of toxicity and complications. Presented at UIP World Congress Chapter Meeting, San Diego, California, 27-31 August 2003.

50. van den Bos R, Arends L, Kockaert M, et al. Endovenous therapies of lower extremity varicosities: a meta-analysis. J Vasc Surg 2009;49:230-239.

51. Raines JK, Garcia de Quevedo W, Jahrmarkt S, et al. Abbreviated method of determining vein volume in balloon-controlled vein ablation. Phlebology 2007;22:40-44.

52. Almeida JI, Raines JK. Comparison of thermal and chemical saphenous endoablation. Poster: American Venous Forum 18th Annual Meeting, Miami, FL, 2006.

53. Almeida JI, Raines JK. Pulse spray sclerotherapy: a pilot study. Poster presented at the American Venous Forum 20th Annual Meeting, Charleston, SC, 2008.

54. Goldman MP. Treatment of varicose and telangiectatic leg veins: double-blind prospective comparative trial between aethoxyskerol and sotradecol. Dermatol Surg 2002;28:52-55.

55. Kern P, Ramelet AA, Wutschert R, et al. Single-blind, randomized study comparing chromated glycerin, polidocanol solution, and polidocanol foam for treatment of telangiectatic leg veins. Dermatol Surg 2004;30:367-372.

56. Guex JJ. Microsclerotherapy. Semin Dermatol 1993;12:129-134.

57. Kern P, Ramelet AA, Wutschert R, et al. Compression after sclerotherapy for telangiectasias and reticular leg veins: a randomized controlled study. J Vasc Surg 2007;45:1212-1216.

58. Fraser IA, Perry EP, Hatton M, et al. Prolonged bandaging is not required following sclerotherapy of varicose veins. Br J Surg 1985;72:488-490.

59. Morrison N, Neuhardt DL, Rogers CR, et al. Comparisons of side effects using air and carbon dioxide foam for endovenous chemical ablation. J Vasc Surg 2008;47:830-836.

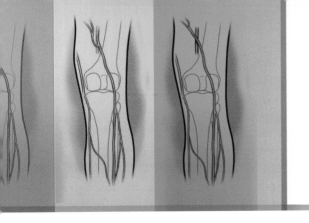

CHAPTER 8

Treatment of Perforating Veins

Jose I. Almeida

HISTORICAL BACKGROUND

Although the role of perforator veins (PVs) in the development of signs and symptoms remains unclear, the number of incompetent PVs and the size of both competent and incompetent PVs have been shown to increase with worsening chronic venous disease (CVD).[1-4] Furthermore, it was recently reported that the duration of outward flow in these veins was longer in patients with ulcers compared with those in lower classes of CVD.[2]

ETIOLOGY AND NATURAL HISTORY OF DISEASE

Reflux in PVs is defined as outward flow from the deep to the superficial veins. It has been suggested that high flow from the deep veins during muscular contraction eventually renders the PVs incompetent.[5] The etiology of venous reflux in superficial veins and PVs is unknown. The most predominant theory is that the weakening of the venous wall eventually leads to valve failure.[6] During early stages of the disease, reflux is most prevalent in the superficial veins.[7-9] Others have also suggested that reflux in the PVs is caused by volume overload at the reentry points of incompetent superficial veins.[10,11] However, direct evidence for both of these theories is lacking because most investigations have been cross-sectional population studies without sufficient longitudinal study regarding disease progression.

Labropoulos et al.[11] identified two other patterns by which previously competent PVs become incompetent—these were ascending development and new sites becoming incompetent. The ascending development of reflux into PVs from previously competent segments of superficial veins was more prevalent. A smaller number of incompetent PVs were detected in new locations that previously did not have reflux in any system PV reflux was always associated with reflux in an adjacent superficial vein and underscores the important role of superficial vein reflux in the development of PV incompetence. Because most limbs in the early stages of CVD exhibit reflux in the superficial veins only, it can be assumed that one of the mechanisms for development of PV insufficiency involves the presence of reflux in an adjacent superficial vein segment that acts as a capacitor for the refluxing PV. As local hemodynamic conditions change and as intravenous pressure increases, the diameter of the PV increases, and the PV valve becomes incompetent. This may be in combination with or separate from primary venous wall disease.

Deep vein reflux is not required for development of PV incompetence in primary venous disease. Rather, deep vein reflux can develop as a result of increased flow from the incompetent superficial veins through the PV, the diameter of which has increased. Labropoulos et al.[11] showed that only five new incompetent PVs were seen in association with juxtaposed reflux in the deep vein. At all five sites, deep vein reflux was not present at the time of the initial duplex study, when the adjacent PV was still competent; the deep venous incompetence developed simultaneously with PV incompetence. Superficial vein reflux was present at all sites.

Finally, this study also suggested that the development of reflux in previously normal PVs was seen in association with worsening of the clinical stage of CVD in 40% of limbs. Although the worsening of the clinical stage cannot be attributed to extension of reflux in the PVs alone, one can assume that the natural history of long-standing reflux in the superficial veins is that of progressive deterioration, with extension of reflux to other previously competent segments of the superficial veins and their associated PVs.[12]

PATIENT SELECTION

In general, PVs should be reserved for specific situations:

1. *When they are found in continuity with the areas of axial (or neovascular) reflux in recurrent varicose vein cases*

2. *When found beneath an ankle ulcer*

3. *When there are large incompetent midthigh PVs that serve as escape points and represent the highest point of reflux*

ENDOVASCULAR INSTRUMENTATION

- For chemical ablation, a 25- or 27-gauge needle is used under ultrasound guidance.
- RF catheters are dedicated devices and enter without sheath support.
- A 16-gauge angiocath (for a 600-μm laser fiber) or a 21-gauge micropuncture needle (for a 400-μm laser fiber) can be used for laser ablation.
- If the anatomy of the PV allows, a wire may be placed into the deep system for better control during access.

OPERATIVE STEPS

Percutaneous ablation of perforators (PAPs) was coined by Elias and Peden.[12] The basic method involves (1) ultrasound-guided intraluminal access; (2) introduction of some ablative element (chemical or thermal); (3) confirmation of initial treatment success; and (4) follow-up of treatment success. Thus far, the techniques used have been either chemical (sodium tetradecyl sulfate [STS], aethoxysclerol, or sodium morrhuate)[13,14] or thermal (radiofrequency [RF] or laser).[15-17]

After access is obtained, the thermal ablation device should be placed at or just below the fascia to minimize deep vessel and nerve injury. This is analogous to subfascial endoscopic perforator surgery (SEPS) where clips are placed just below the fascia level.

The patient is placed in a reverse Trendelenburg position to fully dilate the vein for access. After access, the various modalities differ in energy application. Therefore each technique is discussed separately so that key technical points can be elucidated.

PAPs Technique: Chemical Ablation

Ultrasound-guided sclerotherapy (UGS) (Fig. 8-1) is an effective and durable method of eliminating incompetent PVs and results in significant reduction of symptoms and signs as determined

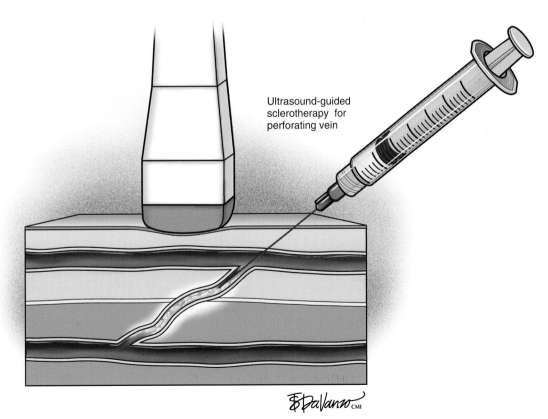

Ultrasound-guided
sclerotherapy for
perforating vein

■ Fig 8–1

by venous clinical scores. As an alternative to open interruption or SEPS, UGS may lead to fewer skin and wound-healing complications. Little has been published regarding the outcomes following UGS for PVs.

In a series by Masuda et al.,[13] patients primarily had isolated perforator disease (83%) without concomitant axial reflux from the thigh to the calf in the saphenous or deep systems. Clinical improvement following UGS was suggested by improvement of the Venous Clinical Severity Score (VCSS) and Venous Disease Severity (VDS) and lack of perforator recurrence with a mean follow-up of 20 months. In this study, successful obliteration of PVs with no recurrent symptoms was 75%. Perforator recurrence occurs particularly in those with ulcerations, and therefore surveillance duplex scanning after UGS and repeat injections may be needed. This study suggests that patients with perforator disease without axial reflux appear to benefit from injection sclerotherapy.

In 1992, Thibault and Lewis[17] reported their early experience with injection of incompetent PVs by using ultrasound guidance and showed that PVs remained successfully obliterated in 84% at 6 months after treatment. In 2000 at the Pacific Vascular Symposium in Hawaii, Jerome Guex[18] from France reported his experience with direct perforator treatment with ultrasound guidance. The sclerosing agent used was sodium tetradecyl sulphate (Sotradecol) (3%) (Bioniche Life Sciences Inc., Belleville, Ontario, Canada) or polidocanol (3%) for veins larger than 4 mm, and a more dilute solution was used for veins smaller than 4 mm. He estimated that 90% of PVs could be eliminated after one to three sessions of injections.

This method also involves ultrasound-guided access and confirmation with aspiration of blood. Many types of sclerosants have been used: sodium morrhuate, STS, and aethoxysclerol. Some advocates use the sclerosant in a liquid state. More recently, foam sclerotherapy has been advocated as being more efficacious. Most studies use STS 3% in the liquid form, injecting 0.5 to 1 ml of sclerosant or sodium morrhuate 5% in a similar manner, with care being taken not to inject the accompanying artery.[14,19] After infusion of the sclerosant, compression is applied with wraps or stockings and direct pressure over the treated PV.

PAPs Technique Using the Radiofrequency System

Ultrasound-guided access can be made by needle, angiocath, or specialized probe. Confirmation of access with ultrasound visualization of the device intraluminally and aspiration of blood are the sine qua non of successful entry. The radiofrequency stylet (RFS) catheter (VNUS Medical, Inc.) also has the ability to measure impedance in ohms.

There are times when the device appears to be intraluminal by duplex imaging, but impedance readings indicate an extraluminal location. An impedance value between 150 and 350 ohms is indicative of intraluminal placement. If the RF device is in soft tissue, then higher values are registered. This feature complements ultrasound visualization. After attaining good placement and good location level relative to the fascia and the deep system, a small amount of tumescent anesthesia is infiltrated around the PV with ultrasound guidance. The patient is placed in the Trendelenburg position. Energy is then applied using a target temperature of 85°C, and pressure is applied with the overlying ultrasound transducer. These maneuvers, tumescence, pressure, and Trendelenburg, are done to exsanguinate the vein and improve device-to-vein wall contact.

The RF energy is applied to all four quadrants of the vein wall for 1 minute each. The catheter is then withdrawn 1 to 2 mm, and a second level of vein is treated. Theoretically, the longer the segment of the vein is treated, the better. After energy delivery, pressure is applied to compress the walls of the treated PV for 1 minute. Immediately posttreatment, a duplex scan should show no flow in the treated section of the PV with normal flow in the deep-paired posterior tibial veins and arteries. If too much anesthetic is infiltrated into the tissues, the PV becomes very difficult to visualize.

PAPs Technique Using the Laser System

As with RF, intraluminal access into the target PV is the key step. There are two methods of laser access: a 21-gauge micropuncture needle or a 16-gauge angiocath. A direct puncture is made using ultrasound guidance with the patient in the reverse Trendelenburg position. Intraluminal placement is confirmed by ultrasonography and aspiration of blood. If a micropuncture needle is used (21 gauge), a 400-μm fiber can be passed directly through the needle into the PV with ultrasound visualization and positioned at or just below the fascial level; this is similar to RF. If a 600-μm fiber is used, then a 16-gauge angiocath or the sheath from the micropuncture access kit is used (Figs. 8-2 to 8-5). A 600-μm fiber diameter is too large to traverse the 21-gauge micropuncture needle.

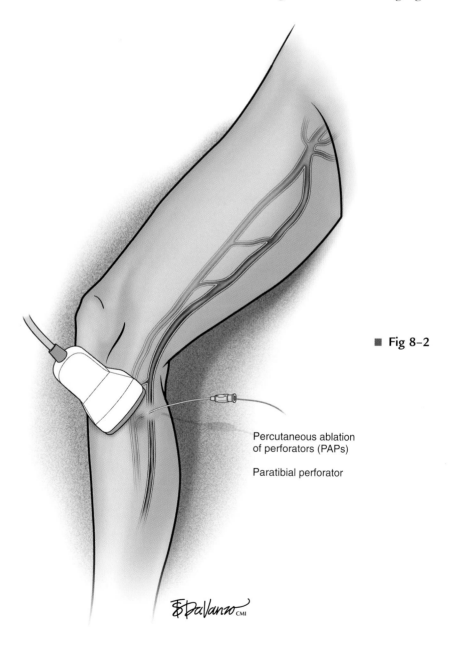

■ Fig 8–2

Percutaneous ablation
of perforators (PAPs)

Paratibial perforator

A

Continued

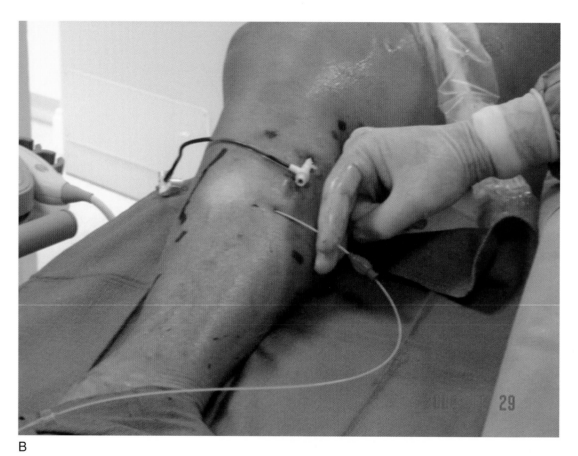

B

■ **Fig 8–2, cont'd B,** Percutaneous ablation of perforators: access to Boyd perforator vein (live).

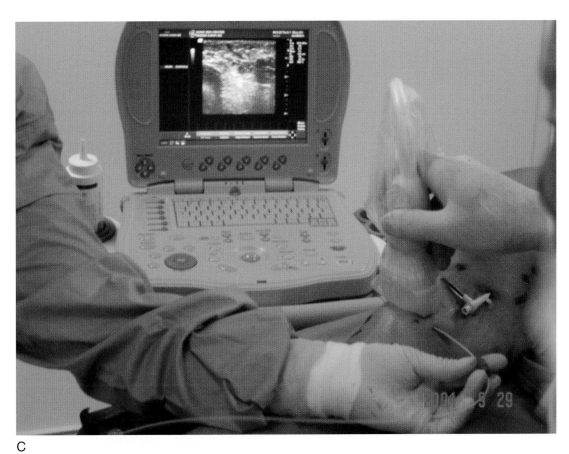

C

■ **Fig 8–2, cont'd C,** Percutaneous ablation of perforators: ultrasound-guided positioning of laser fiber tip at deep muscular fascia.

Tumescent anesthesia is infiltrated around the catheter, and the patient is placed in the Trendelenburg position. Energy is then applied to the segment, with pressure being applied with the ultrasound transducer to ensure fiber–to–vein wall contact. It is advisable to treat as long a segment as possible. Therefore, areas approximately 1 to 2 mm apart should be treated as the fiber is withdrawn with a total of two or three segments.

Pulsed or continuous delivery methods of energy can be used. If pulsed, the laser is set for 15 W with a 4-second pulse interval during laser pullback. Each segment of vein is treated twice, thus administering 120 J to each segment; three segments are usually treated. At Miami Vein Center we use 10 W in the continuous mode and deliver 60 to 80 J/cm (see Figs. 8-2 to 8-5). Often we approach an ankle PV in a retrograde fashion (Fig. 8-3).

Text continued on p. 215

■ **Fig 8–3**

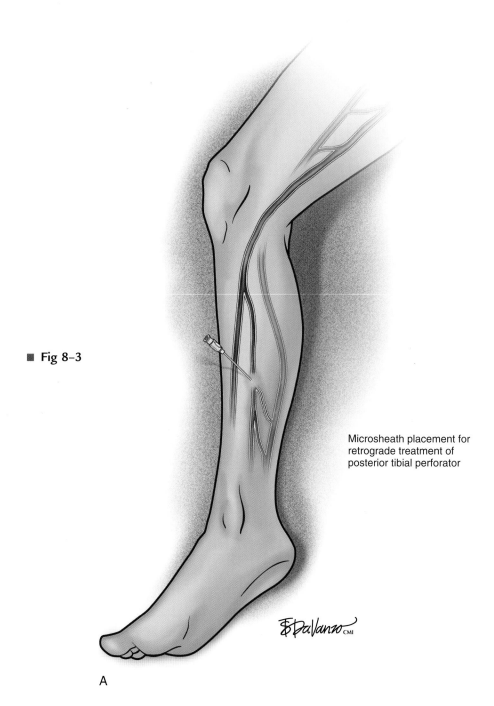

Microsheath placement for retrograde treatment of posterior tibial perforator

A

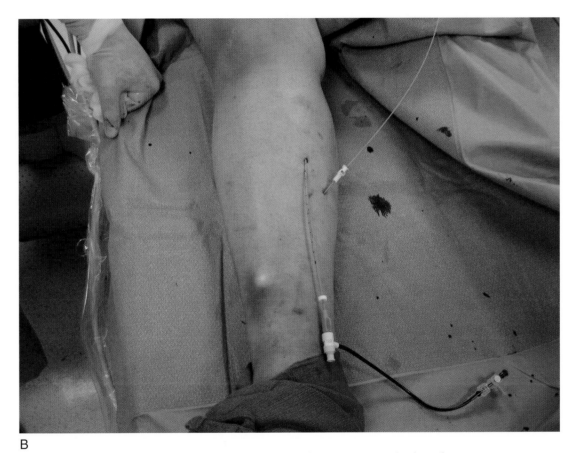

B

■ **Fig 8–3, cont'd B,** Retrograde approach to posterior tibial perforating vein (live).

■ Fig 8–4

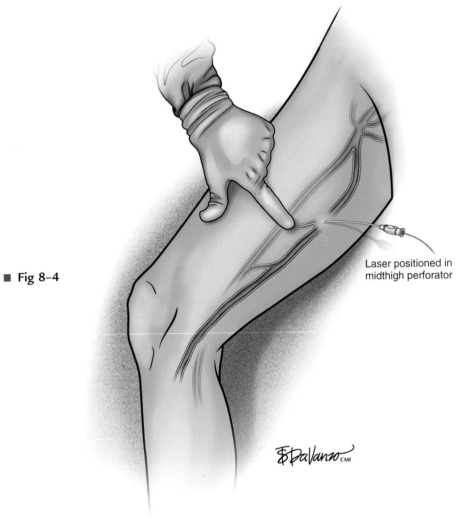

Laser positioned in
midthigh perforator

A

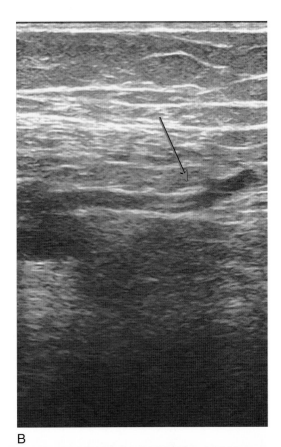

B

C

■ **Fig 8–4, cont'd B,** Midthigh perforator vein ultrasound image. **C,**
Percutaneous ablation of perforators: midthigh perforator vein (access).

Continued

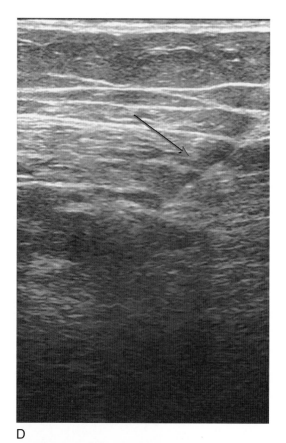

D

■ **Fig 8–4, cont'd D,** Percutaneous ablation of perforators: percutaneous access with 21-gauge needle (ultrasound view). **E,** Percutaneous ablation of perforators: midthigh perforator vein (microsheath placement–ultrasound view).

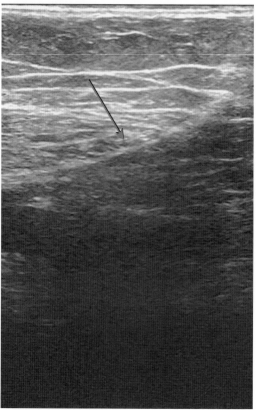

E

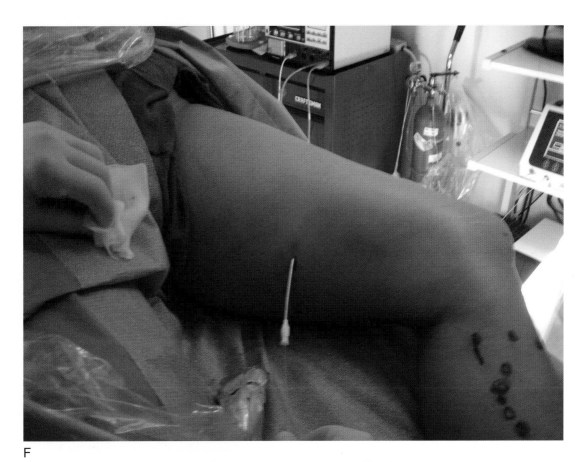

F

■ **Fig 8–4, cont'd F,** Laser pullback.

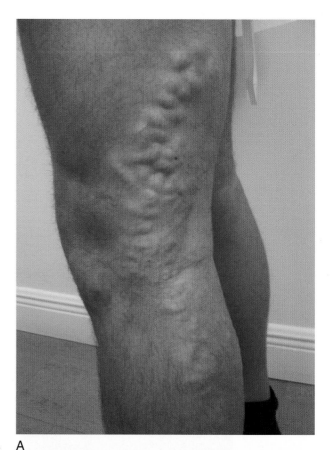

A

■ **Fig 8-5** **A,** Lateral thigh varicose veins originating from lateral thigh perforator vein. **B,** Ultrasound view, lateral thigh perforator vein.

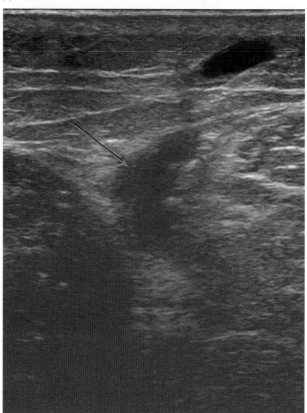

B

Proebstle and Herdemann[16] also attempt to treat three locations within the PV (just below the fascia, at the fascia level, and just above). Each treated segment receives between 60 and 100 J. After energy delivery, an eccentric pressure dressing is applied for 1 minute over the PV, as is done with RF. During wrapping, a pressure bandage is applied with direct pressure over each PV with a cotton ball or something similar. They reported on a total of 67 PVs treated with 1320 nm at 10 W (median of 250 J) or with 940 nm at 30 W (median of 290 J). With the exception of one vein, all others were occluded on postoperative day 1. Side effects were moderate. They concluded that ultrasound-guided endovenous laser ablation of incompetent PVs is safe and feasible.[16]

Rarely, a small incision is made with the patient under local anesthesia to access larger-diameter PVs to ligate them (Fig. 8-6). Confirmation of occlusion is documented with duplex imaging, and patency of the deep vessels is also confirmed. The results have been quite good.

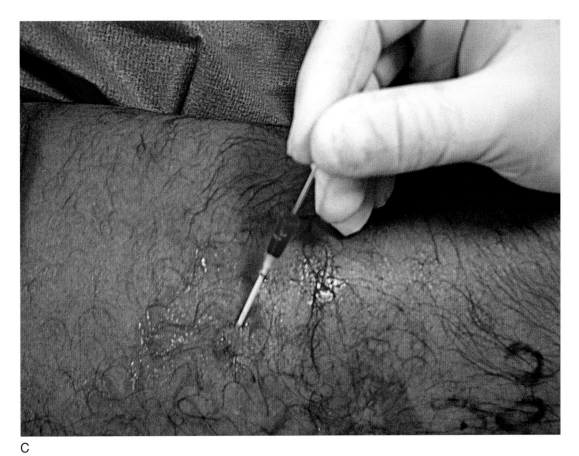

C

■ **Fig 8–5, cont'd   C,** Percutaneous access to lateral thigh perforator vein.

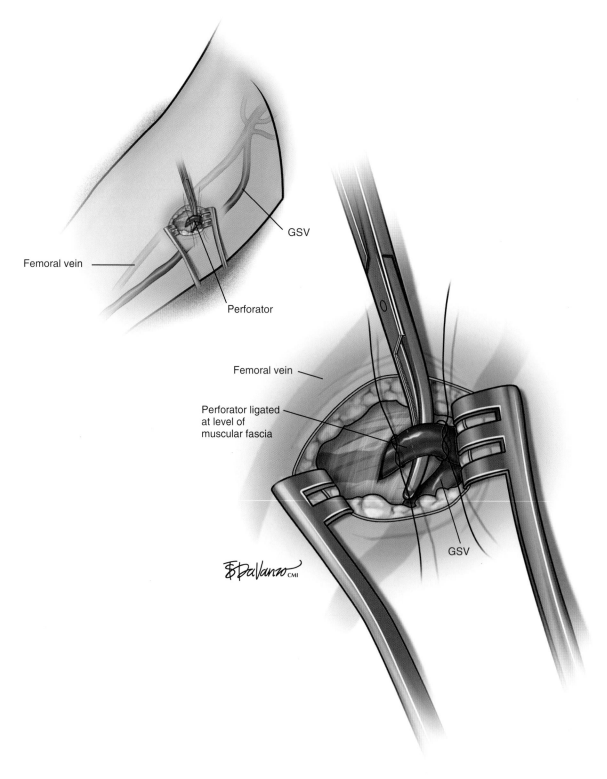

Femoral vein

GSV

Perforator

Femoral vein

Perforator ligated
at level of
muscular fascia

GSV

A

■ Fig 8–6

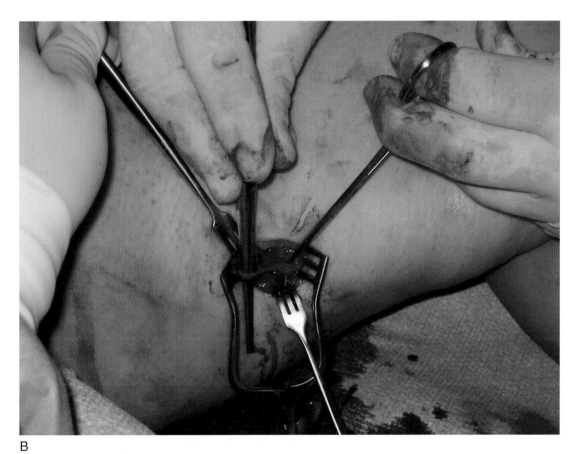

B

■ **Fig 8-6, cont'd B,** Open ligation of midthigh perforator vein (live).

PEARLS AND PITFALLS

The question still exists as to which PVs need treatment. Incompetent PVs are usually associated with superficial venous reflux, and therefore incompetent PVs may not require specific surgical interventions after saphenous truncal ablation. Ninety percent of the patients with C5-C6 disease have incompetent PVs, while less than half of the patients with C2 disease have incompetent PVs. Therefore, incompetent PVs are clearly associated with venous ulcers, and the question is whether these incompetent PVs have any hemodynamic significance and whether they really contribute to the inflammatory changes in these limbs.[20]

COMPLICATIONS

Complications are rare. Wound complications, such as previously seen with the Linton procedure, are virtually nonexistent. Thromboembolic and nervous complications are rare with percutaneous techniques.

COMPARATIVE EFFECTIVENESS OF EXISTING TREATMENTS

Referable to the controversial topic of the role of PV incompetence causing nonhealing venous stasis ulcers, the ESCHAR trial[20] establishes a Grade 1A recommendation that ligation and stripping of the GSV are associated with the prevention of ulcer recurrence. More traditional methods such as the Linton procedure and its modifications of open perforator ligation have a relatively high incidence of wound complication ranging from 20% to 40%.[21-23] At present, there is no compelling Level 1 evidence to provide a Grade A recommendation that the treatment of incompetent PVs alone affects venous ulcer healing or recurrence.

Unfortunately, the treatment of incompetent PVs is blurred by concomitant treatment of GSV incompetence in the two RCTs that putatively explored the role of incompetent PV treatment.[24,25] Moreover, surrogate hemodynamic outcomes, which assess the treatment of incompetent PVs alone as well as the effect of GSV treatment alone on perforator competence, also argue against the importance of treating incompetent PVs. This observation emphasizes the need for a properly designed trial in CEAP C5/C6 patients. Based on the RCTs cited and the results of studies with surrogate endpoints of restoring perforator competence, the current role of incompetent PV treatment can be considered a Grade 2B recommendation.

The effectiveness of treating PVs with isolated reflux was suggested by the randomized trial reported in 1974 by Hobbs[26] comparing compression sclerotherapy with surgery that included saphenous vein stripping and subfascial ligation of PVs. He found that in the face of great or small saphenous vein reflux, surgery proved to have better 6-year results than sclerotherapy alone. On the other hand, when incompetent PVs were present without concomitant saphenous vein disease, sclerotherapy of calf PVs proved to be better than surgery.

REFERENCES

1. Pascarella L, Schmid Schonbein GW. Causes of telangiectasias, reticular veins and varicose veins. Semin Vasc Surg 2005;18:2-4.

2. Labropoulos N, Mansour MA, Kang SS, et al. New insights into perforator vein incompetence. Eur J Vasc Endovasc Surg 1999;18:228-234.

3. Lees TA, Lambert D. Patterns of venous reflux in limbs with skin changes associated with chronic venous insufficiency. Br J Surg 1993;80:725-728.

4. Pierik EG, Wittens CH, van Urk H. Subfascial endoscopic ligation in the treatment of incompetent perforating veins. Eur J Vasc Endovasc Surg 1995;9:38-41.

5. Cockett FB, Elgan-Jones DE. The ankle blow-out syndrome. Lancet 1953;1:17-23.

6. Kistner RL, Eklof B, Masuda EM. Diagnosis of chronic venous disease of the lower extremities: the "CEAP" classification. Mayo Clin Proc 1996;71:338-345.

7. Labropoulos N. CEAP in clinical practice. Vasc Surg 1997;31:224-225.

8. Labropoulos N, Delis K, Nicolaides AN, et al. The role of the distribution and anatomic extent of reflux in the development of signs and symptoms in chronic venous insufficiency. J Vasc Surg 1996;23:504-510.

9. Delis K. Leg perforator vein incompetence: functional anatomy. Radiology 2005;235:327-334.

10. Zamboni P. Pathophysiology of perforators in primary chronic venous insufficiency. World J Surg 2005;29(Suppl 1):S115-S118.

11. Labropoulos N, Tassiopoulos AK, Bhatti AF, et al. Development of reflux in the perforator veins in limbs with primary venous disease. J Vasc Surg 2006;43:558-562.

12. Elias S, Peden E. Ultrasound-guided percutaneous ablation for the treatment of perforating vein incompetence. Vascular 2007;15:281-289.

13. Masuda EM, Kessler DM, Lurie F, et al. The effect of ultrasound-guided sclerotherapy of incompetent perforator veins on venous clinical severity and disability scores. J Vasc Surg 2006;43:551-557.

14. Guex JJ. Ultrasound guided sclerotherapy (UGS) for perforating veins (PV). Hawaii Med J 2000;59:261-262.

15. Peden E, Lumsden A. Radiofrequency ablation of incompetent perforator veins. Perspect Vasc Surg Endovasc Ther 2007;19:73-77.

16. Proebstle TM, Herdemann S. Early results and feasibility of incompetent perforator vein ablation by endovenous laser treatment. Dermatol Surg 2007;33:162-168.

17. Thibault PK, Lewis WA. Recurrent varicose veins. Part 2: injection of incompetent perforating veins using ultrasound guidance. J Dermatol Surg Oncol 1992;18:895-900.

18. Guex JJ. Ultrasound guided sclerotherapy (USGS) for perforating veins (PV). J Vasc Surg 2000;31:1307-1312.

19. Stuart WP, Lee AJ, Allan PL, et al. Most incompetent calf perforating veins are found in association with superficial venous reflux. J Vasc Surg 2001;34:774-778.

20. Barwell JR, Davies CE, Deacon J, et al. Comparison of surgery and compression with compression alone in chronic venous ulceration (ESCHAR study): randomized controlled trial. Lancet 2004;363:1854-1859.

21. Sato DT, Goff CD, Gregory RT, et al. Subfascial perforator vein ablation: comparison of open versus endoscopic techniques. J Endovasc Surg 1999;6:147-154.

22. Pierik EG, Van Urk H, Hop WC, et al. Endoscopic versus open subfascial division of incompetent perforating veins in the treatment of leg ulceration: a randomized trial. J Vasc Surg 1997;26:1049-1054.

23. Stacey MC, Burnand KG, Layer GT, et al. Calf pump function in patients with healed venous ulcers is not improved by surgery to the communicating veins or by elastic stockings. Br J Surg 1988;75:436-439.

24. van Gent WB, Hop WC, van Pragg MC, et al. Conservative versus surgical treatment of venous leg ulcers: a prospective, randomized, multicenter trial. J Vasc Surg 2006;44:563-571.

25. O'Donnell TF. The present status of surgery of the superficial venous system in the management of venous ulcer and the evidence for the role of perforator interruption. J Vasc Surg 2008;48:1044-1052.

26. Hobbs JT. Surgery and sclerotherapy in the treatment of varicose veins, a random trial. Arch Surg 1974;109:793-796.

CHAPTER 9

Ambulatory Phlebectomy

Jose I. Almeida

HISTORICAL BACKGROUND

Ambulatory phlebectomy (AP) is a minor surgical procedure designed to remove varicose vein clusters located close to the skin surface. Originally performed in ancient Rome, the technique was published by Robert Muller in 1966.[1] In many office-based venous surgery practices in the United States, AP is performed with the use of local tumescent anesthesia. The six basic features of the technique are as follows:

1. *Absence of venous ligatures*
2. *Exclusive use of local infiltration anesthesia*
3. *Immediate ambulation after surgery*
4. *Incisions of 2 mm*
5. *Absence of skin sutures*
6. *Postoperative compression bandage kept in place for 2 days, then replaced with daytime compression stockings for 3 weeks*

Complete surgical removal of varicose veins may be achieved in a single session or in separate sessions. Endovenous ablation and AP are suitable for the office and, in the author's practice, are routinely performed together. All procedures are guided with duplex ultrasound to get a "roadmap underneath the skin." The advantage of this combination technique is that patients can expect all varicose veins to disappear after a 1-hour procedure.

ETIOLOGY AND NATURAL HISTORY OF DISEASE

Bulging varicose veins on the surface of the skin can originate from different sources. Identification of these sources is important because the source influences the treatment plan. Varicosities on the medial aspect of the thigh and calf are usually the result of great saphenous vein (GSV) incompetence. To minimize the chance for recurrence, the incompetent GSV must be eliminated from the circulation. This concept has been substantiated in several prospective randomized clinical trials involving patients who were treated with or without saphenectomy by conventional vein stripping.[2-5] The recurrence rates for limbs without saphenectomy were much higher than those for limbs with saphenectomy. Of course, now thermal ablation techniques with either radiofrequency or laser have proved to be the methods of choice for eliminating the GSV from the circulation.[6,7]

Varicosities on the anterior thigh usually result from anterior accessory saphenous vein incompetence. These veins usually course over the knee and into the lower leg. Small saphenous vein (SSV) reflux produces varicosities on the posterior calf. When also present on the posterior thigh, the surgeon must consider a cranial extension of the SSV, which can be identified with duplex ultrasound imaging. Cranial extensions may enter the GSV (Giacomini vein) or enter the femoral vein directly.

In cases where no "feeding source" is found, phlebectomy of the varicosities may be all that is required. Labropoulos et al.[8] have shown that varicose veins may result from a primary vein wall defect and that reflux may be confined to superficial tributaries throughout the lower limb. Without great and small saphenous trunk incompetence, perforator and deep vein incompetence, or proximal obstruction, their data suggest that reflux can develop in any vein without an apparent feeding source. This is often the case when bulging reticular veins are seen along the course of the lateral leg. This lateral subdermic complex and its vein of Albanese are often dilated and bulging in elderly patients. The underlying source of venous hypertension is usually perigeniculate perforating veins, not easily identifiable with duplex imaging. AP using an 18-gauge needle stab incision and a small crochet hook for exteriorization of the vein is an excellent procedure for this clinical problem.

PATIENT SELECTION

AP is indicated for the removal of varicosed venous tributaries, when visible and palpable on the surface of the skin. AP is simple to perform and well tolerated and can be used in conjunction with other treatment modalities. As stated earlier, it is critical to recognize that bulging veins are usually associated with an underlying source of venous hypertension, and treatment of the source is as important as the vein removal. Prior to AP, the treating physician must perform a thorough evaluation with duplex ultrasound imaging to determine whether a source is present for venous hypertension. The source of venous hypertension should be eliminated prior to, or in conjunction with, AP.

Prior to placing the patient in the supine position on the operating table, the veins of interest must be marked in the standing position with an indelible marker. Marking is performed in the standing position because hydrostatic pressure is elevated and the pressurized veins become visible and palpable. Bulging veins literally disappear when patients lie supine because the venous pressure drops to near 0 mm Hg.

ENDOVASCULAR INSTRUMENTATION

AP is not truly endovascular in the purist sense; rather, it is a common and perfect adjunct to an endovascular procedure. The following are tools needed to perform AP:

1. ***Tumescent anesthesia***
2. ***Knife***
3. ***Hook***
4. ***Hemostat***

IMAGING

We prefer mapping these veins using visual inspection and palpation; other investigators might prefer transillumination mapping using specialized vein lights.[9] Ultrasound-guided vein hooking is useful for deeper veins.

HEMOSTASIS AND ANTICOAGULATION

Avulsion of venous segments treated by AP is relatively hemostatic when tumescent anesthesia is used. Hemostasis is augmented by applying gentle pressure over the incision site. The epinephrine in the anesthetic preparation enhances the hemostasis process through vasoconstriction. When extracting larger veins with the stab-avulsion technique, significant force may be required and some minor bleeding may be encountered. Placing the patient in the Trendelenburg position may also help control bleeding if there is more than usual.

Klein[10] has shown through clinical studies that a dose of 35 mg/kg of dilute lidocaine solution is well tolerated and safe. Infiltrating solutions should contain epinephrine in appropriate concentrations to induce vasoconstriction and more gradual absorption of lidocaine into the bloodstream.

Infections are rare after liposuction and venous procedures with tumescent anesthesia and are usually confined to the incision site.[11] The reason for the low rate of infection is not clear, although there are reports of lidocaine concentration–dependent bacteriostatic and bactericidal activity. Pathogens commonly found on the skin may be sensitive to this activity.[12]

Compression bandage: Careful application of the postoperative dressing cannot be overstated because improper dressing placement can lead to bleeding and hematoma, blistering, nerve injury, and ischemia. The limb is wrapped circumferentially from foot to groin with a bulky compression dressing that is removed after 48 hours. The dressing should be applied with graduated pressure; the amount of pressure should decrease as one proceeds from foot to groin. It is critical to place extra padding over the lateral fibular head to avoid pressure-induced injury to the deep that is superficial peroneal nerves.

Deep peroneal nerve injury is quite serious because it is a motor nerve. A patient who develops a foot drop after venous surgery will have a decreased quality of life—a common source of litigation.

All patients are encouraged to ambulate immediately after the procedure to minimize thromboembolic complications.

OPERATIVE STEPS

Tumescent anesthesia (Fig. 9-1): Tumescent anesthesia allows large areas of the body to be anesthetized with minimal effect on intravascular fluid status, avoidance of general anesthesia, and short postoperative recovery. Tumescent anesthesia provides a safe, easy-to-administer technique for use with AP. The technique of tumescent anesthesia involves infiltration of the subdermal compartment with generous volumes of a 0.1% solution of lidocaine with epinephrine. The anesthetic preparation is administered subdermally under pressure. The doctor pushes the fluid until a characteristic peau-d'orange effect is visualized on the skin. The tumescent fluid hydrodissects the subcutaneous fat from the venous tissue as it enters, thus facilitating vein extraction afterward.

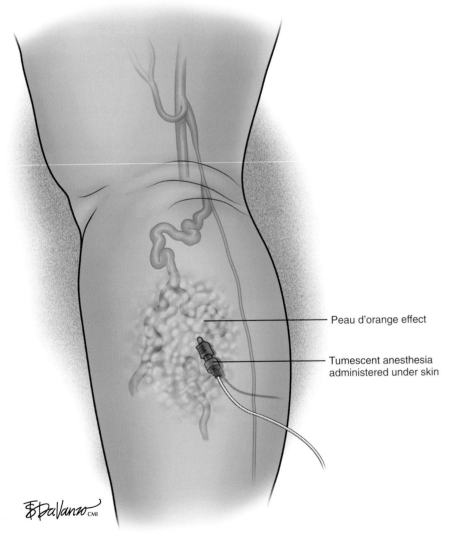

Peau d'orange effect

Tumescent anesthesia administered under skin

■ **Fig 9–1**

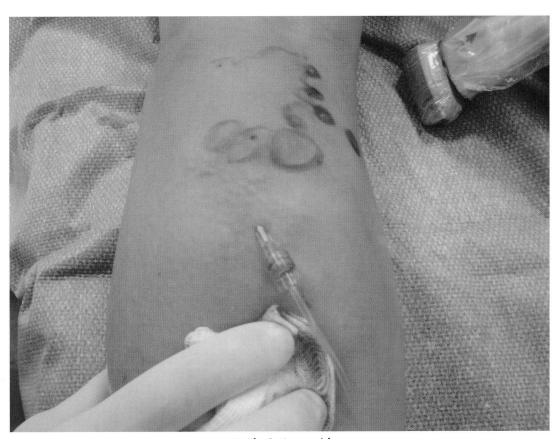

■ Fig 9–1, cont'd

Incisions (Figs. 9-2 and 9-3): The most popular instruments for creating incisions are No. 11 scalpel blades, 18-gauge needles, and 15-degree ophthalmologic Beaver blades. Incision length should correspond to vein size but is usually in the range of 1 to 3 mm. The author removes small varicose veins through an 18-gauge needle hole, while larger veins require slightly larger incisions made with a No. 11 scalpel blade.

Widening of incisions with a hemostat is tempting but should be avoided because this traumatizes wound margins and may lead to increased pigmentation in the postoperative scar. There have been anecdotal reports of "tattooing" the skin when the incision is placed through the indelible ink mark made preoperatively, which is why many operators circle the veins.

The incisions are oriented vertically because this allows wound edges to close solely with the force of a circumferentially placed compression dressing. That is, the dressing approximates the wound edges without the need for sutures or adhesive tapes. Horizontal incisions are preferred around the knees and ankles.

Hooking and extraction (Fig. 9-4): Hooking the target vein through the small incision is the next step. There are multiple instruments available—some are medical and others are manufactured for crochet. The latest available device is disposable and mounts the blade and hook on the same instrument.

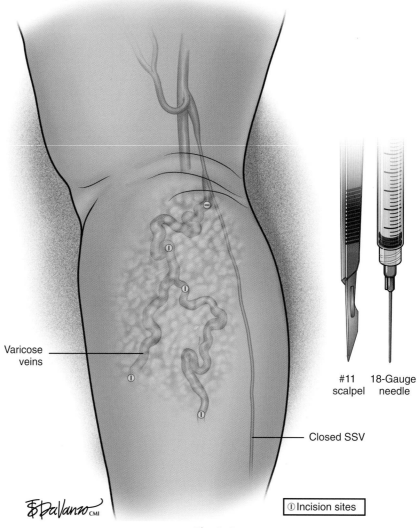

Varicose veins

\#11 scalpel   18-Gauge needle

Closed SSV

① Incision sites

■ **Fig 9–2**

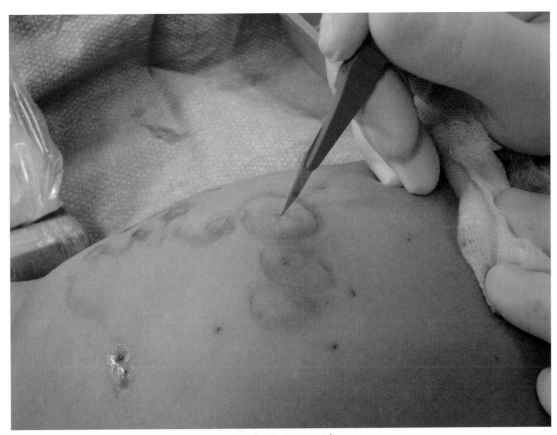

■ **Fig 9-2, cont'd**

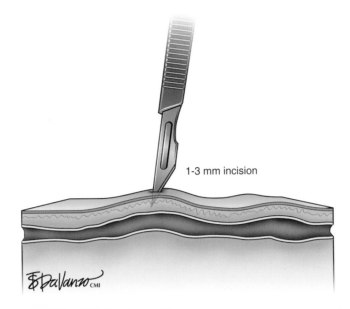

1-3 mm incision

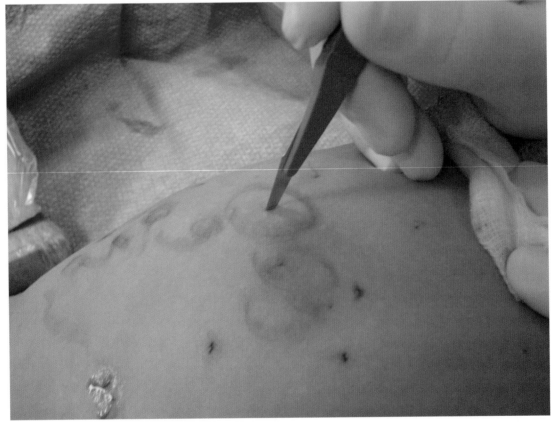

■ **Fig 9–3**

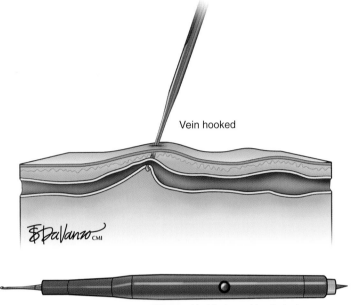

Vein hooked

Disposable blade and hook device

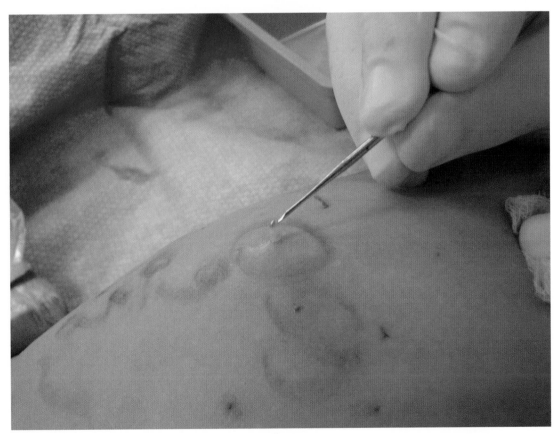

■ Fig 9–4

Using a hook of choice, the vein is exteriorized from the wound. Hooks need not be introduced into the wound deeper than 2 to 3 mm, and they should be inserted gently and deliberately to avoid unnecessary trauma to the wound margins. Gentle probing and "searching" for the target vein with the hook are routinely necessary and should be done with great care. Once a segment of vein is exteriorized from the wound, it is grasped with fine hemostatic clamps (Fig. 9-5). With the use of gentle traction in a circular motion, the vein is teased out of the wound (Fig. 9-6).

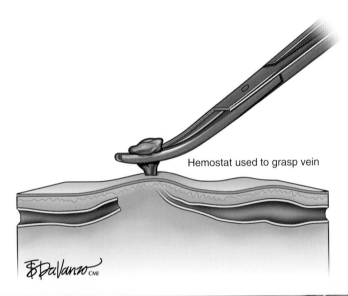

Hemostat used to grasp vein

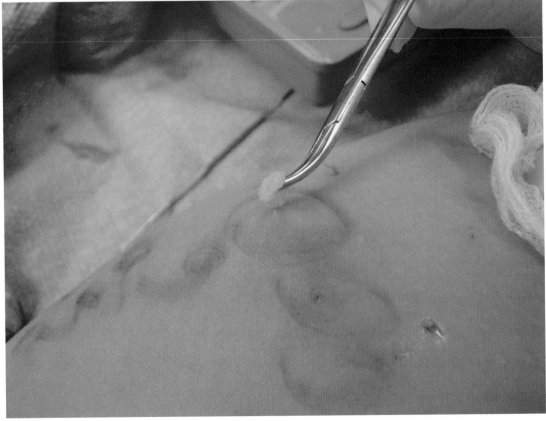

■ **Fig 9–5**

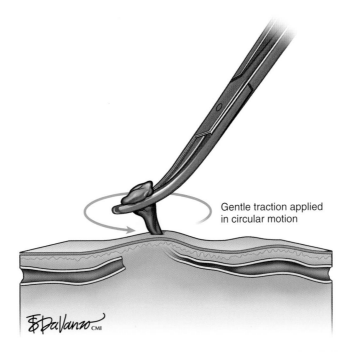

Gentle traction applied
in circular motion

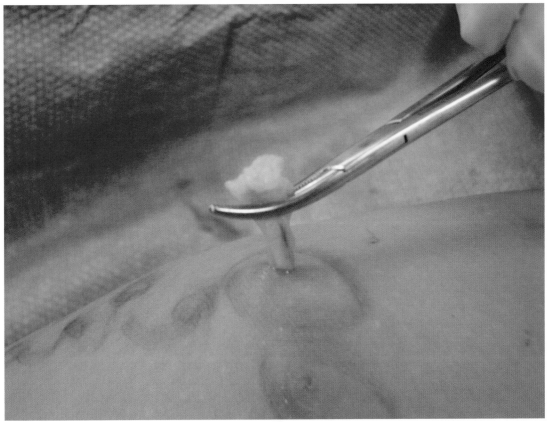

■ Fig 9–6

With experience, one learns to distinguish between the vein wall, which is elastic, and the connective perivenous tissue, which is not elastic. Dissection of the vein from its perivenous investments greatly facilitates its extraction. Perivenous tissue issuing from the wound is excised at the skin level. This tissue should never be forcefully pulled out of the wound.

When traction is applied to the vein, the skin juxtaposed to the incision site will momentarily depress downward. Attention to this detail gives the operator an idea of where to place the next incision. The depression represents the point at which the vein will avulse. The next incision is made near the area of depressed skin, and the process is repeated sequentially until all of the venous bulges have been addressed. Although all bulges should be marked preoperatively, not all of the marks need to be incised if the operator takes care in identifying the skin depressions described earlier. It is very rewarding when a large segment is removed from a single site (Fig. 9-7). On balance, in some cases only small fragments of varicose veins are encountered that can make the operation quite tedious; this frequently cannot be avoided.

If vein exteriorization proves difficult, it is better to make larger incisions rather than induce ischemia at the wound edges from excessive stretching. For the number of incisions to be reduced, the incisions should be made one at a time (Fig. 9-8). If avulsion proves difficult and the vein

■ Fig 9–7

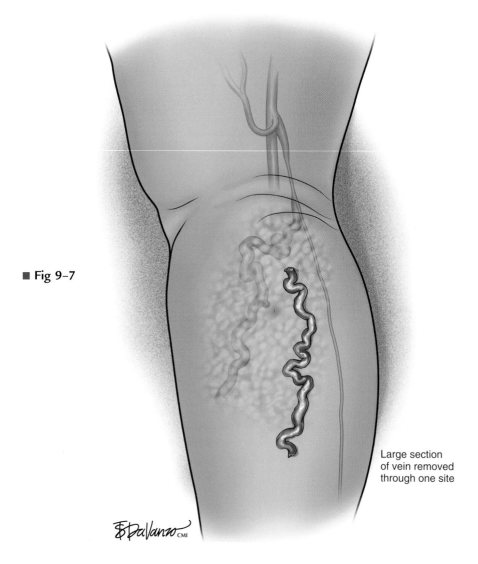

Large section of vein removed through one site

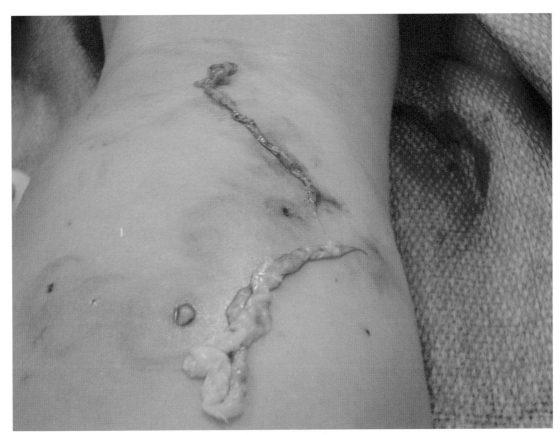

■ **Fig 9–7, cont'd**

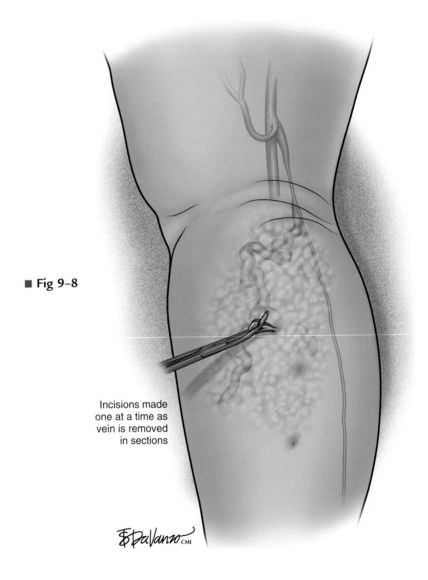

■ **Fig 9–8**

Incisions made
one at a time as
vein is removed
in sections

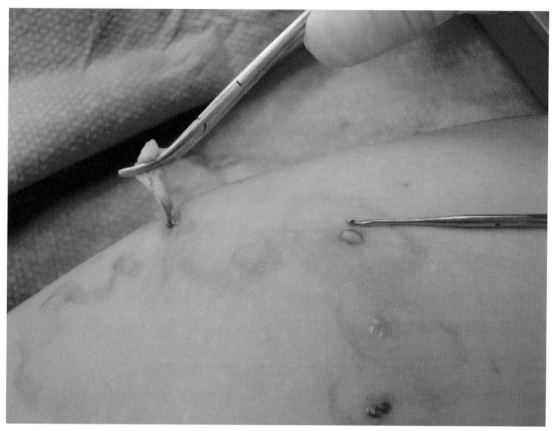

■ **Fig 9–8, cont'd**

breaks, it is more convenient to make more incisions than to waste time trying to retrieve more vein from the same incision (Fig. 9-9).

Areas where there is minimal subcutaneous fat or inflammatory changes can make the procedure more difficult. Typically, the operator will struggle around the knee, pretibial areas, and dorsum of the feet because these areas do not harbor much fat. Areas involved with previous superficial thrombophlebitis or previous surgery have more fibrosis.

Varicose veins sometimes act as outflow tracts for perforating veins; therefore, avulsion of varicose veins can disconnect underlying perforators. A perforator may be recognized by its perpendicular course and by the fact that the patient reports discomfort when traction is applied to the varicosity. The perforator is pulled until it yields, and then avulsed. Bleeding is controlled with digital compression.

Whether to close or not close wounds is a matter of judgment. The wounds may be left open or closed with simple sutures or adhesive tape. Most venous surgeons leave the wounds open and allow spontaneous healing. This technique results in little or no scarring and also has the advantage of allowing drainage of blood and anesthetic fluid into the overlying compressive dressing, obviating the formation of hematomas.

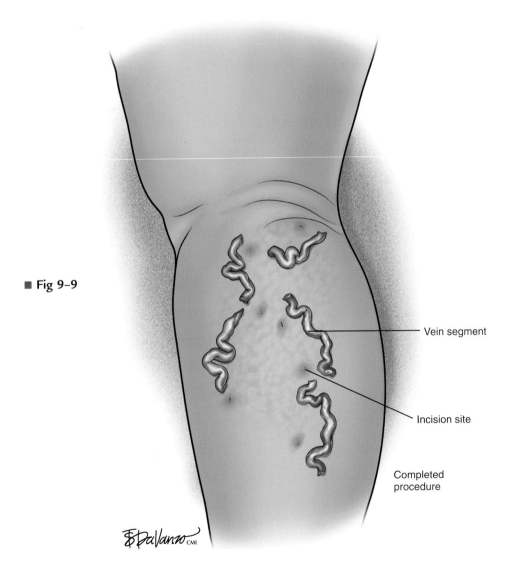

■ **Fig 9–9**

Vein segment

Incision site

Completed
procedure

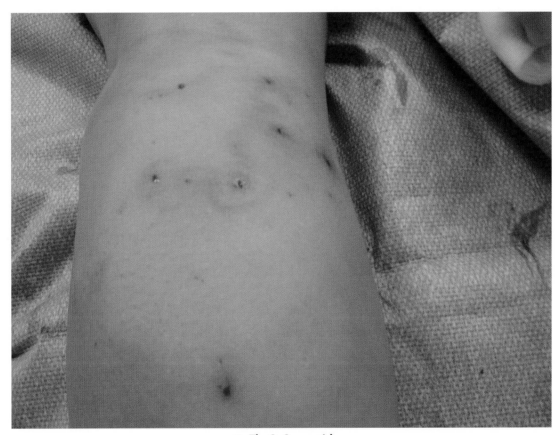

■ Fig 9-9, cont'd

A single suture to close wounds near the foot and ankle may be required because of the elevated venous pressure at these locations in the upright position. Frequent ambulation will aid in decreasing ambulatory venous pressure in these dependent locations. Adhesive tapes are associated with a high incidence of skin blistering; therefore, these must be used with caution.[13]

After 10 minutes of postoperative observation, patients ambulate from the office, with a three-layer compression bandage in place. Minimal postoperative discomfort is the norm, but if it is more intense, it can usually be easily managed with nonsteroidal antiinflammatory agents.

Patients return to the office on postoperative day 2 for dressing removal and for duplex ultrasound to exclude the presence of deep venous thrombosis. Some ecchymosis is to be expected near the treated areas; this rarely results in permanent discoloration of the skin. Some minor leakage of blood and tumescent anesthesia may also drain from the open wounds. Regular adhesive bandages will usually control this satisfactorily. After the compression bandage is removed, patients wear graduated compression stockings (20 to 30 mm Hg) for 2 weeks during the daytime.

Indurated areas are commonly seen at AP incision sites and usually defervesce without incident over a period of several weeks. Firm subcutaneous inflammatory nodules may occasionally form directly under the incision sites; these, too, are self-limiting after several months.

PEARLS AND PITFALLS

Avoiding nontarget tissues: The venous surgeon must have a thorough command of neurovascular anatomy to avoid injury to nontarget tissues such as arteries and nerves. If the treating physician heeds several important suggestions, complications will rarely be encountered. Knowledge of the course of the common femoral artery, superficial femoral artery, popliteal artery, and anterior and posterior tibial arteries will keep the surgeon from injuring these structures while probing to exteriorize a varicose vein. It would be very difficult, although not impossible, to injure the profunda femoris or peroneal arteries during AP. As stated earlier, the hook rarely needs to plunge deeper than 3 mm to contact the target vein.

The saphenous and sural nerves are particularly prone to injury below the knee because of their proximity to the GSV and SSV. If the saphenous or sural nerves are displaced by the hook, the patient will usually complain of shooting pain into the foot. This is a sign for the surgeon to gently release the structure and replace it in situ. Occasionally, hair-sized sensory cutaneous nerves are encountered and inadvertently avulsed during the course of AP. Patients will experience sharp pain that usually dissipates after 2 to 5 minutes without treatment. If this occurs in the ankle and foot area, chances are that the patient will develop postoperative paresthesias or areas of dysesthesia that in most cases will be temporary.[14]

The femoral, obturator, sciatic, tibial, and peroneal (common, deep, and superficial) nerves are deep and generally not disturbed in the hands of a competent surgeon.

Foot: The skin of the foot is thin and fibrotic. Further, there is minimal subcutaneous fat, less protection against trauma of the skin, and important underlying tissues such as tendons, tendon sheaths, and joints. There are more small nerve branches that can be damaged by the hook. As in the popliteal space, there is greater risk of injuring an artery.

Eyelid: AP of the periocular vein avoids the concerns regarding thrombotic phenomena within ocular, orbital, or cerebral veins possibly associated with periocular vein sclerotherapy. Weiss and Ramelet[15] reported excellent results on 10 patients who underwent removal of periocular reticular blue veins via AP. A single puncture with an 18-gauge needle sufficed in most cases. It is important to attempt to remove the entire segment, as partial resection may lead to recurrence. The use of postoperative compression for 10 minutes reduces the incidence of bruising. The puncture sites typically disappear quickly without scarring.

Hands: In general, inquiries about hand vein treatment come from elderly women who find them unsightly. Often, they have had prior facelift surgery and worry that their hands need rejuvenation to complement the face. Our initial consultation stresses the importance of hand veins for reasons of intravenous access; furthermore, removal of these veins may require central venous access should the patient be hospitalized in the future. If attempts to dissuade the patient fail, we recommend AP as the procedure of choice for hand vein removal. AP is identical to leg vein treatment and closely resembles treating the dorsum of foot because of the thin skin overlying the area. Results have been excellent.

COMPLICATIONS

Complications from AP in experienced hands are rare and, when they do occur, are minor.[16] A multicenter study performed in France evaluated 36,000 phlebectomies. The most frequently encountered complications were telangiectasias (1.5%), blister formation (1%), phlebitis (0.05%), hyperpigmentation (0.03%), postoperative bleeding (0.03%), temporary nerve damage (0.05%), and permanent nerve damage (0.02%).

At the Miami Vein Center, we have performed more than 5000 AP procedures in the office environment, and complications have been limited to hyperpigmentation, telangiectatic matting, seroma, transient paresthesia, superficial phlebitis, blistering, and "missed veins" requiring repeat treatment. Each of these complications occurred in less than 0.5% of cases.

COMPARATIVE EFFECTIVENESS OF EXISTING TREATMENTS

We do not look at AP as a solitary procedure but rather as part of our armada in the treatment of venous disease. We usually perform endovenous thermal ablation of the saphenous trunk in the same setting as AP because bulging varicose veins are usually in continuity with a refluxing axial vein such as the GSV. Other operators delay AP until 4 weeks following endovenous ablation. The argument for this strategy is to allow the bed of varicosities distal to a refluxing axial vein to shrink in size and number. Then, fewer incisions will be required for vein removal at the time of AP.

It is important to note that Monahan reported during the follow-up period that complete resolution of visible varicose veins was seen in only 13% of limbs after saphenous ablation alone.[17] Therefore, about 90% of patients require another intervention after saphenous ablation to fully eradicate their visible varicose veins. This has also been our experience.

If the patient returns in the postoperative period and points out veins that were missed during AP, a redo procedure is generally not required. Sclerotherapy, with or without ultrasound guidance, can be performed 4 to 6 weeks postoperatively to "clean-up" any missed veins. If redo phlebectomy is required, we permit 3 months to elapse; this allows the inflammatory response to subside at the original AP sites.

AP versus TriVex: In a published prospective comparative randomized trial comparing AP with the new technique of transillumination powered phlebectomy (TriVex), there was no difference in operating time. Although an incision ratio of 7:1 favored TriVex, there was no perceived cosmetic benefit between the patient groups. There was a higher number of recurrences in the TriVex group (21.2%) compared with the AP group (6.2%) at 52 weeks postoperatively. Assessment of pain scores showed no difference between groups.[18]

AP versus compression sclerotherapy: There is one randomized controlled trial on recurrence rates and other complications after sclerotherapy and AP. One year after sclerotherapy, 25% of

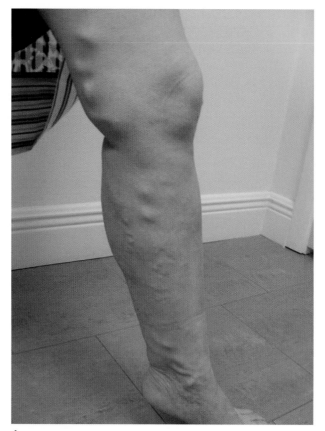

A

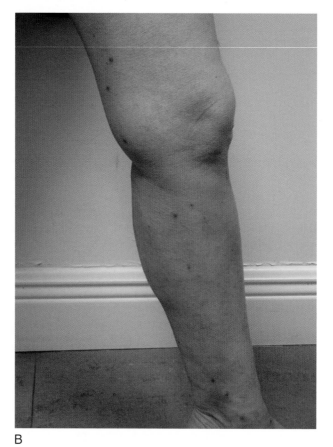

B

■ **Fig 9–10 A,** Before. **B,** After.

varicose veins had recurred versus only 2% recurrence after phlebectomy. After 2 years, the difference in recurrence was even larger: 38% recurrence in the sclerotherapy group and only 2% in the AP group.[19]

CONCLUSION

AP is elegant by its mere simplicity. It is effective and safe with acceptable cosmetic results (Fig. 9-10). AP is a perfect complement to endovenous thermal ablation of the saphenous veins. With this combination, patients can expect all varicose veins to vanish following a 1-hour procedure that used only local anesthesia in the comfort of a physician's office.

REFERENCES

1. Muller R. Traitement des varices par la phlebectomie ambulatoire. Phlebologie 1966; 19:277-279.
2. Jones L, Braithwaite BD, Selwyn D, et al. Neovascularisation is the principal cause of varicose vein recurrence: results of a randomized trial of stripping the long saphenous vein. Eur J Vasc Endovasc Surg 1996;12:442-445.
3. Winterborn RJ, Foy C, Earnshaw JJ. Causes of varicose vein recurrence: late results of a randomized controlled trial of stripping the long saphenous vein. J Vasc Surg 2004;40: 634-639.
4. Dwerryhouse S, Davies B, Harradine K, et al. Stripping the long saphenous vein reduces the rate of reoperation for recurrent varicose veins: five-year results of a randomized trial. J Vasc Surg 1999;29:589-592.
5. Sarin S, Scurr JH, Coleridge Smith PD. Stripping of the long saphenous vein in the treatment of primary varicose veins. Br J Surg 1994;81:1455-1458.
6. Min RJ, Khilnani N, Zimmet SE. Endovenous laser treatment of saphenous vein reflux: long-term results. J Vasc Interv Radiol 2003;14:991-996.
7. Merchant RF, Pichot O, Myers KA. Four-year follow-up on endovascular radiofrequency obliteration of great saphenous reflux. Dermatol Surg 2005;31:129-134.
8. Labropoulos N, Kang SS, Mansour MA, et al. Primary superficial vein reflux with competent saphenous trunk. Eur J Vasc Endovasc Surg 1999;18:201-206.
9. Weiss RA, Goldman MP. Transillumination mapping prior to ambulatory phlebectomy. Dermatol Surg 1998;24:447-450.
10. Klein JA. Tumescent technique for local anaesthesia improves safety in large-volume liposuction. Plast Reconstr Surg 1993;92:1085-1098.
11. Keel D, Goldman MP. Tumescent anaesthesia in ambulatory phlebectomy: addition of epinephrine. Dermatol Surg 1999;25:371-372.
12. Schmid RM, Rosenkranz HS. Antimicrobial activity of local anaesthetics: lidocaine and procaine. J Infect Dis 1970;121:597.
13. Almeida JI, Raines JK. Principles of ambulatory phlebectomy. In: Bergan JJ, ed. The Vein Book. San Diego: Elsevier; 2007:247-256.
14. Ramelet AA. Complications of ambulatory phlebectomy. Dermatol Surg 1997;23: 947-954.
15. Weiss RA, Ramelet AA. Removal of blue periocular lower eyelid veins by ambulatory phlebectomy. Dermatol Surg 2002;28:43-45.
16. Olivencia JA. Complications of ambulatory phlebectomy: review of 1,000 consecutive cases. Dermatol Surg 1997;23:51-54.

17. Monahan DL. Can phlebectomy be deferred in the treatment of varicose veins? J Vasc Surg 2005;42:1145-1149.
18. Aremu MA, Mahendran B, Butcher W, et al. Prospective randomized controlled trial: conventional versus powered phlebectomy. J Vasc Surg 2004;39:88-94.
19. De Roos KP, Nieman FH, Neumann HA. Ambulatory phlebectomy versus compression sclerotherapy: results of a randomized controlled trial. Dermatol Surg 2003;29:221-226.

CHAPTER 10

Endovenous Approach to Recurrent Varicose Veins

Jose I. Almeida

HISTORICAL BACKGROUND

Recurrence rates of varicose veins of 20% are common, with rates as high as 70% at 10 years.[1-3] Up to 25% of procedures for varicose veins are performed for recurrent disease,[4] thus placing considerable demands on health care resources. It is important to note that recurrent varicose vein surgery carries a much greater morbidity risk to the patient than does primary surgery.[3] This risk is reduced markedly with endovenous techniques.

ETIOLOGY AND NATURAL HISTORY OF DISEASE

Patients who have had previous high ligation and stripping typically present with recurrent varicose veins; anatomic distribution of these veins is variable. Neovascularization is commonly seen following traditional stripping procedures and is thought to be secondary to "frustrated" venous drainage from the abdominal wall and perineum.[5] Regardless of the mechanism, the result is recurrent reflux in the thigh or lower leg veins.

Multiple factors contribute in the development of recurrent disease. The weight of each factor has not yet been determined because there are no prospective studies with adequate sample size. The following descriptions are common etiologies seen at Miami Vein Center after clinical and color flow duplex imaging (CFDI) examinations are performed in patients presenting with recurrent varicose veins.

PEARLS AND PITFALLS

Previous High Ligation and Stripping

All patients with recurrent varicose veins should be evaluated with CFDI. Usually findings include neovascularity in the groin from which one or more tributary veins are found to descend the thigh. The tributary may attach to another tributary, a perforator, or a remnant of the great saphenous vein (GSV) in the thigh or calf (Fig. 10-1). The reflux extends into dilated tributaries of the skin; these vessels bulge and are palpable. In most cases, our approach is to enter any straight incompetent axial venous segments deep to the skin with a micropuncture access kit. These kits usually contain 4-Fr microsheaths, through which we place a 400- or 600-μm-diameter

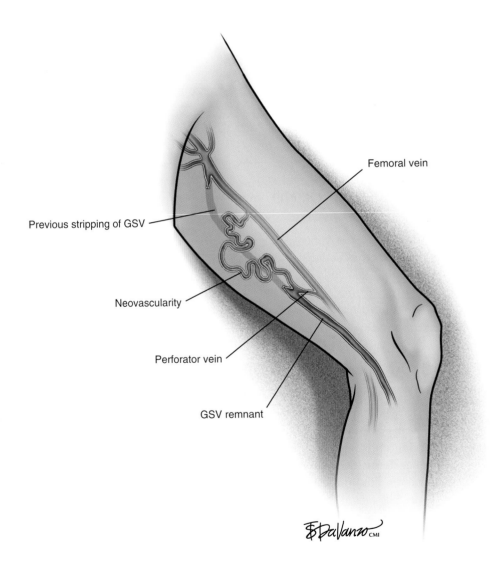

Previous stripping of GSV

Femoral vein

Neovascularity

Perforator vein

GSV remnant

A

■ **Fig 10–1**

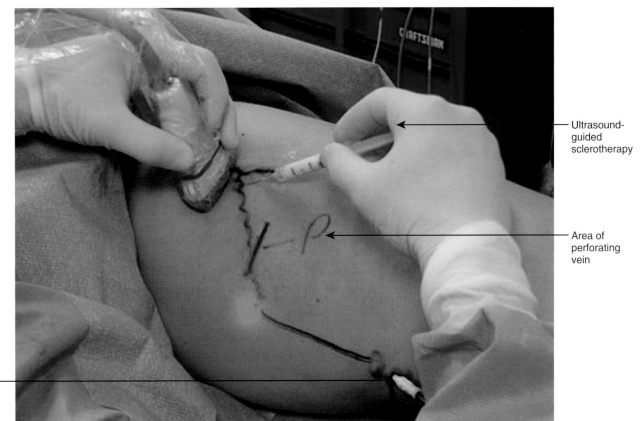

Ultrasound-guided sclerotherapy

Area of perforating vein

Ablation of saphenous vein remnant

B

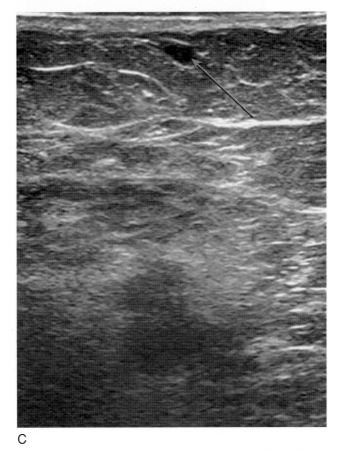

C

■ **Fig 10–1, cont'd** **B,** Treatment of recurrent varicose vein with the use of combination endovenous laser and foam scleropathy. **C,** Cross-sectional view of a subcutaneous tortuous tributary. These tortuous veins are ideal candidates for ultrasound-guided foam sclerotherapy treatment.

Continued

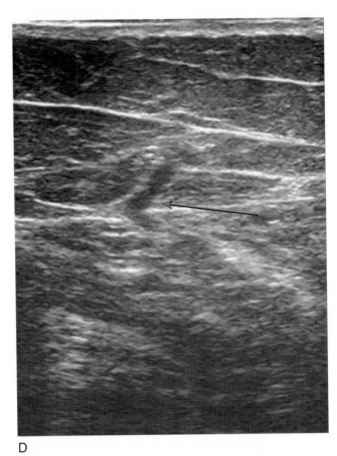

D

■ **Fig 10–1, cont'd D,** Incompetent midthigh perforating vein is the source of the recurrent varicose veins, which is most effectively treated with thermal ablation if anatomically in a straight orientation. If oriented in a tortuous manner, however, ultrasound-guided foam sclerotherapy treatment is preferred.

laser fiber. Perivenous tumescent anesthesia is placed, and the vein or veins are ablated in the usual manner. Because tortuous incompetent venous segments below the level of the skin do not allow the passage of guidewires, these are treated with ultrasound-guided foam sclerotherapy (Fig. 10-2).

Finally, all bulging varicose veins that are palpable on the skin receive treatment with ambulatory phlebectomy. These three techniques, used concomitantly, yield very satisfactory results. These types of patients are told that the treatments are palliative and they likely will need "touch-up" treatments in the future.

Previous Phlebectomy Without GSV Stripping

Also common in our practice are patients presenting with recurrent varicose veins previously treated with phlebectomy only at an outside facility. These limbs, once examined with CFDI, usually have a large incompetent GSV descending from the groin and terminating ultimately in the calf at a site where large varicosities are noted. These patients do very well with routine GSV ablation using either radiofrequency or laser and using ambulatory phlebectomy for associated varicosities.

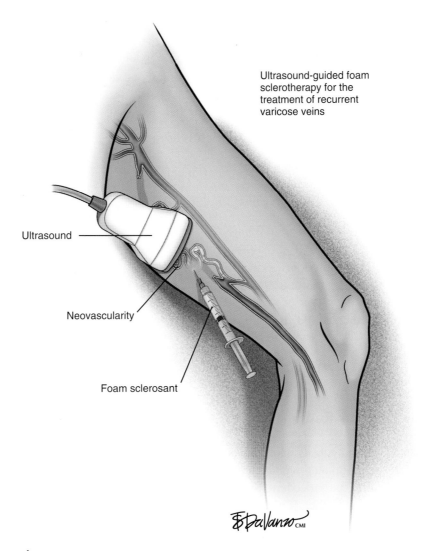

Ultrasound-guided foam sclerotherapy for the treatment of recurrent varicose veins

Ultrasound

Neovascularity

Foam sclerosant

A

■ **Fig 10–2**

Continued

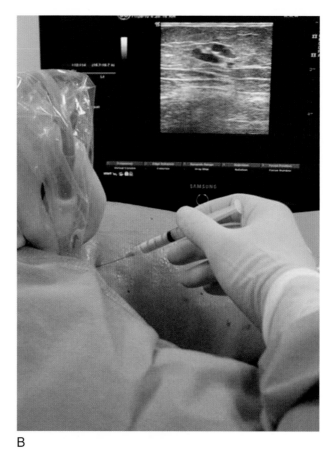

B

■ **Fig 10-2, cont'd B,** Ultrasound-guided foam sclerotherapy for the treatment of recurrent varicose veins; tortuous veins seen on ultrasound are in the background.

Previous Laser or Radiofrequency Ablation Without Phlebectomy

There are individuals who have seen other physicians and come to our practice with a history of GSV ablation that "worked temporarily." That is, the venous cluster on the medial calf improved shortly after the procedure, but with time, the same cluster began filling and dilating. CFDI performed in our office usually shows successful ablation of the target GSV. However, the cluster of varicose veins in these cases has found a connection with an incompetent perforating vein. This is usually a Boyd perforating vein in the upper calf. This concept of an untreated "venous reservoir" dictates that other sources of reflux will eventually connect due to low venous resistance. Treatment involves either ultrasound-guided sclerotherapy or thermal ablation of the perforator (function of size) and ambulatory phlebectomy of the varicose clusters.

We have also seen cases in which two sources of venous hypertension from superficial axial vein reflux were identified preoperatively but only one was treated. In these cases usually only the incompetent GSV was ablated, and the incompetent anterior accessory saphenous vein was left untreated. There may be temporary improvement of the varicosities in direct continuity with the GSV; less direct varicosities may respond with minimal or no improvement. Our approach with these patients is thermal ablation of the anterior accessory saphenous vein followed by ambulatory phlebectomy at the same stage.

Previous GSV Ablation with No Improvement

When a patient has a history of previous GSV ablation performed at an outside facility and no improvement was observed by the patient, this should be a red flag that the patient was initially misdiagnosed. The majority of these cases were straightforward cases with classic SSV incompetence in the limbs; however, the original physician failed to view the posterior calf with CFDI. Ablation of the SSV with laser or radiofrequency energy in combination with ambulatory phlebectomy will quickly rectify this problem.

Gastrocnemial vein incompetence has a prevalence of up to 30% in patients with varicose veins. Most practitioners do not treat this vein. Also, incompetent perforators connecting through this vein at the posteromedial calf may be overlooked or missed. We have seen these as sources of recurrent varicose veins. Depending on the severity of the signs and symptoms of the disease, we may elect to treat gastrocnemius veins with ultrasound-guided sclerotherapy. Obviously, this adds controversy to the dearth of clinical information referable to this vein.

COMPARATIVE EFFECTIVENESS OF EXISTING TREATMENTS

There are no publications available that focus on endovenous treatment of recurrent varicose veins. The aforementioned techniques are self-taught techniques, applying standard endovenous principles. The adage developed by the author is "If an incompetent vein is straight—burn it; if it is tortuous—foam it; if the vein is palpable on the skin (straight or tortuous)—remove it with phlebectomy."

Depicted in Figure 10-3 is an endovenous sheath inside a saphenous vein remnant (to deliver laser energy), with a syringe prepared with a foamed sclerosant attached to the sheath side-arm to deliver foam into an area of neovascularization—and the patient is marked for phlebectomy. We have had no complications with this approach in several hundred recurrent varicose vein cases. Recurrences after endovenous treatment develop secondary to progression of disease and are retreatable with the same approach.

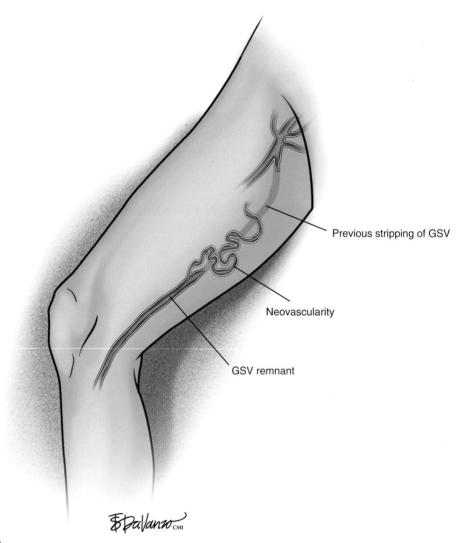

Previous stripping of GSV

Neovascularity

GSV remnant

A

■ **Fig 10–3**

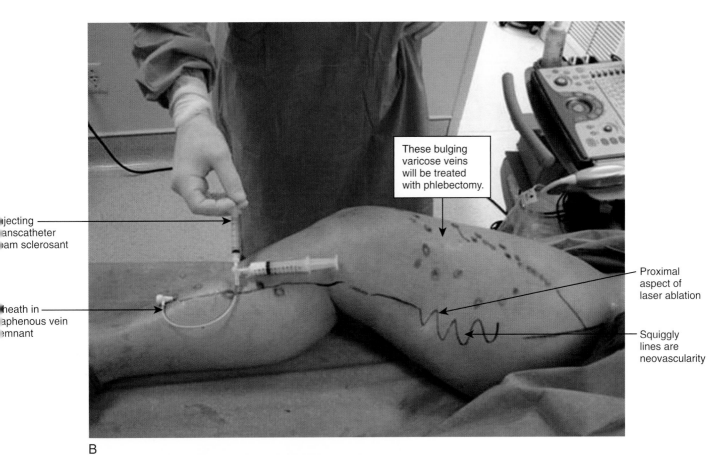

jecting
anscatheter
am sclerosant

heath in
aphenous vein
emnant

These bulging
varicose veins
will be treated
with phlebectomy.

Proximal
aspect of
laser ablation

Squiggly
lines are
neovascularity

B

C

■ **Fig 10–3, cont'd B,** Recurrent varicose veins from neovascularity in upper thigh and a refluxing saphenous vein remnant. Treatment with a combination of ultrasound foam sclerotherapy, endovenous laser ablation, and ambulatory phlebectomy. **C,** Arrow points to saphenous vein remnant.

Continued

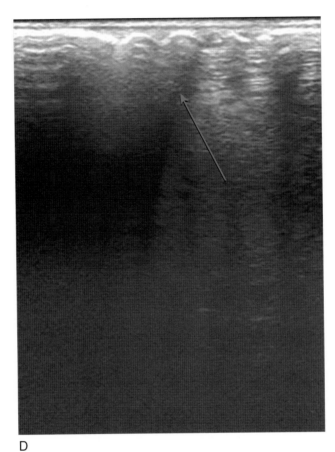

D

■ **Fig 10–3, cont'd D,** Arrow points to foam-filled varicose veins just below skin surface.

REFERENCES

1. Negus D. Recurrent varicose veins; a national problem. Br J Surg 1993;80:823-824.
2. Rivlin S. The surgical cure of primary varicose veins. Br J Surg 1975;62:913-917.
3. Royle JP. Recurrent varicose veins. World J Surg 1986;10:944-953.
4. Hayden A, Holdsworth J. Complications following re-exploration of the groin for recurrent varicose veins. Ann R Coll Surg Engl 2001;83:272-273.
5. Chandler JG, Pichot O, Sessa C, et al. Treatment of primary venous insufficiency by endovenous saphenous vein obliteration. Vasc Surg 2000;34:201-214.

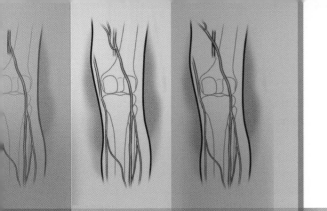

CHAPTER 11

Treatment of Spider Telangiectasias

Edward G. Mackay

HISTORICAL BACKGROUND

Although the treatment of varicose veins was in the phase of further refinement, the treatment of telangiectasias was not seriously attempted until the 1930s. It was Biegeleisen who is credited with initially attempting injection into the perivascular space around telangiectatic areas. Later, he implemented intravascular injections using homemade microneedles.[1] These early efforts led to disappointing results, primarily because the sclerosing solutions, such as sodium morrhuate, were very caustic. It was not until the 1970s that others attempted to treat spider telangiectasias with intravascular injection using less caustic solutions such as sodium tetradecyl sulfate (STS) (Sotradecol) and hypertonic saline. It was these agents that propelled the treatment of telangiectasias forward. The enthusiasm for these treatments increased steadily as Foley's publication, relating to this new technique, gained momentum.[2]

Etiology

Although research continues to be done in this area, there is consensus today that telangiectasias result from a number of causes, alone or more likely in combination with other etiologic factors. Telangiectatic leg veins, according to the contemporary research, arise as a result of venous hypertension secondary to a number of different causes and conditions. The etiology of varicose veins and telangiectasias, for the most part, is similar. The pathophysiology of telangiectasias is usually broadly categorized as genetic/congenital, acquired and iatrogenic. Some of the genetic causes of telangiectasias include nevus flammeus (port-wine stains), nevus araneus (spider telangiectasia, which can also result from acquired diseases), and Klippel-Trenaunay syndrome. Congenital conditions associated with telangiectasias include Maffucci syndrome and Rothmund-Thomson syndrome (poikiloderma). Acquired causes of telangiectasias can arise from a primary cutaneous disorder, such as varicose veins and keratosis lichenoides chronica, or the result of a disorder with a secondary cutaneous component, such as lupus erythematosus, a collagen disorder, and mastocytosis (telangiectasia macularis eruptiva perstans). Hormonal influences (estrogen and progesterone) also play a role in the pathogenesis of telangiectasia. Pregnancy places the person at risk for the development of telangiectasia as early as a couple of weeks after conception. Birth control pills, menses, and the time just before ovulation are also associated with the development or worsening of telangiectasia, and increased venous dispensability. Topical steroids, particularly at high doses, have also been identified as a possible causative factor. Last, physical insults, like trauma (contusions) and infection, have also been implicated as causal forces. See Box 11-1 for a comprehensive listing of the many causes of lower leg cutaneous telangiectasia.

Telangiectasia is also associated with a number of other conditions and traits. These include, but are not limited to, those listed here:

- Age (peaks during one's 50s and 60s)
- Female gender
- Occupation and lifestyle: sedentary occupations and lifestyles are associated with telangiectasia
- Diseases such as cirrhosis
- Excessive exposure to the sun
- Therapeutic radiation (Figs. 11-1 through 11-8)

Patient Selection

Patients with spider telangiectasias typically present with primarily cosmetic complaints. Patient selection for the treatment of spider telangiectasias, as with all medical treatments, begins with a thorough assessment that includes not only an assessment of the person's telangiectasia, but also the medical history, chief complaint, family history, and the patient's expectations relating to his or her possible spider telangiectasias. On the basis of this assessment, the physician must determine whether or not the treatment can resolve the patient's cosmetic complaints. At times, the telangiectasia is the result of a more generalized, systemic problem such as venous insufficiency. If venous insufficiency is present, it must be treated prior to the treatment of the spider telangiectasia; otherwise, the venous hypertension would likely thwart the desired outcome. Second, it must be determined whether the patient's expectations are realistic and achievable. The patient must clearly understand that the treatment is elective and that it is not likely to produce any significant health benefits. The patient should also understand that multiple treatments are often necessary for optimal results. Some patients may not be willing to do this. As with all invasive procedures, the patient must be educated about the benefits, risks, and alternatives to treatment. He or she must be thoroughly aware of all potential adverse sequelae and possible complications. Last, the patient must be informed that the treatment of spider telangiectasias is not curative and that further development of telangiectatic areas is likely.

Although there are no absolute contraindications to this treatment, people taking certain medications and/or patients with some chronic illnesses, especially those that could affect the occurrence of sclerotherapy complications, should be approached with extreme caution. For example, conditions such diabetes and peripheral vascular disease may lead to serious complications, such as ulcers. Some medications, such as minocycline or isotretinoin, can lead to adverse reactions if not discontinued prior to the treatment.

Text continued on p. 260

BOX 11–1 CAUSES OF CUTANEOUS TELANGIECTASIA OF THE LOWER EXTREMITIES

Genetic/Congenital Factors
Vascular nevi
Nevus flammeus
Klippel-Trenaunay syndrome
Nevus araneus
Angioma serpiginosum
Bockenheimer syndrome

Congenital Neuroangiopathies
Maffucci syndrome
Congenital poikiloderma (Rothmund–Thomson syndrome)
Essential progressive telangiectasia
Cutis marmorata telangiectatica congenita
Diffuse neonatal hemangiomatosis
Acquired disease with a secondary cutaneous component

Collagen Vascular Diseases
Lupus erythematosus
Dermatomyositis
Progressive systemic sclerosis
Cryoglobulinemia

Other
Telangiectasia macularis eruptiva perstans (mastocytosis)
Human immunodeficiency virus (HTLV-III)

Component of a Primary Cutaneous Disease
Varicose veins
Keratosis lichenoides chronica

Other Acquired/Primary Cutaneous Diseases
Necrobiosis lipoidica diabeticorum
Capillaritis (purpura annularis telangiectodes)
Malignant atrophic papulosis (Degos disease)

Hormonal Factors
Pregnancy
Estrogen therapy
Topical corticosteroid preparations

Physical Factors
Actinic neovascularization and/or vascular dilation

Trauma
Contusion
Surgical incision/laceration

Infection
Generalized essential telangiectasia
Progressive ascending telangiectasia
Human immunodeficiency virus (HTLV-III)
Radiodermatitis
Erythema ab igne (heat/infrared radiation)

Modified from Goldman MP, Bennett RG. J Am Acad Dermatol 1987;17:167.

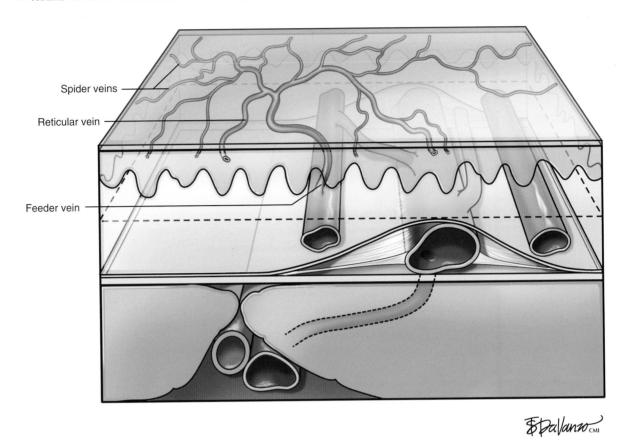

Spider veins

Reticular vein

Feeder vein

■ **Fig 11–1** Normal subcutaneous venous anatomy.

■ **Fig 11–2** Patient with Klippel-Trenaunay syndrome.

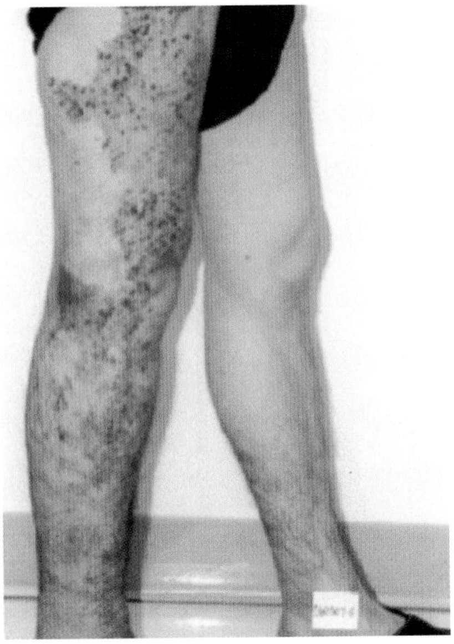

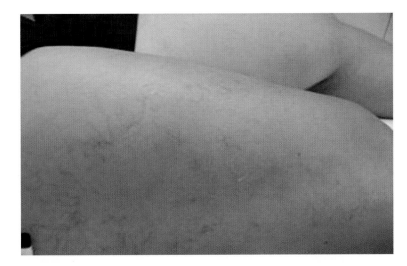

■ **Fig 11-3** Spider vein.

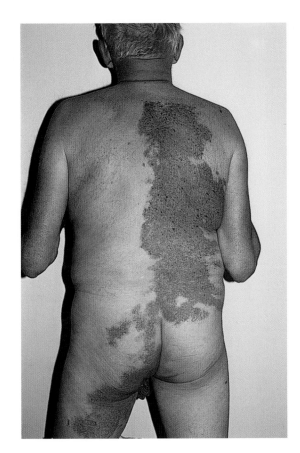

■ **Fig 11-4** Nevus flammeus. *(From Weiss RA, Goldman MP, Bergan JJ, et al. Sclerotherapy: Treatment of Varicose and Telangiectatic Leg Veins. St Louis: Elsevier, 2007, Fig. 4.6, p. 76.)*

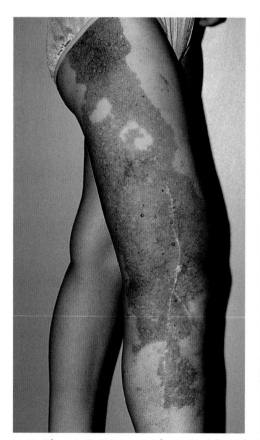 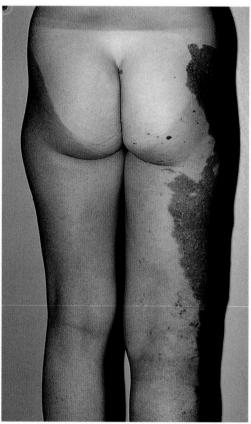

■ **Fig 11–5** Woman, 16 years old, with Klippel-Trenaunay syndrome and associated varicose veins and nevus flammeus of the right lower extremity from the toes to the buttock. *(From Weiss RA, Goldman MP, Bergan JJ, et al. Sclerotherapy: Treatment of Varicose and Telangiectatic Leg Veins. St Louis: Elsevier, 2007, Fig. 4.17, p. 84.)*

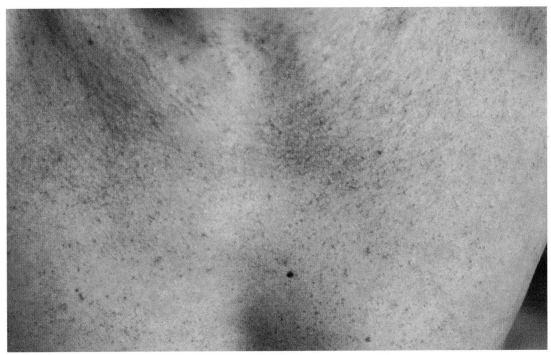

■ **Fig 11–6** Extensive fine red telangiectasia on the chest of a severely sun-damaged 50-year-old woman. *(From Weiss RA, Goldman MP, Bergan JJ, et al. Sclerotherapy: Treatment of Varicose and Telangiectatic Leg Veins. St Louis: Elsevier, 2007, Fig. 4.19, p. 85.)*

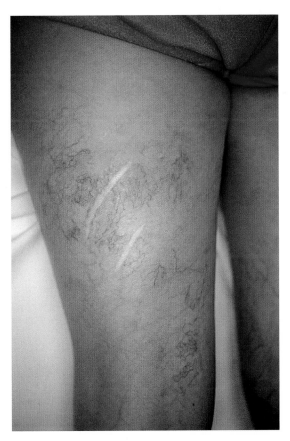

■ **Fig 11–7** This woman underwent an extensive ligation and stripping of her varicose veins at 18 years of age. She developed extensive telangiectasia around all of the surgical sites within weeks of the surgical procedure. This photograph was taken 22 years after the surgical procedure. *(From Weiss RA, Goldman MP, Bergan JJ, et al. Sclerotherapy: Treatment of Varicose and Telangiectatic Leg Veins. St Louis: Elsevier, 2007, Fig. 4.20, p. 86.)*

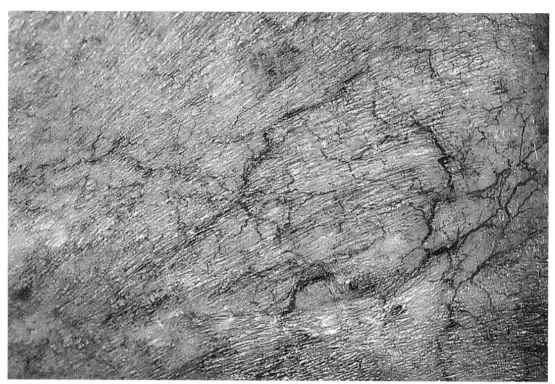

■ **Fig 11-8** Appearance of telangiectasis occurring as a result of radiation treatment on the lateral neck for laryngeal carcinoma 20 years previously. *(From Weiss RA, Goldman MP, Bergan JJ, et al. Sclerotherapy: Treatment of Varicose and Telangiectatic Leg Veins. St Louis: Elsevier, 2007.)*

Endovascular Instrumentation

The basic endovascular instrumentation used for the treatment of spider telangiectasias includes needles for access and syringes to deliver the sclerosant to the affected areas. The needles used for telangiectasia are typically 30 gauge, although a 27-gauge butterfly needle may be used sometimes for larger reticular veins. Smaller needles, as small as a 33 gauge, can also be used but they tend to bend too easily when they are penetrating the skin (Fig. 11-9).

The syringes that are typically used vary from a 1-mL tuberculin syringe to a 3-mL syringe. Most prefer a 3-mL syringe because it exerts the lowest pressures during injection, and it is also manually manipulated more precisely by the practitioner than a 1-mL syringe, especially if it is only filled to 2 mL.

The environment of care for sclerotherapy should include a comfortable table for the patient, a comfortable room temperature, and ample lighting. The treatment table height should permit the physician to sit comfortably on a stool with his or her legs under the table without having to lean over the table and the patient for access. Environmental lighting should be bright and capable of providing adequate indirect illumination without any glare on the patient's skin (Fig. 11-10).

General supplies would include alcohol swabs, cotton balls, tape, and compression supplies such as Ace wraps or Coban. Patients can supply their own stockings or they can be provided by the practice, which would require keeping a fairly large inventory (Figs. 11-11 and 11-12).

Last, but also most important, is emergency equipment. Fortunately, life-threatening complications are very rare; however, they are always possible. Basic emergency equipment must minimally include oxygen, airway equipment, epinephrine, steroids, and antihistamines (Fig. 11-13).

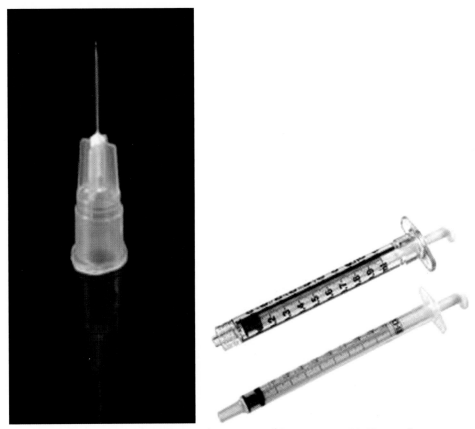

■ **Fig 11–9** Needles and syringes. *(Courtesy Dr. M. Nerney.)*

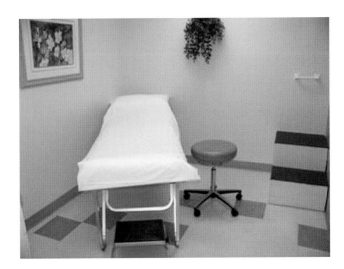

■ **Fig 11–10** Table and chair.

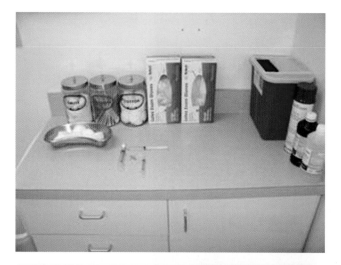

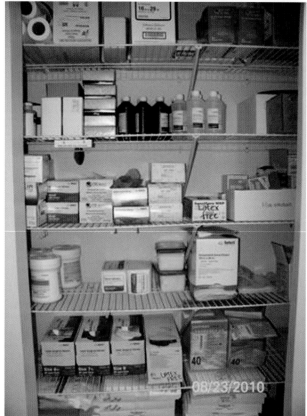

■ **Fig 11–11** Surgical supplies.

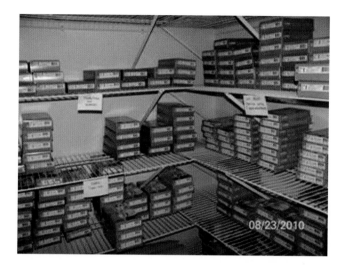

■ **Fig 11-12** Compression stockings.

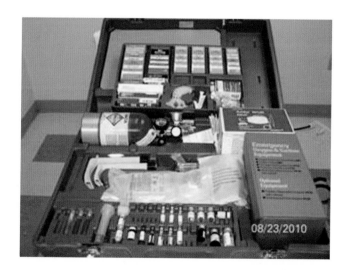

■ **Fig 11-13** Emergency equipment.

Imaging

Spider telangiectasias are primarily a cosmetic, aesthetic concern for the patient; therefore, they are primarily treated visually. Several things can be used to aid in the visualization.

First and foremost are magnifying glasses or loupes. These aids help to visualize the insertion of the needle into the smaller veins, particularly those that are less than 1 mm in diameter. Because loupes typically have 2½ times the magnification, they facilitate good visualization while the needle pierces the skin and enters the vein (Fig. 11-14).

A number of lighting systems are used for visualization of veins to be treated. Vein lights provide visualization of vessels just under the skin that are sometimes too deep for normal visualization. These lights create a "shadow" from the absorption of the blood in the vein. Polarized lights are also used to provide better visualization through the skin (Fig. 11-15).

Syris polarized lights with magnification (Syris, Gray, ME) also provide better visualization through the skin (Fig. 11-16).

Infrared visualization is also done. Infrared lights allow the practitioner to see veins a few millimeters under the skin because these lights provide infrared images of the hemoglobin contained within the red cells circulating in the vessel that is then projected back onto the skin using the VeinViewer or a camera. This is particularly helpful for identifying "feeding" reticular veins that could be causing the telangiectasias (Fig. 11-17).

Duplex imaging is also an invaluable tool. This imaging is primarily used for the diagnostic workup of venous insufficiency. It is also used for directing that treatment, including varicose veins. New high-frequency probes, in the 15- to 17-mHz range, can identify very small veins, as small as 1 to 2 mm, such as reticular "feeding" veins. These reticular feeding veins may demonstrate reflux that may contribute to spider telangiectasias.

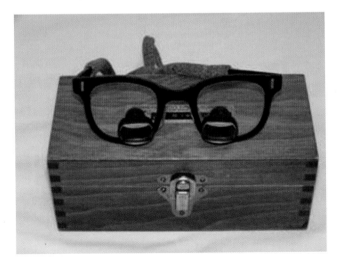

■ **Fig 11–14** Loupes.

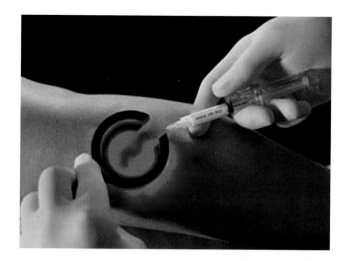

■ **Fig 11–15** Vein light. *(Courtesy Dr. M. Nerney.)*

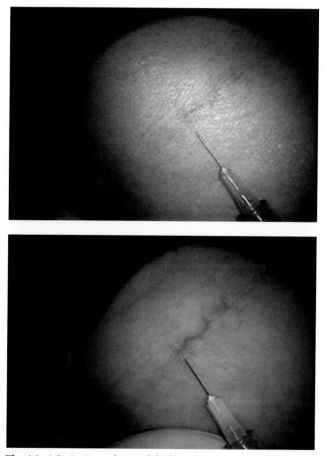

■ **Fig 11–16** Syris polarized light. *(Courtesy Dr. M. Nerney.)*

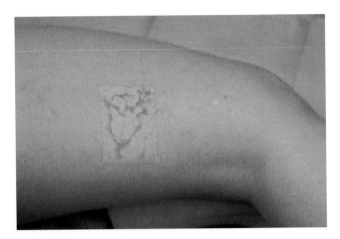

■ **Fig 11-17** Vein viewer. *(Courtesy Dr. M. Nerney.)*

Sclerosants

Sclerosants used for the treatment of spider telangiectasias can be divided into three main groups: detergents, hyperosmolar, and chemical irritants. This section will cover the most frequently used sclerosants for treatment of telangiectasias in the United States.

The detergent solutions are primarily sodium tetradecyl sulfate (STS) (Sotradecol) and polidocanol (POL). These solutions work by attacking the endothelial cells at their cell surface lipids. STS has been around since 1946. It is manufactured in the United States by BionichePharma. STS is used for the treatment of spider telangiectasias in various concentrations from 0.05% to 0.5%. It can be foamed if desired. POL, used for the treatment of spider telangiectasias, comes in concentrations of 0.25% to 1% and it, too, can be used as a foam. POL just recently became approved by the U.S. Food and Drug Administration (FDA), so experience with it is not nearly as extensive as it is in Europe.

The hyperosmolar, or hypertonic, sclerosant group consists primarily of hypertonic saline (HS), hypertonic dextrose, sodium salicylate, and a combination of hypertonic saline and hypertonic dextrose. These agents work by dehydrating the endothelial cells. Hypertonic saline is used in concentrations of 11.7% to 23.4%. Hypertonic dextrose comes in a concentration of 75% that can be diluted. The combination of 10% saline and 25% dextrose is sold as Sclerodex manufactured by Omega laboratories in Canada.

Chemical irritant sclerosants that are currently used in the United States are primarily limited to glycerin 72%. It works as a caustic agent on the vessel wall. Glycerin can be diluted, most frequently with lidocaine 1% with or without epinephrine (Fig. 11-18).

ACCESS AND CLOSURE

As previously stated, access is primarily done through visualization with aspiration for the larger vessels. Smaller vessels are located by palpation alone because these veins are too small for aspiration. These smaller vessels are accessed by direct visualization while maintaining slight pressure on the plunger. Access is then confirmed when the sclerosing solution is seen going through the vein. Pressure should be light so as not to cause a bleb under the skin. The injection should be stopped and a different site used if a bleb is seen. Larger veins, such as reticular veins, can be aspirated before being injected. This aspiration and injection should be effortless and without any resistance. The injection should be stopped if any resistance is met because this may indicate that the needle has come out of the vein. Closure, or hemostasis, is accomplished with

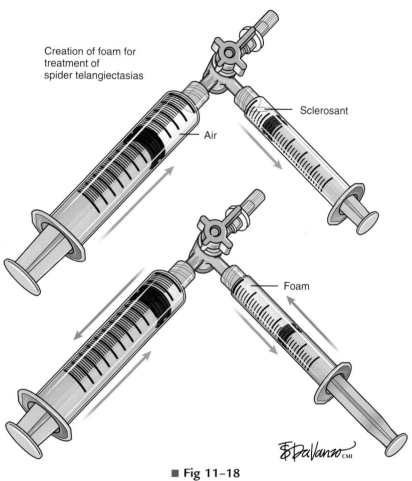

Creation of foam for
treatment of
spider telangiectasias

Air

Sclerosant

Foam

■ Fig 11–18

digital pressure after the removal of the needle. A cotton ball can be applied with atraumatic tape, such as paper tape, over the puncture site for additional compression.

OPERATIVE STEPS

After appropriate informed consent is obtained and patient education is complete, the next step is to obtain photographic documentation of the areas being treated to establish a baseline for later posttreatment comparison. This comparison is useful to both the physician ant the patient. Minimally, four views should be obtained with additional close-up views as indicated.

After this photographic documentation, the patient is then placed in the supine position, preferably with the head slightly lower than the legs. As previously mentioned, the height of the table itself should be comfortable for the person performing the injections. Good indirect lighting, without glare on the skin, is also necessary. The skin should be cleansed with alcohol, not only for asepsis but also to remove the outermost dead layer of skin in order to make the veins more visible to the practitioner.

Treatment should begin at the source of reflux, if the source has been determined, or proximal to it if the precise location is not known. In the latter case, the larger veins are treated prior to the treatment of the smaller ones. It can be assumed that the source of reflux is the perigeniculate perforators, located usually just above the knee, for the lateral venous plexus area (Fig. 11-19).

Complete treatment of the reticular feeding veins is performed in a given area before moving to the treatment of the smaller spider telangiectasias in the same area. Sclerosant injected into the feeder vein often travels into the spiders, thus effectively treating both the feeding veins and the spider veins. Access with the needle, as described earlier, is done with aspiration to confirm placement into the larger reticular feeder veins. The method of injection should be smooth and with very little pressure on the plunger. The volume of the injection solution depends on the size of the reticular vein. By definition, reticular veins range from 1 mm to 3 mm in diameter. Using 2 mm as an average, the volume of a 5-cm segment is 0.16 mL. Therefore a 15-cm segment would require 0.5 mL of sclerosant. Imaging with vein lights, a vein viewer, and polarized lights is sometimes very helpful (Figs. 11-20 through 11-22).

The practitioner has a choice of sclerosant and concentration for reticular veins. Typically chosen is 0.5% to 1.0% STS liquid or 0.25% to 0.5% foamed STS. When POL is chosen, it is generally 0.75% to 1% liquid or 0.5% to 0.75% foam. Other choices may include 23.4% HS or 66% dextrose.

Following the reticular feeding vein treatment, the spider telangiectasia can immediately be treated during the same visit or postponed for a later date. When the spider veins are ready for treatment, these veins are accessed with visual cues or with the tactile feel of the needle and plunger. As the needle enters the vein there is a lessening of resistance and, with a light touch on the plunger, the sclerosant will clear the vessel. If there is any evidence of extravasation, the injection must be stopped immediately.

The volume of injection is dependent on the size of the vein being treated. It is important to keep in mind that a 1-mm vein has only 0.1 mL of volume for every 13 cm of length. The injection of the appropriate volume of the solution is often ascertained by a visual determination by the experienced practitioner. Gentle positive pressure on the plunger and the injection of the sclerosing solution continue until the segment of vein fills with approximately 0.1 mL.

After the injection is stopped, the needle is then held in position for several seconds, up to 30 seconds. This increases the contact time of the sclerosant with the vein wall. The choice and concentration of sclerosant for spider veins are based on the size of the spider vein and practitioner preference, with ranges from 0.05% to 0.25% for STS and from 0.25% to 0.5% for POL,

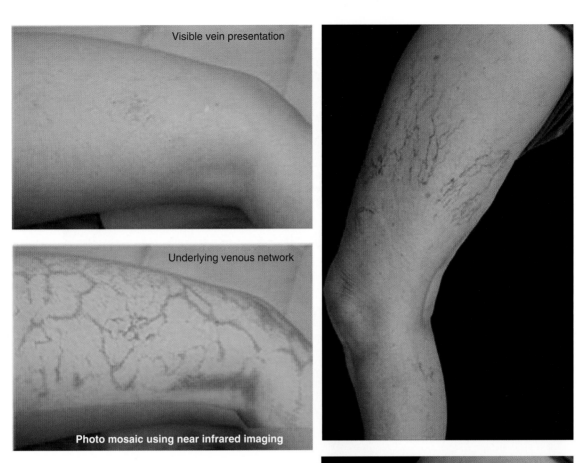

Visible vein presentation

Underlying venous network

Photo mosaic using near infrared imaging

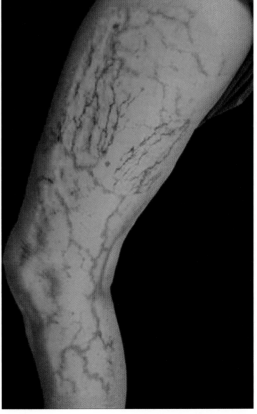

■ **Fig 11-19** Lateral venous plexus with and without a composite vein viewer. *(Courtesy Dr. M. Nerney.)*

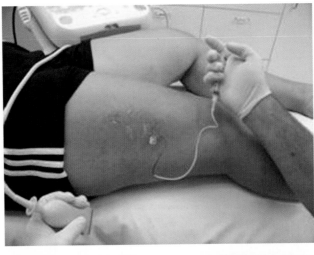

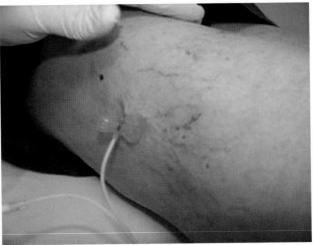

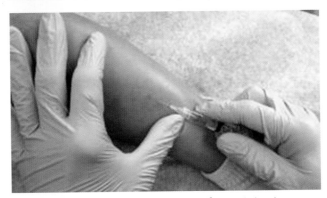

■ **Fig 11–20** Lateral venous plexus injection.

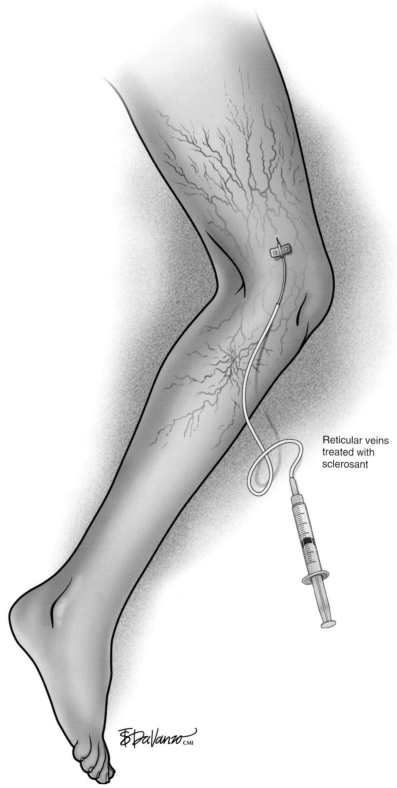

Reticular veins
treated with
sclerosant

■ **Fig 11–21** Illustration of a lateral venous plexus injection.

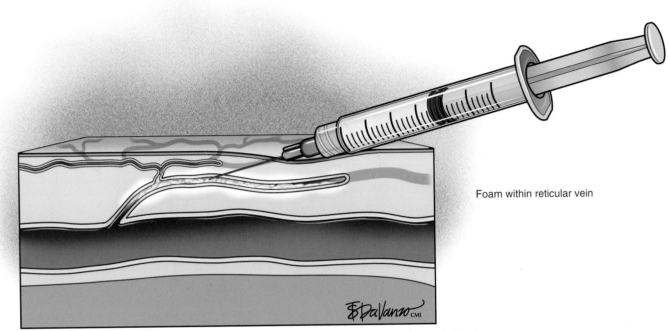

Foam within reticular vein

■ **Fig 11–22** Illustration of a lateral venous plexus injection.

11.7% HS, and 48% glycerin diluted with lidocaine. The total volume of the injection depends on which type and concentration of sclerosant are being used. For example, the maximum dose for STS is 10 mL of 3%, so if one is injecting a 0.25% solution, the total volume would be 120 mL (Figs. 11-23 and 11-24).

Many recommend placing a cotton ball over the injection site immediately after each injection to achieve hemostasis, to compress the vein walls together, and to prevent the filling of the vein with blood, which would lead to a clot. Atraumatic tape, such as paper tape, is used to hold the cotton ball in place when it is used. Further compression may be accomplished with foam pads, Ace wraps, or compression stockings. There is some data to suggest that compression stockings worn for several weeks after treatment can decrease adverse events, such as staining, but there are no data to suggest that compression stockings enhance the effectiveness of the treatment.[3]

Many practitioners recommend that patients elevate their legs, ambulate frequently, and avoid hot showers after treatment to decrease venous pressure or to avoid vasodilatation, although there is no research to support these posttreatment recommendations.

Follow-up treatments can be scheduled from a few days to several months later. There is concern that frequent treatments within a few weeks to the same area can increase the risk of inflammation in the area and possibly increase adverse effects. Again, there are no data that statistically support this concern.

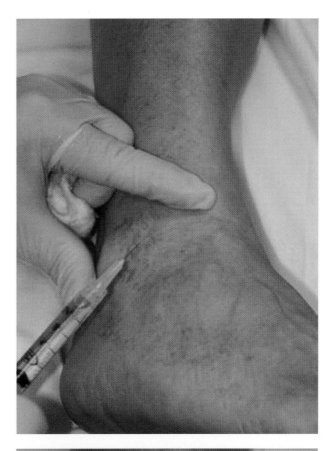

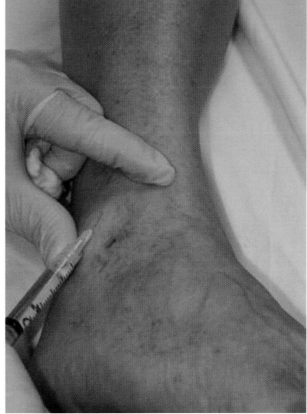

■ **Fig 11–23** Injections.

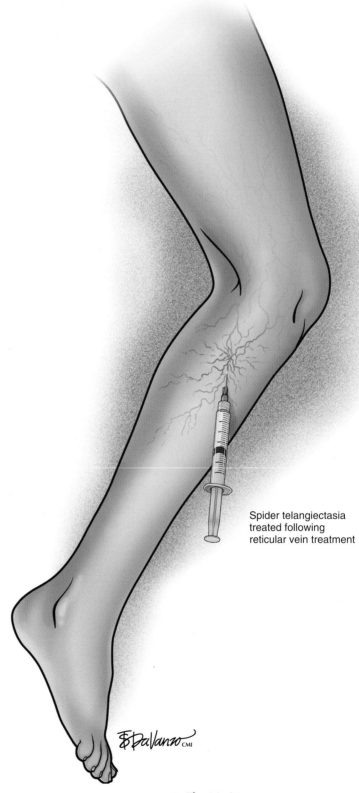

Spider telangiectasia
treated following
reticular vein treatment

■ Fig 11–24

PEARLS AND PITFALLS

Foam sclerotherapy has greatly improved the outcome of varicose vein sclerotherapy.[4] However, its merits in terms of the treatment of spider telangiectasias are less clear. The foam actually increases the surface area of contact by displacing the blood as opposed to injecting the sclerosing agent only, which is diluted by the blood. The foam then thickens the blood vessel wall, causing less blood to pass through. The same effect of foaming can be achieved with the use of only the sclerosing agent by keeping the needle within the vein after injection and maintaining slight pressure on the plunger. The reticular feeding veins may benefit from foam because they are larger and more difficult to visualize.

Foam sclerotherapy is also associated with greater risk in terms of potential complications because air is added to the vascular system. Several reports of neurologic events have been noted. These risks may be reduced by using CO_2 as the gas rather than air. CO_2 rapidly dissolves in blood, whereas the nitrogen in air does not.[5]

Sclerotherapy therapy may not improve spider telangiectasias if matting develops in the vasculature. Matting is the formation of new, fine spider veins in an area previously injected. This area may improve with additional treatments or may need further evaluation. Various imaging devices may be used to assess for venous hypertension caused by an incompetent saphenous or perforator vein. Ultrasound may show an underlying refluxing vein that should be treated. Vein lights and infrared imaging, such as the vein viewer and polarized light, may help to identify the reticular vein feeding the spider complex (Fig. 11-25).

Pain is one of the most common complaints during the procedure, and several methods have been used in an attempt to allay and reduce the pain. Adding lidocaine to the solution or pretreating the area with a topical anesthetic, such as topical lidocaine or EMLA, can reduce the pain from the needle stick but these measures do not typically reduce the pain from the sclerosing solution itself. Alternative pain minimization procedures are consistently being investigated. One method, popular in South America, uses hypertonic solutions that are cooled to −30°C while cold air is blown onto the area being injected with this cold solution. The cold solution acts not only as an anesthetic but also increases contact time with the vein walls as it is more viscous than solutions at room temperature. Advocates of this method believe that these colder solutions improve the outcomes of the procedure as well.

If, after several weeks posttreatment there is no significant improvement of the affected area(s), a different, stronger, and/or higher concentration of the sclerosant can be attempted for better results. Before this is done, however, it must be determined if there is some overlooked underlying problem, such as venous insufficiency, that must be addressed. Additionally, the feeder veins must be assessed to determine whether they were adequately treated. A repeat ultrasound may reveal an underlying problem that was missed on the initial assessment and examination. The imaging techniques previously described may also reveal feeder veins that must be addressed before the spider veins can be successfully treated.

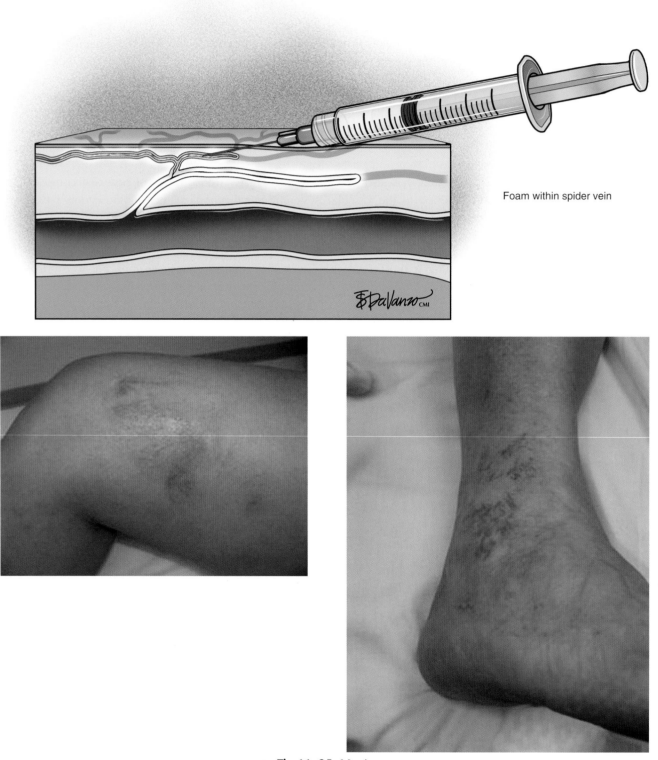

Foam within spider vein

■ **Fig 11–25** Matting.

COMPLICATIONS AND ADVERSE SEQUELAE

The potential complications of sclerotherapy for telangiectatic veins and varicosities are numerous and varied, but most often they are temporary in nature and not serious. Some of the most commonly occurring and less severe complications and adverse sequelae of these treatments include the following:

- Injection site pain
- Edema
- Urticaria localized over the injection site
- Tape compression blisters and folliculitis
- Hyperpigmentation
- Recurrence of treated vessels
- Other conditions such as staining and matting

Included among the more serious and less commonly occurring complications and adverse sequelae associated with these procedures are the following:

- Nerve damage
- Superficial thrombophlebitis
- Pulmonary emboli and deep venous thrombosis (DVT)
- Air emboli
- Distal necrosis resulting from an inadvertent injection of a sclerosing agent into an artery
- Allergic reactions
- Cutaneous necrosis

Pain

Pain and soreness are sometimes experienced; however, there are a number of interventions that can be used to minimize and eliminate this discomfort. The pain and discomfort are a function of several variables including the treatment site, the injection technique, the sclerosing agent, and the needle itself. The level of discomfort is typically greatest when the feet, ankles, medial knees, and/or medial upper thighs are treated. Pain and discomfort can be prevented or diminished with the use of the smallest possible gauge bevelled needle that is silicone coated, sclerosing agents with a lidocaine additive, and slow infusion followed immediately by massage.

The hypertonic solutions used for sclerotherapy are synonymous with pain and discomfort; however, the pain can be decreased without any compromise in terms of desired outcome when a 2% solution of nonacidified lidocaine is added to the sclerosing agent and no more than 0.1 mL is slowly injected into each site followed by massage. Although the effectiveness of the treatment is not compromised, the addition of lidocaine may increase the risk of an allergic response. The addition of 1% lidocaine and a limitation of no more than 0.1 mL per site are recommended for glycerin sclerosing solutions to prevent pain and cramping. STS and POL are virtually painless with proper technique; however, STS can lead to pain when it is accidentally injected into perivascular areas.

Any transient pain or discomfort can be effectively treated with properly fitting graduated compression stockings for a week or two after the treatment. The presence of severe and/or unrelieved pain signals the need to assess the patient for venous thrombosis and inflammation.

Edema

Temporary swelling can result from a number of factors, including the nature of the treated site, perivascular and intravascular space differentials, endothelial permeability, the strength of the sclerosing solution, the volume of the sclerosing solution, and the lack of proper graduated compression after the treatment (tourniquet effect).

Posttelangiectasia treatment edema is most often associated with treatment areas below the ankle; however, edema can be present in other areas as well. Limiting volume to no more than 1 mL for each ankle can prevent or minimize swelling in this area. The extent of inflammation and resulting edema in the perivascular area is affected by the strength of the sclerosing agent and the client's unique status in terms of mast cells (sensitivity), medication profile (e.g., non-steroidal antiinflammatory drugs [NSAIDs], corticosteroids), and a history of sclerosing agent sensitivity. The application of graduated compression stockings for up to 3 weeks posttreatment may be helpful for some patients, as is the application of a topical corticosteroid to enhance the antiinflammatory response. Patients must be educated about the proper application of their graduated compression stockings and about the signs of edema that can occur as a result of their poor application.

Urticaria

Localized urticaria, typically occurring over the injection site and lasting only a few minutes, is a result of transient irritation and the release of histamine. This transient complication, however, must be scrupulously differentiated from sensitivity and the onset of a systemic allergic response, which can be very serious.

The intensity of the localized itching tends to be positively correlated with the strength of the sclerosing agent. The incidence of urticaria is most often associated with the use of POL and STS as well as a failure to limit the volume of the agent. Prevention and treatment consist of the application of a topical corticosteroid to the injection sites immediately after treatment and limiting the volume of the solution for each injection site.

Blisters and Folliculitis

Blisters and folliculitis usually occur as the result of tape used to secure dressing pads. Blisters most commonly occur

- During the summer months (perspiration and moisture)
- Among those who are thin
- Among the elderly and other people who have fragile skin
- On areas behind the knee, the interior aspect of the thigh, and other areas where there is tissue movement

Tapes with the greatest adhesiveness place patients at more risk for blisters than less adhesive tapes like paper tape. Although blisters are relatively harmless, they must be assessed in order to determine whether these lesions are an allergic response, infection, or a sign of early cutaneous necrosis. Blisters can be prevented with the use of a tubular support bandage, rather than tape, over the pad for stability as the compression stocking is applied. An occlusive hydroactive dressing can be placed over the blister if it does not resolve on its own.

Folliculitis, like a blister, most commonly occurs during the summer months and as a result of a tape dressing. The treatment consists of the application of a topical antibiotic, such as clindamycin or erythromycin, and/or an antibacterial cleanser such as Hibiclens. This complication is often self-limiting or effectively treated with topical antimicrobials. Folliculitis rarely requires the use of a systemic antimicrobial drug.

Hyperpigmentation

Hyperpigmentation, or cutaneous pigmentation, is a relatively common occurrence after treatment, regardless of the sclerosing agent that is used (Fig. 11-26). Hyperpigmentation is often very temporary in nature; however, rare persistence can occur for a small number of patients 1-year posttreatment. Most areas of pigmentation occur along the linear aspect of the treated vein. These areas indicate that the vein is no longer functioning. Less commonly encountered occurrences, such as those found at the injection site(s), can also occur as the result of the sclerosing agent's endothelial damage, inflammation, and red blood cell extravasation into the area. Areas below the knee and vessels from 0.6 to 1.2 mm in diameter are at greatest risk. Affected areas usually resolve within 6 to 12 months after sclerotherapy.

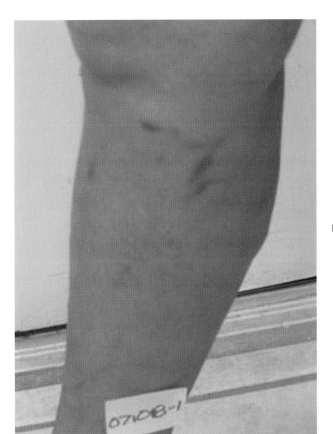

■ **Fig 11–26** Hyperpigmentation.

Hyperpigmentation results from a number of factors, including the type of sclerosing agent, the concentration of the agent, the technique used, the postprocedure treatment(s), the diameter of the vessel, and pressures (gravitational and intravascular). Additionally, the risk of hyperpigmentation increases with some unique patient characteristics, including an innate predisposition for hyperpigmentation, and medication(s), particularly minocycline (Dynacin, Minocin), taken at the time of the treatment.

Prevention aims to minimize necrosis and to avoid total endothelial destruction as well as accompanying red blood cell extravasation. The incidence of hyperpigmentation can be decreased with a number of preventive measures including, but not limited to, those listed next.

> Use sclerosing agents that have been scientifically associated with the least incidence of hyperpigmentation and inflammation. These solutions include sodium salicylate, glycerin, and chromated glycerin (CG).
>
> Keep the concentration of the sclerosing agent to the minimum necessary for effectiveness. Liquid agents are less potent than foams, so when a foam is used, it is necessary to modify the concentration, particularly when spider veins are treated.
>
> Inject the agent with a 3-ml syringe, rather than a smaller one, because injection pressure increases proportionately with smaller piston diameters. Red blood cell extravasation and vessel rupture are more apt to occur with increased injection pressures.
>
> Remove posttreatment coagulation using a gentle rocking expression of the clot via a small incision made with a 21-gauge needle (Fig. 11-27).

Although a number of hyperpigmentation treatments have been used, it appears that many have limited and/or questionable effectiveness, other than treatment with a Q-switched laser.

Recurrence of Treated Vessels

The recurrence of treated veins is common but also troublesome, particularly for the patient who has undergone the treatment. The practitioner may be able to rule out suspected recurrence with a thorough examination 1-year posttreatment that identifies the area(s) as new or previously untreated telangiectasia, rather than a recurrence of the treated vessels.

When it is present, the degree and extent of recurrence are positively correlated with the degree of intravascular thrombosis; therefore, the most important preventive measures aim to limit intravascular thromboses. Adequate compression for an adequate duration of time is necessary to prevent recurrence.

Other Minor Conditions

Other complications and adverse sequelae include harmless suntan fading, telangiectatic matting (as discussed earlier), staining, vasovagal reflex (stress related), localized hypertrichosis, and transient urticaria, which warrants attention because it may signal a systemic allergy.

Nerve Damage

Temporary paresthesia and permanent nerve damage can occur because of the proximity of some nerves to the sclerotherapy injection sites. Temporary paresthesia, most often lasting less than 6 months, can occur when the local inflammatory process affects superficial sensory nerves.

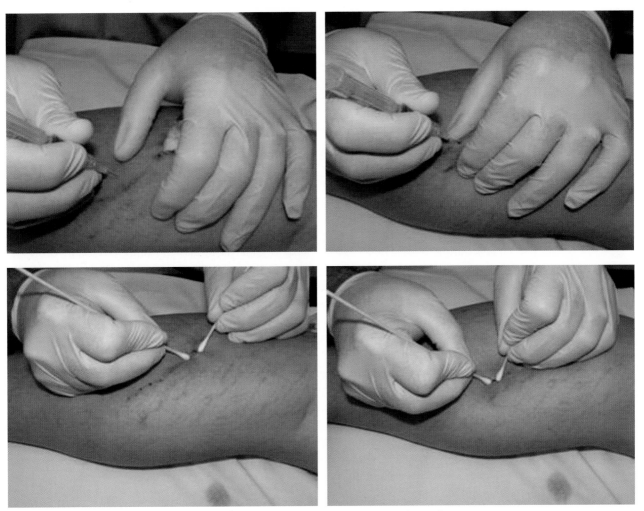

■ **Fig 11-27** Incision and drainage (I & D).

Treatment consists of the administration of NSAIDs. Major nerve damage, although very rare, can occur. This damage occurs from poor technique and malformations or anomalies of the patient's venous system.

Superficial Thrombophlebitis

The advent of posttreatment graduated compression has greatly diminished the incidence and prevalence of thrombophlebitis; however, it does occur on some occasions for a variety of reasons. Some patients are at risk for thrombophlebitis because they are predisposed to it as a result of an innate state of hypercoagulopathy. Other examples of predisposition are conditions and disorders such as pregnancy, genetic excesses of coagulation factor VII, and a protein C deficiency.

Superficial thrombophlebitis presents as an induration that is tender and reddened or an area of hyperpigmentation along the vein, usually from 1 to 3 weeks after treatment. For the most part, this complication can be prevented with posttreatment compression over the entire leg (not just the treated area), which is adequate in terms of both duration and degree.

When prevention is not successful, the treatment of thrombophlebitis consists of maintaining adequate compression, NSAIDs, drainage, frequent ambulation, and, at times, low-molecular-weight heparin.

Emboli and Deep Venous Thrombosis

Fortunately, pulmonary emboli and deep venous thrombosis (DVT) are rare occurrences subsequent to sclerotherapy. Nonetheless, the incidence of DVT is probably grossly underestimated because it is often overlooked and not diagnosed as such. Although many cases are not properly or promptly diagnosed, there are clinical signs that should alert the practitioner. Among these signs are the cardinal signs of inflammation (redness, heat, swelling, pain, loss of function), dilated superficial veins, some laboratory markers, such as plasma D-dimers, as well as venous Doppler and impedance phlebography results. DVT usually presents 8 to 10 hours after treatment, particularly during times when vascular stasis is greatest. Pulmonary emboli typically occur from 5 to 7 days after thrombus formation. Because the mortality rate from a DVT and pulmonary emboli, without treatment, is alarmingly high, a thorough assessment of the patient and his or her risk factors as well as careful posttreatment monitoring are essential components of care. Patient education is also important. The patient and family members must be informed about the signs and symptoms of DVT and emboli and the importance of immediately reporting their observations to the physician.

Although the cause of DVT is largely unknown, it appears that both intrinsic patient-related factors (a hypercoagulability predisposition) and extrinsic treatment-related factors (vascular stasis and endothelial damage) have an impact on the occurrence of DVT. Limiting the volume of the sclerosing agent to only 0.5 to 1 mL per site, adequate compression with properly fitted graduated support hose (30 to 40 mm Hg pressure), and encouraging physical activity (muscular movement) immediately after the procedure will reduce thromboembolic complications. Additionally, use extreme caution when the patient has a thrombophilia to prevent this serious postsclerotherapy complication.

The treatment of DVT must be immediate, decisive, and highly effective. A rapid reduction of clots can be accomplished with peripheral or direct infusions of a thrombolytic agent such as urokinase or a tissue plasminogen activator (t-PA). Alternative treatment consists of the administration of anticoagulation therapy using intravenous heparin, which is then followed by warfarin, heparin subcutaneously, or a low-molecular-weight heparin (LMWH) preparation, such as enoxaparin sodium (Lovenox).

Air Embolism

Small amounts of air entering the venous system do not pose a threat because these minimal amounts usually absorb into the blood, without ill effect, before the bloodstream reaches the pulmonary circulation. Larger amounts of air, however, such as may occur when using foams, can potentially lead to air emboli that manifest with migraines, nausea, and visual disturbances, all of which are usually self-limiting and without any long-term adverse effects.

Distal necrosis may occur from an inadvertent injection into an artery. This complication is quite rare but it perpetually plagues the thoughts of the physician because no sclerosing treatment is totally risk free of this complication, a complication that mandates intense immediate action. Arterial injection of a sclerosing agent can lead to emboli, occlusion, blood flow stasis, and necrosis. The most vulnerable areas include the groin, the medial or posterior malleolar area, and the back of the knee.

This complication requires instantaneous action. The sclerosing agent and blood should be aspirated immediately upon the realization that this inadvertent injection has occurred. This action

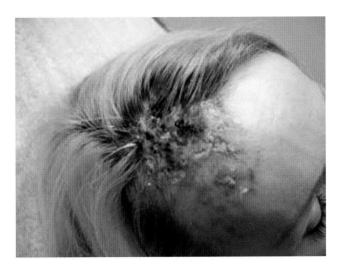

■ **Fig 11-28** Arterial injection.

should be immediately followed by an injection of heparin (10,000 units) using the same needle kept in place with only the replacement of the syringe containing heparin, often a feat for only the ambidextrous, particularly when the patient is experiencing acute and severe pain. Ongoing treatment consists of the application of ice to the affected area, a heparin regimen for 6 or more days, IV dextran 10% for 3 days, and nifedipine, hydralazine, or prazosin orally for 30 days. At times, direct thrombolytic therapy is indicated.

An inadvertent injection into an artery is best prevented with arterial visualization using duplex imagery and having the patient in an upright position when the challenging malleolar area is injected (Fig. 11-28).

Allergic Reactions

Systemic allergic reactions are rare; nonetheless, they can occur. Some allergic reactions are minor and transient, whereas others can be severe and life threatening. Nonetheless, all patients with even minor allergic reactions must be assessed and monitored for any signs of a more serious reaction, including bronchospasm, angioedema, anaphylaxis, pulmonary toxicity, renal toxicity, and cardiac toxicity.

Minor allergic reactions, such as urticaria, are typically treated with an antihistamine, such as hydroxyzine (Atarax) or diphenhydramine (Benadryl). Prednisone may also be added for a brief course of therapy. Angioedema, with and without respiratory stridor, is treated with an oral antihistamine and intramuscular diphenhydramine in combination with intravenous corticosteroids, respectively. Aminophylline intravenously, an inhaled bronchodilator, corticosteroids, and antihistamines usually successfully treat bronchospasm without any further intervention; however, the practitioner must be aware of the fact that bronchospasm may signal the onset of anaphylaxis.

The earliest warning signs of impending anaphylaxis include urticaria, angioedema, itching, rising levels of anxiety, wheezing, coughing, and other more subtle warnings. The three classic signs of actual anaphylaxis, a severe life-threatening condition that requires immediate attention, are bronchospasm, respiratory airway edema, and vascular collapse (systemic vasodilation and cardiac failure). Emergency treatment and transport to an acute care facility in the community are most often necessary. This condition is treated with epinephrine to maintain blood pressure, intubation, theophylline, and oxygen to establish and maintain adequate oxygenation as well as other medications such as corticosteroids and diphenhydramine.

Some of the sclerosing agents that are most often associated with an allergic reaction include:

- Ethanolamine oleate
- Sodium morrhuate
- STS
- Chromated glycerin
- Plain glycerin
- POL
- Polyiodinated iodine
- Hypertonic saline
- Heparin
- Sodium salicylate
- Lidocaine (an additive to glycerin and hypertonic saline)

Cutaneous Necrosis

This most often self-limiting complication can occur, albeit rarely, irrespective of sclerosing agent type. Several factors impact on the occurrence of cutaneous necrosis. These include extravasation, injection into an arteriole, reactive vasospasm, lymphatic injection, and excessive compression.

The extent and degree of extravasation are functions of both the type of the sclerosing agent and the concentration given. Despite good technique, a small amount of the sclerosing solution may leak into the surrounding tissue as the needle is withdrawn or when numerous punctures are necessary, thus leading to extravasation. More toxic solutions pose greater threats to subcutaneous damage than less toxic ones. For example, glycerin and CG are less toxic to tissue than is STS.

Inadvertent arteriolar injection may occur as a result of a rapid, large volume injection of a sclerosing agent into telangiectasias with microshunts. Glycerin solutions are believed to be the least offensive in terms of arteriolar injection and subsequent tissue ulceration. Likewise, lymphatic vessel injection can also lead to cutaneous necrosis, particularly if the patient has lymphovenous anastomoses and the solution is caustic. Reactive arterial vasospasm also plays a role in terms of cutaneous necrosis. Some people, for unknown reasons, tend to have a predisposition to these vasospasms. Vigorous massage, in combination with a topical nitroglycerin ointment, may alleviate or eliminate this problem. Last, cutaneous ulceration, as a result of tissue ischemia and anoxia, may occur when there is excessive localized compression. It is therefore recommended that the patient wear a graduated compression stocking of no more than 40 mm Hg when in the supine position for long durations of time. Other preventive measures include the use of double stockings during non–bed rest times and the removal of the outer one during periods of bed rest so that the pressure can be lowered to an acceptable level.

Cutaneous necrosis can be prevented with the dilution of sclerosing solutions and the injection of hyaluronidase into multiple sites around the extravasation within 60 minutes of the episode, should extravasation occur (Fig. 11-29).

Summary of Complications and Adverse Sequelae

The adverse sequelae and complications associated with sclerotherapy of telangiectatic veins and varicosities can often be prevented; however, these procedures can never be devoid of inherent

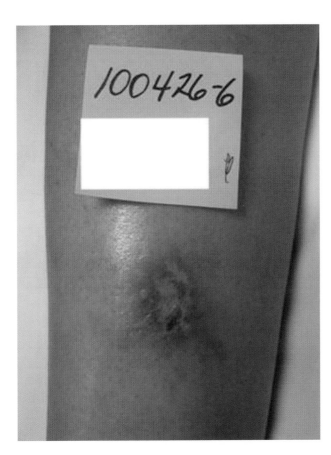

■ **Fig 11-29** Ulcer.

risks despite all preventive measures and superior technique. Some of these untoward events are minor, transient, and self-limiting, but some are life threatening and serious. Patients must be given complete information about the procedure, its benefits, risks, follow-up care, and alternatives for them to give informed consent prior to the procedure.

Comparative Effectiveness

Comparative research studies have been conducted to determine the relative effectiveness of the various sclerosants that are used for spider telangiectasias. Curlin and Ratz compared the effectiveness of STS 0.5%, POL 0.25%, and HS 20% with heparin. The results of this research indicated that POL was best tolerated while HS and STS showed fastest clearing. In terms of effectiveness, there were no statistically significant differences among STS 0.5%, POL 0.25%, and HS 20% with heparin.[6]

Goldman[7] compared STS 0.25% and POL 0.5% and found little difference in terms of effectiveness. Another study, comparing 100% CG, POL 0.25% solution, and POL 0.25% foam, indicated that CG was associated with higher degrees of pain, better clearance, and no staining or matting, while foam POL caused the most staining and matting.[8] Another study, by Leach and Goldman, compared 72% glycerin diluted 2:1 with 1% lidocaine with epinephrine and STS 0.25%. This study showed significantly better and more rapid clearance with the glycerin and less staining than the STS.[9]

LASER TREATMENT OF SPIDER TELANGIECTASIAS

Historical Perspective

The laser is a relative newcomer to the treatment domain of lower extremity spider vein treatment; however, it is gaining increased popularity and refinement. This technological newcomer's popularity is, interestingly, primarily driven by the consumer, not the practitioner, unlike most other new advances. Lasers are particularly useful for lower extremity spider veins that arise from matting or are refractory to sclerotherapy treatment. They treatments are also useful for people who have phobias, fears, and concerns relating to needles. Despite its advantages, however, laser use has some limitations, including the fact they are an adjunctive and complementary therapy after sclerotherapy, rather than a substitute for it.

Basic Concepts and Terminology

"Laser," an acronym for *l*ight *a*mplification by *s*timulated *e*mission of *r*adiation, produces a beam of monochromic, coherent, collimated light of a specific wavelength. "Pumping" is a term used to describe the process of supplying the amount of energy necessary for the amplification of the laser beam. This energy can be delivered as light, of varying wavelengths, or as an electrical current, which is measured in terms of joules (J). The amount of energy delivered to an area is referred to as "fluence," and it can be represented as J/cm^2. The power with which the energy is delivered is referred to as "watts." A watt is equivalent to one joule per second. The number of watts (W) that are delivered to a given unit area, typically indicated as W/cm^2, is called "irradiance." Last, "pulse width" is the duration of laser exposure and it is documented in terms of milliseconds.

The therapeutic usefulness as well as the possible untoward effects of laser treatments are based on the fact that as a laser beam strikes the skin, it leads to four reactions: scattering, absorption, transmission, and reflection. Scattering is a function of wavelength and the presence of substances such as collagen, both of which can potentially have an impact on the occurrence of collateral, unintended tissue damage. For example, shorter wavelengths are associated with increased scattering compared to longer wavelengths. Laser photons are absorbed, and thus therapeutic, when they are not impeded by reflection, scattering, or transmission. The challenges to the practitioner arise from the fact that veins vary in terms of their ability to absorb the laser's energy and each laser generator delivers only one wavelength without any built-in mechanisms to vary it, with one exception—the tunable dye laser. In other words, deeper veins require a longer wavelength than more superficial ones, but the wavelength of a specific generator is fixed; therefore, no variation of wavelength is possible. Only power, spot size, and pulse width can be manipulated in order to attack the full thickness and circumference of the vein wall.

Lasers work by emitting the pulse of light that is absorbed by the hemoglobin in the blood vessel with just enough heat to the vein to cause irreparable, desired, damage to the vein but not enough to damage the skin as a result of the laser's absorption by melanin.

Ideally, the laser should deliver the precise amount of energy needed to damage the intended vein target but not cause any damage to the surrounding tissue, including the skin. It should also be capable of delivering this energy for precisely the correct duration in order to slowly coagulate the vessel's full thickness and entire circumference without rupturing it. In the real world, however, perfect techniques and equipment are not a reality, so the typical laser wavelength used is between 600 and 900 nm.

The shape of the beam and the wavelength of the emitted light for each type of laser give it its unique and specific characteristics. The use of lasers has some advantages in terms of telangiectasias treatment, and many of the complications that are associated with sclerotherapy are not likely to occur with noninvasive laser treatment. Furthermore, this diminished risk is not solely limited to the drug introduced into the body.

Shorter wavelength lasers have very good hemoglobin absorption but they do not penetrate very deeply. They also have higher melanin absorption, something that competes with the hemoglobin. Longer wavelengths have both less hemoglobin absorption and less melanin absorption. They penetrate the skin more deeply. Deeper and larger spider telangiectasias respond better to longer, rather than shorter, wavelength lasers, and they are much better tolerated by darker skin tones, which are more tolerant and more forgiving than lighter skin tones.

Other factors are also important for the practitioner's consideration. For example, how much energy should be given (joules), and how will that energy be delivered? Will it be given using a short burst or using a long pulse? Lasers also offer us a limited number of other variables that can be manipulated to optimize results. For example, stacking pulses allow cooling of the skin between pulses to take full advantage of the different heat specificities between skin and hemoglobin. Additionally, there are methods to cool the skin in order to protect it from burns (cold air, ice packs, cold solutions through clear glass, and a cryogen spray).

Many different lasers have been used for the treatment spider veins, but this section briefly addresses the most common lasers used today.

Types of Lasers

With rare exception, the primary lasers used today for leg veins are light sources and pulsed lasers. Included in these categories are the following types of lasers.

- Potassium titanyl phosphate (KTP 532 nm)
- Yellow pulsed dye laser (585 nm to 605 nm)
- Alexandrite or infrared 755-nm laser
- Diode or infrared 810-nm, 940-nm, and 980-nm laser
- Neodymium:yttrium-aluminium-garnet (Nd:YAG) laser infrared to 1064 nm
- Intense pulsed light (IPL) broadband light source laser with 515 to 1200 nm

KTP and frequency-doubled Nd:YAG 532 nm lasers provide a very short pulse that works exceptionally well on the fine red spider veins. The shorter wavelength, however, does not penetrate very deeply, and it is absorbed by the melanin in the skin, making it NOT the treatment of choice among patients with darker skin types.

Diode lasers come in multiple wavelengths. The wavelengths used for the treatment of spider veins are 810 nm, 940 nm, and 980 nm. These spectrums have considerable hemoglobin absorption, lesser degrees of melanin absorption, and deeper penetration; thus, they are suitable for the treatment of veins up to 1 mm in diameter.

The Nd:YAG 1064-nm laser has become the most widely used laser for the treatment of leg telangiectasias. It provides deeper penetration and less melanin absorption than the other wavelengths. It also has less hemoglobin absorption; however, it also increases water absorption. Higher energies are required with this laser, but these energies are well tolerated because they absorb low levels of melanin. Pain is a commonly occurring phenomenon, however, with this laser. A cooling intervention, such as cold air, cold water between glass, or cryogen spray, is

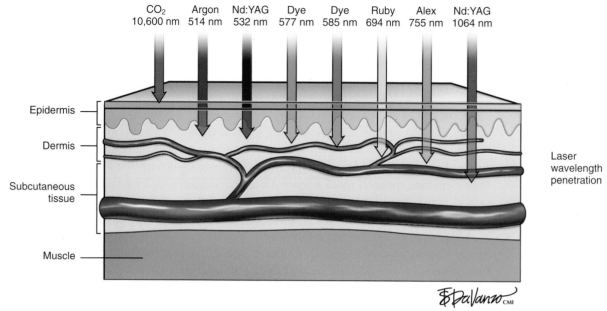

◾ **Fig 11–30** Laser wavelength penetration.

frequently used to reduce any patient's discomfort. A topical anesthetic with lidocaine, for vaso-dilation, is also effective to combat the pain.

Regardless of the laser equipment used, however, there are some pitfalls and concerns that are common to all; therefore, the physician should resist the temptation of overtreating the vessels by delivering unnecessary passes and/or greater than necessary fluences. These actions may lead to blanching, hypopigmentation, and/or necrosis with hyperpigmentation (Fig. 11-30; see Fig. 6-1).

Operative Steps

As previously discussed, the initial steps in laser treatment include a patient assessment, a thorough discussion of the benefits and potential risks of treatment, and photographic documentation. Next, the practitioner must decide which laser to use and what settings should be used for the particular patient.

As discussed previously, smaller red spider veins are typically very superficial veins; therefore, shorter wavelength lasers are the treatment of choice. For example, the KTP 532-nm laser has been used successfully on these fine red spider veins. On the other hand, the Nd:YAG 1064-nm laser works better than the KTP 532-nm laser on larger veins up to, and including, the small reticular veins.

The next decision-making point is determining spot size or the diameter of the laser beam needed to treat the area. The smaller the spot diameter, the more concentrated is the energy—therefore, less energy is needed. Smaller veins can be treated with small spot sizes as low as 1 mm. Larger spider veins, of about 1 mm, require a 2- to 4-mm spot size in order to effectively cover the vein. Larger veins, that is, those over 1 mm, are best treated with 6-mm spot size.

Following are determinations regarding the best pulse duration, the best duration between pulses, and the amount of energy to use. Pulse duration is another variable that can be manipulated in order to achieve optimal results based on the particular vein that will be treated. Smaller veins heat up more quickly than larger veins; therefore, very short pulses are necessary to alleviate this potential hazard when treating the smaller veins. Larger veins take longer to heat up so longer pulses are needed to achieve desired outcomes.

Some lasers will stack pulses allowing for cooling intervals between pulses; therefore, a delay time between pulses may be part of the settings, something that may have to be adjusted according to the unique needs of the patient. Darker skin tones have to cool longer between pulses then lighter skin tones. Energy settings can be by watts or by joules; joules take into account the pulse duration while watts do not. Most lasers are set by joules. Again, larger veins need more energy.

Finally there are different cooling devices from which the practitioner must choose. Some of these choices include cooled air blown on the skin, ice packs, and cryogen air. Regardless of choice, however, each alternative must be carefully implemented either just before and/or just after the pulse of laser light. Pulsed cryogen air timing has to be scrupulously managed because too liberal use may lead to vasospasm and a decrease in the amount of hemoglobin necessary for light absorption. Because cooling prevents or alleviates patient discomfort and it also provides protection against skin injury, it should be a routine aspect of laser treatment.

The most frequently encountered complication associated with cutaneous lasers is a skin burn that could result in a blister, pigmentary changes, and/or scarring. The extent of any burn is affected by several factors, including the wavelength used, the amount of energy delivered, the patient's skin type, and sun exposure prior to the treatment. Shorter wavelengths are more likely to injure the skin than are longer ones because shorter wavelengths have a higher degree of melanin absorption. For this reason, short wavelength lasers should be used with caution in darker skin types.

The amount of energy delivered is also a factor that impacts on the occurrence and extent of any skin injury. Enough energy at virtually all wavelengths will cause skin injury. Joules, again, are calculated as watts per second; therefore, 100 J given in over 100 msec is very different than 100 J given over 20 msec. More optimal results are sometimes achieved by treating darker skinned individuals with the long pulsed 1064-nm Nd:YAG laser, especially for larger spider veins.

Darker skin types have more melanin, and melanin absorbs energy from light as well as hemoglobin. People with darker skin tones are more likely to have an injury from laser treatment and therefore should be approached with caution. Possibly even more important than skin type, however, is recent sun exposure. Sun exposure stimulates melanin production, so even people with light-colored skin may have increased melanin after sun exposure, thus increasing the risk of injury with laser treatment. The patient should be advised to avoid sun exposure for at least 2 weeks before the anticipated treatment and to continue sun avoidance for at least 2 weeks postprocedure.

Eye injury, for both the patient and the practitioner, is also a potential complication of laser treatment. It is essential, therefore, that adequate protective eyewear be worn in order to block the laser wavelength. Lead shields are also used, especially if the laser is used near the eyes (Figs. 11-31 to 11-33)

Comparative Effectiveness

To date, there have been only a few studies comparing cutaneous laser treatment of spider telangiectasia and sclerotherapy. In 2002, research supported the fact that lasers were more effective for sclerotherapy than for spider telangiectasia.[10] A second study led to similar results, but a greater degree of patient satisfaction was observed with sclerotherapy.[11] In 2004, a sequential study comparing Nd:YAG 1064-nm laser treatment followed by sclerotherapy and sclerotherapy followed by laser treatment. The results of this research suggested that the best results were achieved with sclerotherapy followed by laser treatment.[12]

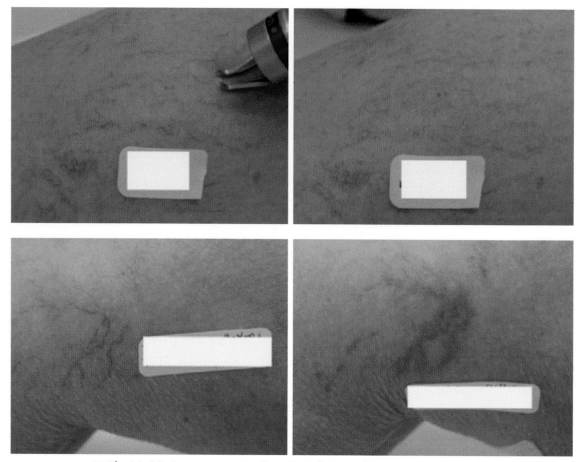

■ **Fig 11–31** Laser treatment Dornier 940 nm. *(Courtesy Dr. R. Bush.)*

■ **Fig 11–32** Sciton Nd:YAG laser.

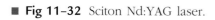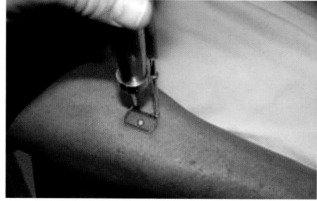

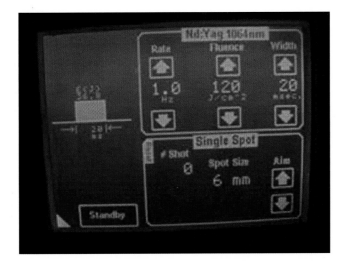

■ **Fig 11–33** Sciton screen settings.

The current consensus is that sclerotherapy remains the primary treatment of choice for leg telangiectasias, but some are convinced that a combination of sclerotherapy and laser may have synergistic effects. This belief was challenged, however, in 1990 by Golman and Fitzpatrick.[13] This research indicated that there were no statistically significant improvements in terms of outcome with this combination. Furthermore, increased complications were observed when compared with the complications encountered with sclerotherapy alone.

In summary, current data do not support laser treatment as the preferred modality for the treatment of leg telangiectasias when compared with sclerotherapy. It can and should be used as an adjunct to it or with "needle phobic" patients and those with allergies to the commonly used sclerosants.

REFERENCES

1. Biegeleisen HI. Telangiectasia associated with varicose veins: treatment by microinjection technique. JAMA 1934;102:2092.
2. Foley WT. The eradication of venous blemishes. Cutis 1975;15:665.
3. Nootheti PK, Cadag KM, Magpantay A, et al. Efficacy of graduated compression stockings for an additional 3 weeks after sclerotherapy treatment for reticular and telangiectatic leg veins. Dermatol Surg 2009;35:53-57.
4. Rao J, Wildemore JK, Goldman MP. Double-blind prospective comparative trial between foamed and liquid polidocanol and sodium tetradecyl sulfate in the treatment of varicose and telangiectatic leg veins. Dermatol Surg 2005;31:631-635.
5. Morrison N, Neuhardt DL, Rogers CR, et al. Comparison of side effects using air and carbon dioxide foam for endovenous chemical ablation. J Vasc Surg 2008;47:830-836.
6. Curlin MC, Ratz JL. Treatment of telangiectasia: comparison of sclerosing agents. J Dermatologic Surg Oncol 1987;13:1181.
7. Goldman MP. Treatment of varicose and telangiectatic leg veins: double-blind prospective trial between aethoxysclerol and sotradecol. Derm Surg 2002;28:52.
8. Kern P, Ramelet AA, Wutschert R, et al. Single-blind, randomized study comparing chromated glycerin, polidocanol solution and polidocanol foam for treatment of telangiectatic leg veins. Dermatol Surg 2004;30:367-372.
9. Leach B, Goldman MP. Comparative trial between sodium tetradecyl sulfate and glycerin in the treatment of telangiectatic leg veins. Dermatol Surg 2003;29:612.
10. Lupton JR, Alster TS, Romero P. Clinical comparison of sclerotherapy vs long pulsed Nd:YAG laser treatment of lower extremity telangiectasia. Derm Surg 2002;28:694-697.

11. Coles MC, Werner RS, Zelickson BD. Comparative pilot study evaluating the treatment of leg veins with a long pulse Nd:YAG laser and sclerotherapy. Lasers Surg Med 2002;30: 154-159.

12. Levy J, Elbahr C, Jouve E, Mordon S. Comparison and sequential study of long pulsed Nd:YAG 1064 nm laser and sclerotherapy in leg telangiectasia treatment. Lasers Surg Med 2004;34:273.

13. Goldman MP, Fitzpatrick RE. Pulsed-dye laser treatment of leg telangiectasia with and without simultaneous sclerotherapy. J Derm Surg Oncol 1990;16:338-344.

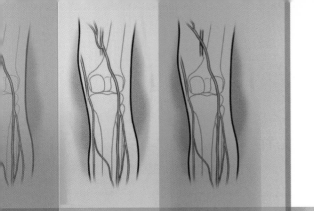

CHAPTER 12

Thromboembolic Disease

Timothy K. Liem and Jose I. Almeida

HISTORICAL BACKGROUND AND EPIDEMIOLOGY OF ACUTE VENOUS THROMBOEMBOLIC DISEASE

The incidence of deep venous thrombosis (DVT) ranges from 5 to 9 per 10,000 person-years in the general population, and the incidence of venous thromboembolism (DVT and pulmonary embolism [PE] combined) (VTE) is about 14 per 10,000 person-years.[1,2] This equates to more than 275,000 new cases of VTE per year in the United States.[3] The number of identifiable risk factors that predispose to the development of VTE has steadily grown. This information has allowed physicians to provide more effective thromboembolism prophylaxis that is evidence-based and stratified according to the number of risk factors present. In patients with established DVT and PE, there has been a relatively recent emphasis evaluating the rate of recurrence and the clinical factors that predispose to recurrent VTE. In turn, the type and duration of long-term anticoagulation also continue to be stratified, based on the number of risk factors for recurrence.

Physicians from a variety of medical and surgical specialties participate in the care of these patients, and vascular surgeons often are called on to assist in their care and should therefore be familiar with the risk factors for VTE and the optimal medical therapy for these patients. This chapter describes risk factors for a first episode of VTE and the options for initial anticoagulation. An increasing number of risk factors and associated conditions that increase the predilection for recurrent VTE continue to be identified. The optimal duration and type of longer-term antithrombotic therapy are also covered, and the role of adjunctive vena cava filters is discussed briefly. VTE prophylaxis, modalities for the diagnosis of VTE, and thrombolytic therapy for VTE are beyond the scope of this chapter and are not discussed in detail.

ETIOLOGY AND NATURAL HISTORY OF ACUTE VENOUS THROMBOEMBOLISM

Etiology

Venous thrombosis may develop as a result of endothelial damage, hypercoagulability, and venous stasis (Virchow triad). Of these risk factors, relative hypercoagulability appears most important in most cases of spontaneous DVT, whereas stasis and endothelial damage play a greater role in secondary DVT following immobilization, surgery, or trauma. Identifiable risk factors for VTE may be classified as inherited, acquired, and those with a mixed etiology (Table 12-1).

When multiple inherited and acquired risk factors are present in the same patient, a synergistic effect may occur. Clinically manifest thrombosis most often occurs with the convergence of multiple genetic and acquired risk factors.[4] Hospitalized patients have an average of 1.5 risk factors per patient, with 26% having three or more risk factors.[5] Multiple risk factors often act synergistically to increase risk dramatically above the sum of individual risk factors. For example, patients who are heterozygous for factor V Leiden are at only moderately increased risk for VTE (4- to 8-fold). However, when combined with the additional risk of oral contraceptive use, the risk for VTE increases to approximately 35-fold, the same order of magnitude as for someone who is homozygous for factor V Leiden. The concomitant presence of obesity, advancing age, and factor V Leiden increases the thrombosis risk associated with hormone replacement therapy

TABLE 12–1 Common Inherited and Acquired Risk Factors for Venous Thrombosis

Acquired	Inherited
Advanced age	Factor V Leiden
Hospitalization/immobilization	Prothrombin 20210A
HRT and OCP	Antithrombin deficiency
Pregnancy and puerperium	Protein C deficiency
Prior VTE	Protein S deficiency
Malignancy	Factor XI elevation
Major surgery	Dysfibrinogenemia
Obesity	
Nephrotic syndrome	**Mixed Etiology**
Trauma/spinal cord injury	
Long-haul travel (>6 hours)	Homocysteinemia
Varicose veins	Factor VII, VIII, IX, XI elevation
Antiphospholipid antibody syndrome	Hyperfibrinogenemia
Myeloproliferative disease	APC resistance without factor V Leiden
Polycythemia	
Central venous catheters	

APC, Activated protein C; *HRT,* hormone replacement therapy; *OCP,* oral contraceptives; *VTE,* venous thromboembolism.

alone. In symptomatic outpatients, the odds ratio for an objectively documented DVT increases from 1.26 for one risk factor to 3.88 for three or more risk factors.[6]

Other factors associated with venous thrombosis include traditional cardiovascular risk factors (obesity, hypertension, diabetes), and there is a racial predilection among whites and African Americans compared with Asians and Native Americans. Certain gene variants (single nucleotide polymorphisms) are associated with a mild increased risk for DVT, and their presence may interact with other risk factors to increase the overall risk for venous thrombosis. However, testing for these polymorphisms is not common in clinical practice.

Natural History

Overt venous injury appears to be neither a necessary nor sufficient condition for thrombosis, although the role of biologic injury to the endothelium is increasingly apparent. Under conditions favoring thrombosis, the normally antithrombogenic endothelium may become prothrombotic, producing tissue factor, von Willebrand factor, and fibronectin. Stasis alone is probably also an inadequate stimulus in the absence of low levels of activated coagulation factors.[7]

The rate of VTE recurrence in patients with untreated isolated calf DVT is approximately 20% to 30%. In contrast, the rate of recurrence in patients with untreated proximal DVT is more difficult to determine, since the majority of patients with proximal DVT receive therapeutic anticoagulation. Limited older data suggest that about 50% of patients with inadequately treated proximal DVT will develop symptomatic PE.

Therapeutic anticoagulation effectively stabilizes venous thrombus, prevents propagation, and promotes dissolution by endogenous plasmin and its mediators. However, there is a low rate of VTE recurrence, even with adequate dosages of heparin, low-molecular-weight heparin, pentasaccharides, and/or vitamin K antagonists. Most VTE recurrence takes place in the first few weeks after anticoagulant therapy is initiated, and it is dependent upon the location of the original DVT. Extension of isolated calf DVT is effectively attenuated by anticoagulation. However, even adequately treated proximal DVTs have a low rate of recurrence.

DIAGNOSIS AND IMAGING

The patient presentation varies widely, depending on the extent of the venous thrombosis and the presence of concurrent medical and surgical problems. In some, the DVT will be discovered during routine screening of patients who are at high risk for VTE.

Laboratory Testing for Venous Thromboembolism

There are no laboratory tests that confirm or exclude the presence of DVT or superficial venous thrombosis (SVT).

D-dimer testing may be useful in two clinical settings. In the first of these situations, a negative D-dimer testing in combination with a low probability clinical scoring criteria in combination with D-dimer testing has a negative predictive value for excluding DVT. However, D-dimer testing is a poorer predictor for the presence of DVT or PE. In the setting of patients with established DVT who have received a course of anticoagulation, D-dimer testing may be used to help guide the duration of anticoagulation.

Imaging

The *venous duplex scan* is the most commonly performed test for the detection of infrainguinal DVT, both above and below the knee, with sensitivity and specificity of greater than 95% in symptomatic patients. In a venous duplex examination performed with the patient supine, spontaneous flow, variation of flow with respiration, and response of flow to the Valsalva maneuver, all are assessed. Continued improvements in ultrasound technology also have improved the ability to visualize color flow within the tibial veins. However, the primary method of detecting DVT with ultrasound is demonstration of the lack of compressibility of the vein with probe pressure on B-mode imaging. Normally, in transverse section, the vein walls should coapt with pressure (Figs. 12-1 and 12-2). Lack of coaptation indicates thrombus.

Venography is the most definitive test for the diagnosis of DVT in both symptomatic and asymptomatic patients. Diagnostic venography involves placement of a small catheter in the dorsum of the foot, with injection of radiopaque contrast to produce projections in at least two views. Venography is not used routinely for the evaluation of lower extremity DVT because of associated complications. More commonly, it is used for imaging prior to operative venous reconstruction or catheter-based endovenous therapy.

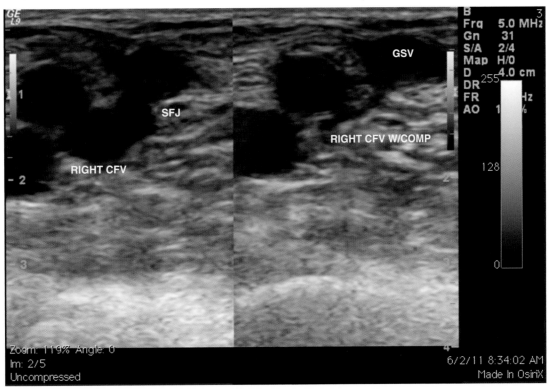

■ **Fig 12-1** Common femoral vein without and with compression. Complete vein wall coaptation indicates absence of deep vein thrombosis.

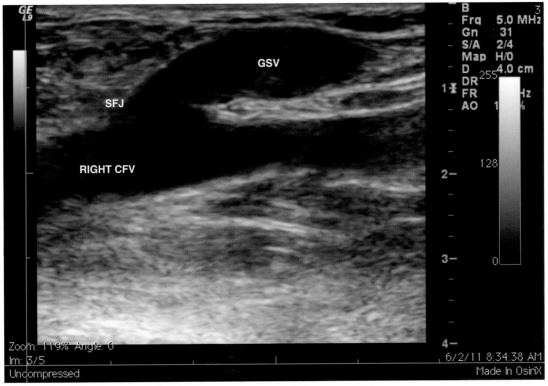

■ **Fig 12-2** Normal saphenofemoral junction.

INITIAL ANTITHROMBOTIC THERAPY FOR ACUTE VENOUS THROMBOEMBOLISM

Once the diagnosis of VTE has been made, antithrombotic therapy should be initiated promptly. The following dosing protocols are the more commonly used treatment regimens, but they are not applicable to all patient populations. In patients who require anticoagulation for acute VTE disease, *initial anticoagulation* usually is administered parenterally with one of the medications listed in Table 12-2. Initial anticoagulation should be continued for at least 5 days, and most patients may begin warfarin therapy on the same day they begin parenteral anticoagulation. Parenteral anticoagulation may be discontinued once the prothrombin time–to–international normalized ratio (PT/INR) is in the therapeutic range (INR goal 2.5, range 2.0 to 3.0) for longer than 24 hours (i.e., two consecutive daily INR values of 2.0 to 3.0).

In patients who have contraindications to anticoagulation, the treatment algorithm will vary, depending upon the location of the original DVT (Fig. 12-3).

LONG-TERM ANTITHROMBOTIC THERAPY

The purpose of long-term anticoagulation is the prevention of recurrent VTE. The recommended duration of anticoagulation is outlined in Table 12-3.

TABLE 12–2 Approved Parenteral Medications for Initiation of Anticoagulation

Medication	Route	Dose and Duration
Unfractionated heparin (UH)	IV SC	5000 U or 80 U/kg bolus IV, then 1300 U/h or 18 U/kg/h IV continuous infusion adjusted to prolong the aPTT corresponding to a plasma heparin of 0.3-0.7 IU/mL Adjusted dose SC UH is an effective alternative
Low-molecular-weight heparin (LMWH)	SC	Once or twice daily, dose is brand dependent No monitoring required (usually) Renal excretion
Fondaparinux	SC	5 mg daily if body weight <50 kg 7.5 mg daily if body weight 50-100 kg 10 mg daily if body weight >100 kg No monitoring required (usually) Renal excretion

IV, Intravenous; *SC,* subcutaneous.

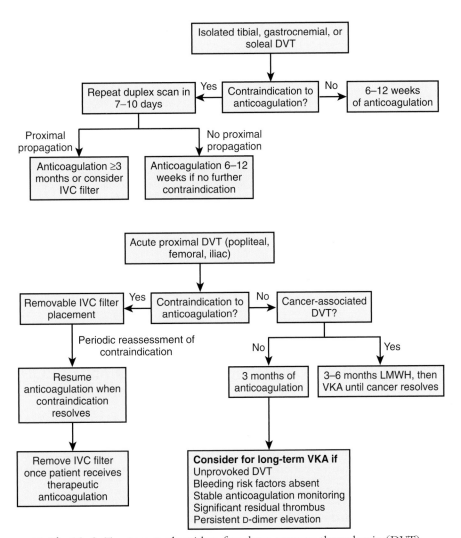

■ **Fig 12-3** Treatment algorithm for deep venous thrombosis (DVT).

TABLE 12–3 Recommended Duration of Anticoagulation

Clinical Subgroup	ACCP Treatment Recommendations
First episode LE DVT/transient risk	VKA for 3 months
First episode LE DVT/unprovoked	VKA at least 3 months
	Then evaluate for long-term therapy if:
	First unprovoked VTE
	Proximal DVT
	Bleeding risk factors absent
	Good anticoagulation monitoring
Distal LE DVT/unprovoked	VKA for 3 months
Second episode VTE/unprovoked	VKA long-term therapy
LE DVT and cancer	LMWH SC for 3-6 months
	Then VKA or LMWH
	Indefinitely or
	Until cancer resolves

Adapted from Kearon C, et al. Antithrombotic therapy for venous thromboembolic disease. American College of Chest Physicians Evidence-Based Clinical Practice Guidelines (8th Edition). Chest 2008;133:454-545.
This assumes that the patient has received a 5- to 10-day course of parenteral medications.
ACCP, American College of Chest Physicians; *DVT,* deep venous thrombosis; *LE,* lower extremity; *LMWH,* low-molecular-weight heparin; *SC,* subcutaneous; *VTE,* venous thromboembolism.

THROMBOPHILIC CONDITIONS: INHERITED AND ACQUIRED

Testing for Thrombophilia

Currently, the American Society of Hematology Education Program Book suggests that testing for thrombophilia for patients with VTE is indicated for those in the following clinical settings:

1. ***Idiopathic first event***

2. ***Secondary, non–cancer-related first event and age younger than 50, including thrombosis on contraceptives or postmenopausal hormones***

3. ***Recurrent idiopathic or secondary noncancer events***

4. ***Thrombosis at an unusual site***

Most authorities include cerebral, renal, portal, or hepatic vein thrombosis as unusual sites. However, the association with upper extremity thrombosis or retinal vein thrombosis is less certain (Table 12-4).

In patients with visceral vein thrombosis, testing for *paroxysmal nocturnal hemoglobinuria* (PNH) and *myeloproliferative syndromes* should be performed. PNH is screened for with a flow cytometry assay, and myeloproliferative syndromes are detected with DNA testing for the *JAK2* mutation. Testing for *heparin-induced thrombocytopenia (HIT)* should be considered in patients

TABLE 12–4 Common Laboratory Assays That Are Performed in the Evaluation of Patients with Suspected Thrombophilia

Test	Approximate Reference Range (Adults)	Test Affected by					
		Heparin	Warfarin	Liver Disease	Acute Thrombosis	DIC	Other
Activated protein C resistance ratio	2.0-5.0						FV deficiency, Ratio ≤0.61 suggests APC resistance
Prothrombin 20210 variant	Negative						
Antithrombin activity	0.86-1.18 U/mL	Yes		Yes	Yes	Yes	
Protein C activity	0.82-1.54 U/mL	Yes	Yes	Yes	Yes	Yes	
Protein S antigen, free	74%-147% male 55%-123% female		Yes	Yes	Yes	Yes	
Factor VIII activity	0.60-1.50 U/mL	Yes	Yes				Acute phase reactant, pregnancy, OCP
Fasting homocysteine	4-12 µmol/L						
Lupus anticoagulant screening	aPTT (26-36 sec) Hexagonal PL (<8.0 sec) DVVT (29.2-45.4 sec)	Yes (no) (no)	No yes	Yes			
Anticardiolipin antibodies	IgG (<9-19 PL units) IgM (<9-19 PL units) IgA (<9-14 PL units)						Low (+) 12-19 units Med (+) 20-79 units High (+) >80 units

Given are the reference ranges for the Pathology Lab at Oregon Health and Science University. Other lab references may vary.
DIC, Disseminated intravascular coagulopathy; *OCP*, oral contraceptives.

who have had recent exposure to heparin or low-molecular-weight heparin and unexplained thrombocytopenia or a 30% to 50% decrease in their platelet count.

The timing for the performance of testing for inherited thrombophilia varies widely. Acute thrombosis, inflammation, and a large thrombus burden may cause transient depression of antithrombin, protein C, and protein S levels. Concomitant administration of oral vitamin K antagonists also decreases protein C and protein S activity. If abnormal results are obtained under these conditions, then repeat testing should be performed once the acute thrombosis has resolved and after discontinuation of the vitamin K antagonist. To avoid the need for repeat lab draws, many clinicians do not perform the thrombophilia testing until after 6 months of warfarin therapy, waiting 4 weeks after the vitamin K antagonists have been discontinued. It is also important to remember that many antiphospholipid antibodies are transient, and the official criteria for antiphospholipid antibody syndrome require two positive tests at least 12 weeks apart.

Superficial Thrombophlebitis

It has been reported that acute SVT occurs in approximately 125,000 people in the United States per year.[8] Traditional teaching mistakenly suggests that SVT is a self-limiting process of little consequence and small risk.

CLINICAL PRESENTATION

Approximately 35% to 46% of patients with SVT are males (average age 54 years). The average age for females is about 58 years.[9,10] Factors associated with SVT include varicose veins (most frequent), age older than 60 years, obesity, tobacco use, and a history of DVT or SVT. Factors associated with extension of SVT include age older than 60 years, male sex, and a history of DVT. SVT of the great saphenous vein (GSV) is most common; however, SVT of the small saphenous vein (SSV) should not be overlooked because it may progress to popliteal DVT.

ETIOLOGY

To determine whether a hypercoagulable state contributes to the development of SVT, a number of markers were determined in a population of patients with acute SVT.[11] All patients had a coagulation profile performed that included (1) protein C antigen and activity, (2) activated protein C (APC) resistance, (3) protein S antigen and activity, (4) antithrombin (AT), and (5) lupus-type anticoagulant. Among 29 enrolled patients, 12 (41%) were found to have abnormal results consistent with a hypercoagulable state. Five of the patients (38%) with combined SVT/DVT and seven of the patients (44%) with isolated SVT were found to be hypercoagulable. These findings suggest that patients with SVT are at an increased risk of having an underlying hypercoagulable state.

DIAGNOSIS

The physical diagnosis of superficial thrombophlebitis is based on the presence of erythema and tenderness in the distribution of the superficial veins, with the thrombosis identified by a palpable cord.

Duplex ultrasound scanning is now the initial test of choice for the evaluation of SVT as well as the diagnosis of DVT. The extent of involvement of the deep and superficial systems can be accurately assessed with this modality because routine clinical examination may not be able to precisely evaluate the proximal extent of involvement in either system.

Duplex imaging has shown concomitant DVT to be present in 5% to 40% of patients with SVT.[12-14] It is important to note that up to 25% of these DVTs may not be contiguous with the SVT and may be in the contralateral lower extremity.

TREATMENT

The goals of treatment are two-fold: reduction in local symptoms and prevention of thrombus propagation into the deep venous system. Frequently used treatment options include:

- High ligation of the saphenofemoral junction (SFJ), with or without GSV stripping and/or anticoagulation with low-molecular-weight heparin or pentasaccharides
- Treatment of SVT localized in tributaries and the distal GSV consists of ambulation, warm soaks, and nonsteroidal antiinflammatory agents

The progression of isolated SVT to DVT has been evaluated. Among 263 patients with isolated SVT by duplex ultrasonography, 30 (11%) patients had documented progression to deep venous involvement.[15] Progression from the GSV in the thigh into the common femoral vein (21 patients) was most common, with 18 of these extensions noted to be nonocclusive and 12 having a free-floating component.

Because of the recognized potential for extension into the deep system and embolization, high saphenous ligation with or without stripping is often recommended for SVT within 1 cm of the SFJ. In a series of 43 patients who underwent ligation of the SFJ with and without local CFV thrombectomy and stripping of the GSV, two patients were found with postoperative contralateral DVT, one of whom had a PE[16-19] (Figs. 12-4 through 12-6).

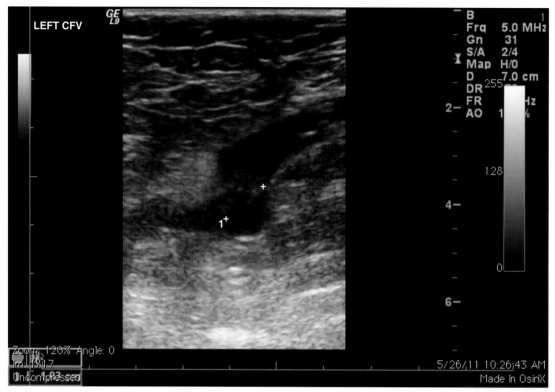

■ **Fig 12–4** Superficial venous thrombosis: thrombus at saphenofemoral junction extends into common femoral vein.

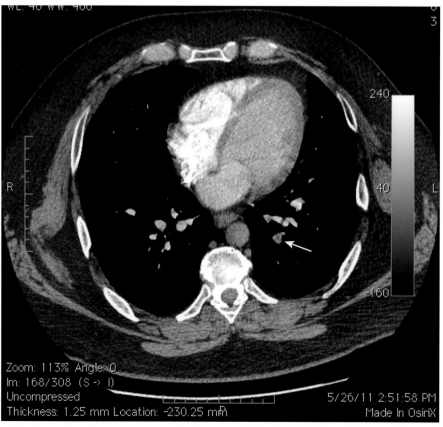

■ **Fig 12–5** Pulmonary artery embolus to left lower lobe (cross-sectional view).

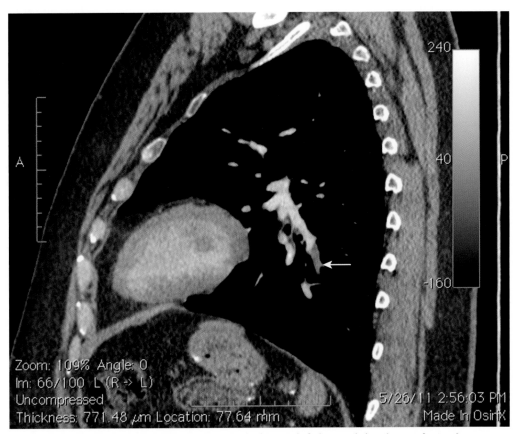

■ **Fig 12–6** Pulmonary artery embolus to left lower lobe (sagittal view).

Ligation was initially proposed to avert the development of DVT by preventing extension through the SFJ. Since issues of noncontiguous DVT and postligation DVT with PE are not addressed by this therapy, alternative treatment options need to be explored.

A prospective nonrandomized study was conducted to evaluate the efficacy of anticoagulation in the management of SFJ thrombophlebitis (SFJT).[20] Duplex ultrasonography was performed before admission, both to establish the diagnosis and to evaluate the deep venous system. Patients were hospitalized, given a full course of heparin treatment, and evaluated with duplex ultrasound 2 to 4 days after admission. Patients with SFJT alone and resolution of SFJT as documented by duplex ultrasound scans were maintained on warfarin for 6 weeks. Those patients with SFJT and DVT were maintained on warfarin for 6 months. Among 20 enrolled patients, 8 (40%) had concurrent DVT, including 4 with unilateral DVT, 2 with bilateral DVT, and 2 with development of DVT despite anticoagulation. DVT was contiguous with SFJT in 5 patients and noncontiguous in 3 patients. Seven of 13 duplex ultrasound scans obtained at 2 to 8 months' follow-up demonstrated partial resolution of SFJT, 5 had complete resolution, and 1 demonstrated no resolution. There were no episodes of PE, recurrence, or anticoagulation complications at maximum follow-up of 14 months. Anticoagulation therapy to manage SFJT was effective in achieving resolution, preventing recurrence, and preventing PE within the follow-up period.

Meta-analysis of surgical versus medical therapy for isolated above-knee SVT has been attempted but has not been feasible because of the paucity of comparable data between the two groups.[21] This review suggested that although stripping provides superior symptomatic relief, medical management with anticoagulants is somewhat superior with respect to minimizing complications and preventing subsequent DVT and PE. Based on these data, the authors suggest that anticoagulation is appropriate in patients without contraindications.

Although proximal GSV SVT occurs frequently, the best treatment regimen based on its underlying pathophysiology and resolution rate remains controversial. More recent investigations do offer some guidelines suggesting that anticoagulation is more effective than venous ligation in preventing DVT and PE.[22] Further examination of the unresolved issues involving SVT is fundamental.

EHIT (endothermal heat-induced thrombosis) was briefly covered in Chapter 5. The following is a typical example of the natural course of an SFJT after thermal ablation treatment. This series of ultrasounds demonstrates a generous thrombus at SFJ retracting over time from postoperative day 3 (initial ultrasound) to postoperative day 5, where retraction has begun. At 3 weeks postoperative, the thrombus extension is no longer visualized. No anticoagulation or platelet therapy was used. Notice that no contiguous thrombotic lesions were identified in the deep system. This situation is very different from the ultrasound and CT scans shown previously (see Figs. 12-4 through 12-6), in which case the patient presented with spontaneous GSV thrombosis extending into the SFJ and developed a PE (Fig. 12-7).

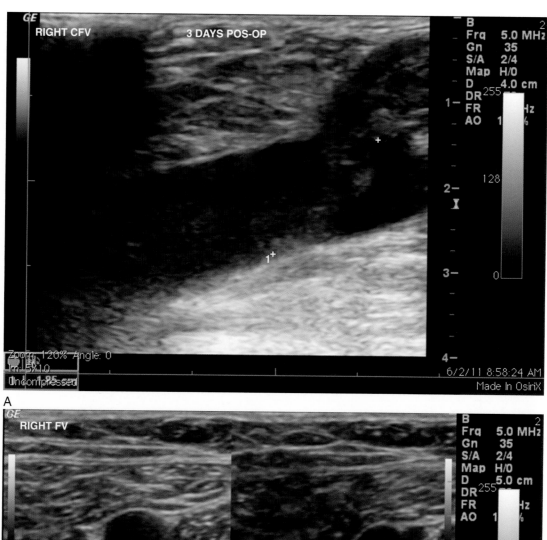

A

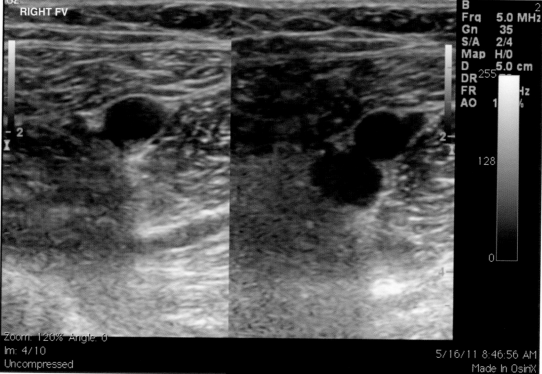

B

■ **Fig 12–7** **A,** Thrombus extension (EHIT) seen on postoperative day 3 at the saphenofemoral junction. **B,** Fully compressed femoral vein (*left panel*) demonstrating no femoral vein thrombosis.

Continued

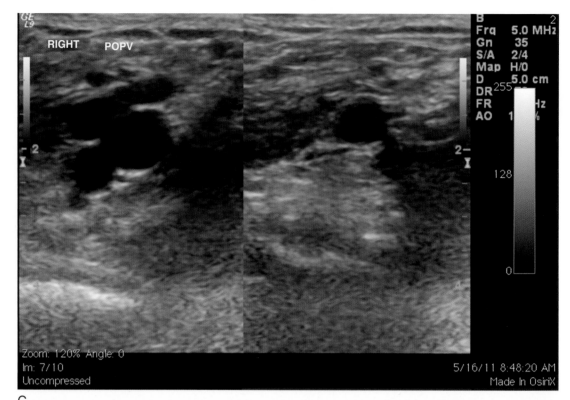

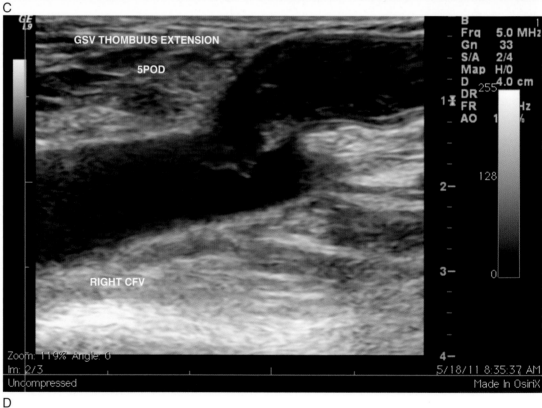

■ **Fig 12-7, cont'd C,** Fully compressed popliteal vein (*right panel*) demonstrating no evidence of popliteal vein thrombosis. **D,** Onset of thrombus retraction (EHIT) seen on postoperative day 5.

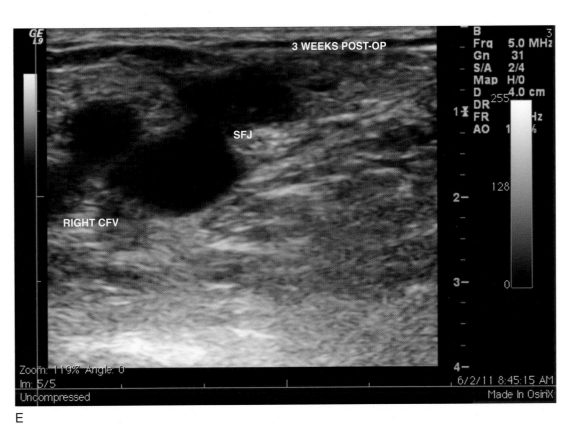

E

■ **Fig 12–7, cont'd** **E,** Completely retracted thrombus extension (EHIT) seen postoperatively at 3 weeks.

REFERENCES

1. Kearon C, Kahn SR, Agnelli G, et al. Antithrombotic therapy for venous thromboembolic disease. American College of Chest Physicians Evidence-Based Clinical Practice Guidelines (8th Edition). Chest 2008;133:454-545.
2. Kearon C. Natural history of venous thromboembolism. Circulation 2003;107:I22-I30.
3. Decousus H, Prandoni P, Mismetti P, et al. Fondaparinux for the treatment of superficial-vein thrombosis in the legs. N Engl J Med 2010;363:1222-1232.
4. Rosendaal FR. Venous thrombosis: a multicausal disease. Lancet 1999;353:1167-1173.
5. Anderson FA, Wheeler HB, Goldberg RJ, et al. The prevalence of risk factors for venous thromboembolism among hospital patients. Arch Intern Med 1992;152:1660-1664.
6. Oger E, Leroyer C, LeMoigne E, et al. The value of risk factor analysis in clinically suspected deep venous thrombosis. Respiration 1997;64:326-330.
7. Thomas DP, Merton RE, Hockley DJ. The effect of stasis on the venous endothelium: an ultrastructural study. Br J Haematol 1983;55:113-122.
8. De Weese MS. Nonoperative treatment of acute superficial thrombophlebitis and deep femoral venous thrombosis. In: Ernst CB, Stanley JC, editors. Current Therapy in Vascular Surgery. Philadelphia: BC Decker; 1991:952-960.
9. Lohr JM, McDevitt DT, Lutter KS, et al. Operative management of greater saphenous thrombophlebitis involving the saphenofemoral junction. Am J Surg 1992;164:269-275.
10. Lutter KS, Kerr TM, Roedersheimer LR, et al. Superficial thrombophlebitis diagnosed by duplex scanning. Surgery 1991;110:42-46.
11. Hanson JN, Ascher E, DePippo P, et al. Saphenous vein thrombophlebitis (SVT): a deceptively benign disease. J Vasc Surg 1998;27:677-680.
12. Bjorgell O, Nilsson PE, Jarenros H. Isolated nonfilling of contrast in deep vein segments seen on phlebography, and a comparison with color Doppler ultrasound to assess the incidence of deep venous thrombosis. Angiology 2000;51:451-461.
13. Jorgensen JO, Hanel KC, Morgan AM, et al. The incidence of deep venous thrombosis in patients with superficial thrombophlebitis of the lower limbs. J Vasc Surg 1993;18:70-73.
14. Skillman JJ, Kent KC, Porter DH, et al. Simultaneous occurrence of superficial and deep thrombophlebitis in the lower extremity. J Vasc Surg 1990;11:818-823; discussion 823-824.
15. Chengelis DL, Bendick PJ, Glover JL, et al. Progression of superficial venous thrombosis to deep vein thrombosis. J Vasc Surg 1996;24:745-749.
16. Gjores JE. Surgical therapy of ascending thrombophlebitis in the saphenous system. Angiology 1962;13:241-243.
17. Husni EA, Williams WA. Superficial thrombophlebitis of lower limbs. Surgery 1982;91:70-74.
18. Lofgren EP, Lofgren KA. The surgical treatment of superficial thrombophlebitis. Surgery 1981;90:49-54.
19. Plate G, Eklof B, Jensen R, et al. Deep venous thrombosis, pulmonary embolism and acute surgery in thrombophlebitis of the long saphenous vein. Acta Chir Scand 1985;151:241-244.
20. Leon L, Giannoukas AD, Dodd D, et al. Clinical significance of superficial vein thrombosis. Eur J Vasc Endovasc Surg 2005;29:10-17.
21. Sullivan V, Denk PM, Sonnad SS, et al. Ligation versus anticoagulation: treatment of above-knee superficial thrombophlebitis not involving the deep venous system. J Am Coll Surg 2001;193:556-562.
22. Neher JO, Safranek S, Greenwald JL. Clinical inquiries. What is the best therapy for superficial thrombophlebitis? J Fam Pract 2004;53:583-585.

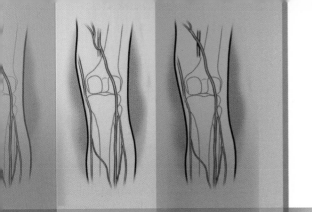

CHAPTER 13

Endovenous Placement of Inferior Vena Caval Filters

Timothy K. Liem

HISTORICAL BACKGROUND

Venous interruption for the prevention of pulmonary embolism was introduced by Homans in 1934. Although his initial description involved ligation of the femoral vein, surgical techniques soon evolved, focusing on interruption at the level of the inferior vena cava (IVC). Complete ligation of the IVC was performed in 1959, but the resulting cardiovascular complications and venous sequelae led to the development of alternative strategies for either temporary interruption or plication. These included temporary ligation of the IVC using absorbable suture, plication of the IVC using interrupted mattress suture, and partially occluding externally applied PTFE clips (Moretz clip, Adams-DeWeese clip). These techniques required retroperitoneal exposure and general anesthesia, which are distinct disadvantages, particularly in patients who are often ill with significant comorbidities.

The Mobin-Uddin umbrella, introduced in 1967, was the first IVC filter that could be inserted via a transjugular approach under local anesthesia. The apex of this device was oriented inferiorly, and the original design incorporated a solid fabric membrane with the intent of causing caval thrombosis. Fenestrations were added later, with the purpose of causing delayed thrombosis, supposedly increasing the development of collaterals. However, some patients maintained a patent IVC, and yet they had a low rate of pulmonary embolization. These observations led to significant design advances, such that IVC thrombosis was no longer the desired outcome. The superior design of the Greenfield filter (Boston Scientific, Natick, MA), with its low rate of caval thrombosis, allowed it to rapidly supplant prior filter designs. The Greenfield (and the ensuing iterations) could be placed via a transjugular or transfemoral approach, and it became the standard caval interruption device to which newer filters were compared for the next few decades.

PATIENT SELECTION

The accepted and relative indications[1] for placement of an IVC filter are shown in Table 13-1. Although anticoagulation is the mainstay of therapy in patients with acute deep venous thrombosis (DVT) or pulmonary embolism, it may be contraindicated for several reasons. Active internal bleeding is an absolute contraindication to therapeutic anticoagulation. However, an increased risk of bleeding due to recent trauma or major surgery (especially neurologic or ocular surgery) more often is a relative contraindication that is subject to clinical judgment. In the era when unfractionated heparin and vitamin K antagonists were the only available antithrombotic agents, nonhemorrhagic complications of anticoagulation (e.g., heparin-induced thrombocytopenia, warfarin-induced skin necrosis) were more common indications for IVC filter insertion. Currently, however, several alternative anticoagulants are available, and they should be considered prior to insertion of an IVC filter. Direct-thrombin inhibitors are very effective antithrombotic alternatives to heparin or low-molecular-weight heparin in patients who develop heparin-induced thrombocytopenia. Subcutaneously injected low-molecular-weight heparins and pentasaccharides, as well as oral direct-thrombin inhibitors, are potential alternatives in patients with warfarin-induced skin necrosis.

An often-cited indication for IVC filter insertion is "failure of anticoagulation." Significant proximal DVT extension and pulmonary embolism may occur in up to 4% to 11% of patients who receive anticoagulation for acute lower extremity DVT. Over 70% of these failures occur in the first 3 weeks after initiation of therapy. However, there should be a distinction between patients who are receiving adequate versus those receiving inadequate antithrombotic therapy. Patients should be carefully questioned, and the anticoagulation records should be reviewed to determine whether dosages and frequency of antithrombotic medications were adequate (Table 13-2; Fig. 13-1; see also Table 13-1).

TABLE 13–1 Indications for Placement of an Inferior Vena Cava Filter

Common Indications for IVC Filter Placement

- Contraindication to anticoagulation in a patient with an acute proximal LE VTE
- Recurrent VTE despite *adequate* antithrombotic therapy. Recurrence may include significant proximal DVT extension in an ipsilateral LE, development of a new proximal DVT in a contralateral LE, or pulmonary embolism.
- Massive pulmonary embolism with residual LE DVT

Relative Indications for IVC Filter Placement

- Patients with pulmonary embolism and significant pulmonary disease (pulmonary hypertension, cor pulmonale)
- Prophylactic IVC filter placement in a patient at high risk for VTE in whom antithrombotic therapy is contraindicated and in whom adequate diagnostic imaging cannot be performed (e.g., trauma patient with lower extremity injuries)
- During catheter-directed pharmacomechanical thrombolysis
- "Free-floating" thrombus in the proximal deep veins of the lower extremities

DVT, Deep venous thrombosis; *IVC,* inferior vena cava; *LE,* lower extremity; *VTE,* venous thromboembolism.

TABLE 13–2 Guidewires and Catheters

Name	Diameter	Length
Guidewires		
Bentson/Rosen	.035 in	150-180 cm
Angled glidewire	.035 in	150-180 cm
Catheters		
Pigtail (with 2-cm calibration)	5-Fr	65-90 cm
Kumpe (or other angled catheter)	5-Fr	65-90 cm
Ancillary Supplies		
Heparinized saline	1000 units/ 1000 mL of normal saline	
Syringes (2)	20 mL, Luer Lock	
Dilators	5-Fr and 6-Fr	
Injectable nonionic contrast, high-flow power injector		

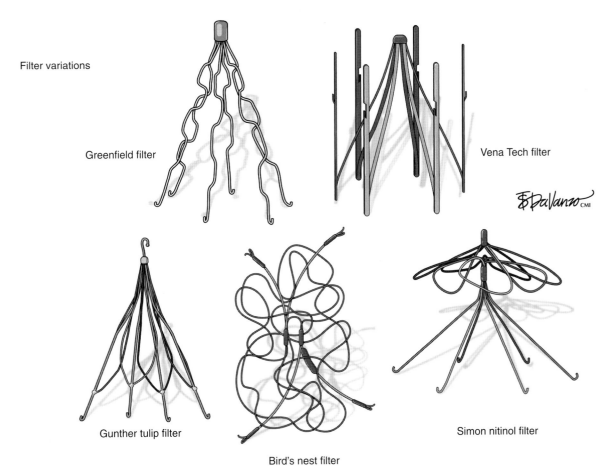

Filter variations

Greenfield filter

Vena Tech filter

Gunther tulip filter

Bird's nest filter

Simon nitinol filter

■ **Fig 13–1**

IMAGING

Venous Duplex Imaging

Most patients who are referred for placement of an IVC filter have had recent ultrasound confirmation of a lower extremity DVT. The proximal extent of the thrombus should be noted, since this may affect potential access sites for venography and filter insertion. If the patient has an acute iliofemoral DVT or if the thrombus extends above the level of the proximal femoral vein, then cannulation of the adjacent common femoral vein should be avoided if possible.

Venography

IVC venography should be performed in most patients prior to insertion of a filter. This imaging is done for several reasons: the location of the renal veins may be determined, the presence of anomalies of the IVC may be detected, the diameter of the IVC may be measured, and the presence of thrombus in the IVC may be visualized. If thrombus is present in the infrarenal IVC, then the filter may need to be placed proximal to the renal veins.

In patients with normal anatomy, the common iliac vein confluence occurs at the L4-L5 vertebral body, and the renal veins insert into the IVC at the L1 vertebral body. Kaufman et al.[2] performed a detailed magnetic resonance imaging analysis of the anatomy of the IVC. The average length of the infrarenal IVC is 94 mm in females and 110 mm in males. However, these lengths vary significantly, especially in patients who have anomalous venous return. Retroaortic and circumaortic left renal veins are found in 7% and 5%, respectively, and multiple right renal veins are present in 8%. Prior literature indicates that the prevalence of duplicate IVCs ranges from 0.7% to 3% based on radiographic investigations and cadaver dissections. A left-sided vena cava is even less common (0.2% to 0.5%). In this latter setting, the infrarenal IVC ascends on the left lateral aspect of the aorta. After insertion in the left renal vein, it then crosses anterior to the aorta to assume its usual anatomic position.

ACCESS AND OPERATIVE STEPS

Inferior vena cavography usually is performed via an internal jugular or common femoral approach (right is preferable to left in both instances). The site for access is often left up to the physician. However, certain clinical situations dictate an optimal strategy. A right internal jugular approach is commonly used, and it usually will not disturb thrombi in the iliac or femoral veins. It also may be used to cannulate either of the common iliac veins in the event that further imaging is needed to visualize potential IVC anomalies. All currently available IVC filters also may be inserted via a jugular approach. A common femoral venous approach may be more advantageous in patients who are intubated or have central venous catheters in place. However, the physician should confirm with duplex imaging that the access site is not involved with the venous thrombosis.

Right Internal Jugular Approach

The internal jugular vein should be cannulated using a combination of anatomic landmarks and ultrasound guidance. The internal jugular vein is located deep to the confluence of the two heads of the sternocleidomastoid muscle. More specifically, it is located deep to the clavicular head of the SCM, about one third of the distance from the medial border to the lateral border of the muscle. A subcutaneous wheel of local anesthetic is injected, and a No. 11 blade is used to incise the dermis. The subcutaneous tissue is spread gently with a mosquito clamp.

An 18-gauge single-wall puncture needle connected to a 5-mL or 10-mL syringe is used to access the vein with ultrasound guidance. The syringe should freely aspirate dark blood, and a .035-inch guidewire is passed into the IVC under fluoroscopic guidance. Occasionally, an angled catheter may be required to steer the wire into the IVC. Alternatively, a 21-gauge needle, .018-in guidewire, and 5-Fr catheter/dilator set (Micropuncture Introducer Set; Cook Medical, Bloomington, IN) may be used to avoid using the larger needle (Table 13-3; Figs. 13-2 through 13-10).

Text continued on p. 324

TABLE 13–3 Right Internal Jugular Approach

- Patient supine, slight Trendelenburg positioning if possible
- Slight neck rotation away from the site of access (overrotation beyond 30 to 60 degrees may increase the risk of carotid cannulation)
- Internal jugular access about 2 cm superior to the sternoclavicular junction, between the two heads of the sternocleidomastoid muscle, needle directed laterally.
- A standard 5- to 10-MHz ultrasound probe is placed transverse to the jugular vein. The syringe is gently aspirated as the needle is used to indent and puncture the anterior wall of the vein.
- The guidewire should pass without resistance and fluoroscopy should be used to confirm wire placement into the superior vena cava.

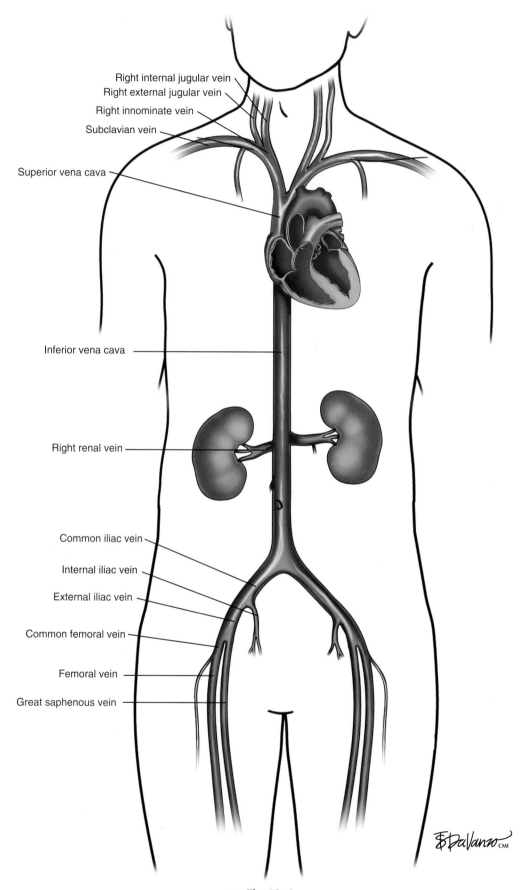

■ **Fig 13–2**

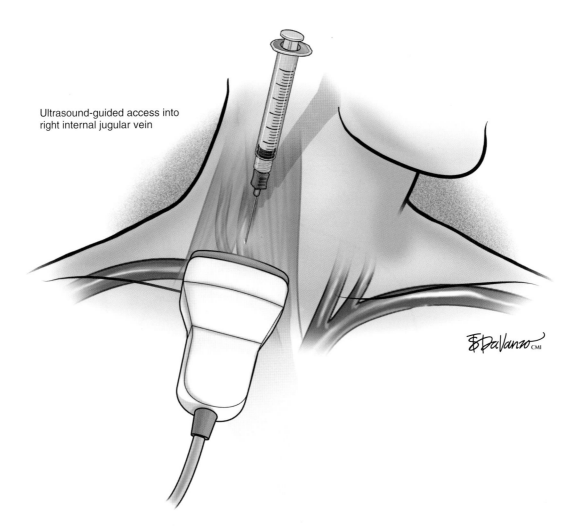

Ultrasound-guided access into
right internal jugular vein

■ **Fig 13–3**

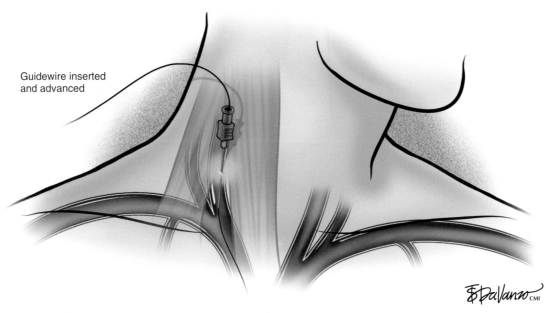

Guidewire inserted
and advanced

■ **Fig 13–4**

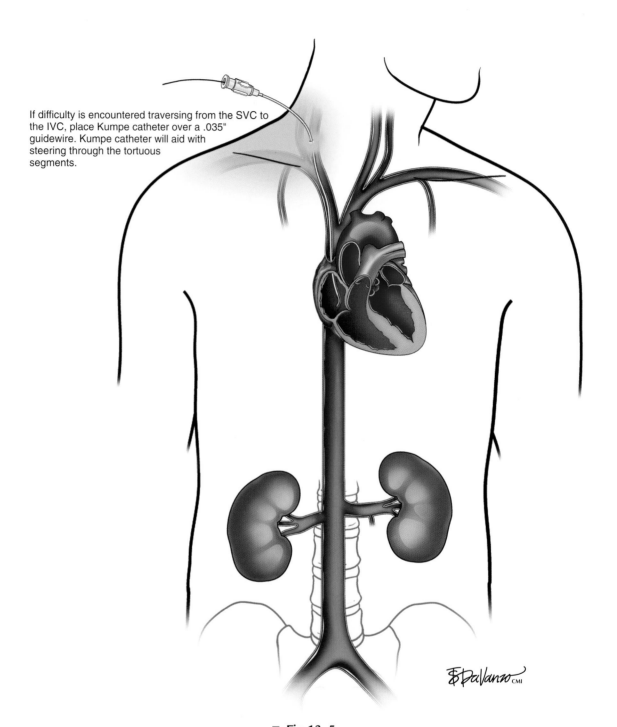

If difficulty is encountered traversing from the SVC to the IVC, place Kumpe catheter over a .035" guidewire. Kumpe catheter will aid with steering through the tortuous segments.

■ Fig 13–5

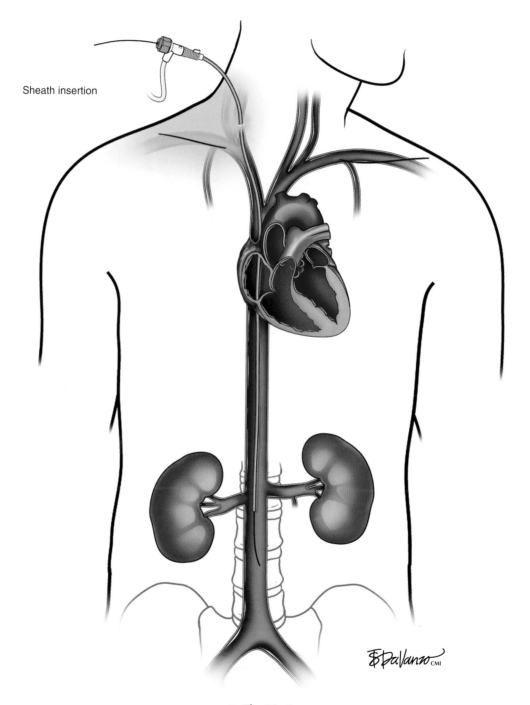

Sheath insertion

■ **Fig 13–6**

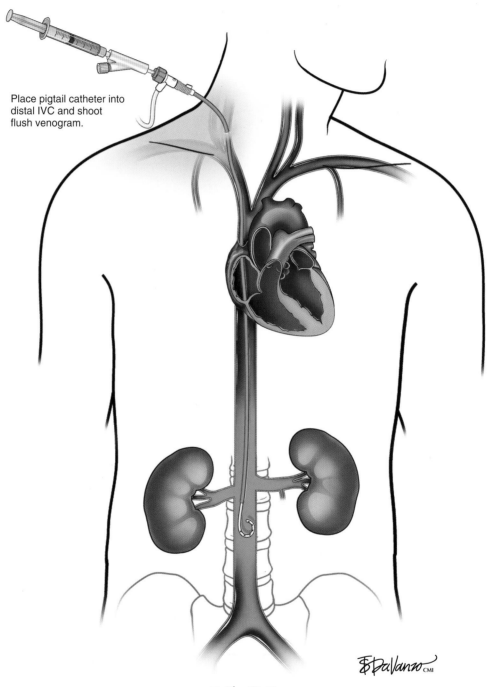

Place pigtail catheter into distal IVC and shoot flush venogram.

■ **Fig 13–7**

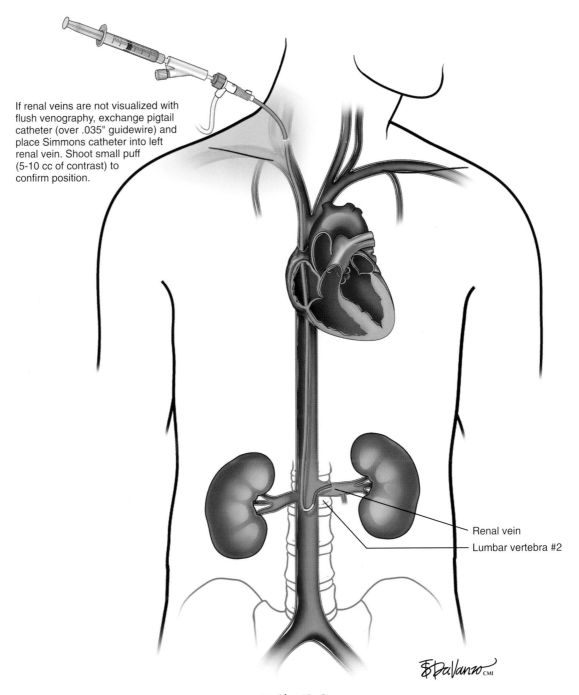

If renal veins are not visualized with flush venography, exchange pigtail catheter (over .035" guidewire) and place Simmons catheter into left renal vein. Shoot small puff (5-10 cc of contrast) to confirm position.

Renal vein

Lumbar vertebra #2

■ **Fig 13–8**

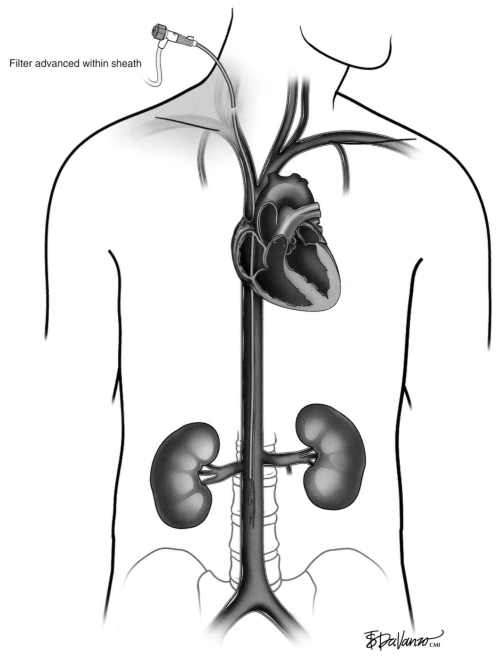

Filter advanced within sheath

■ **Fig 13–9**

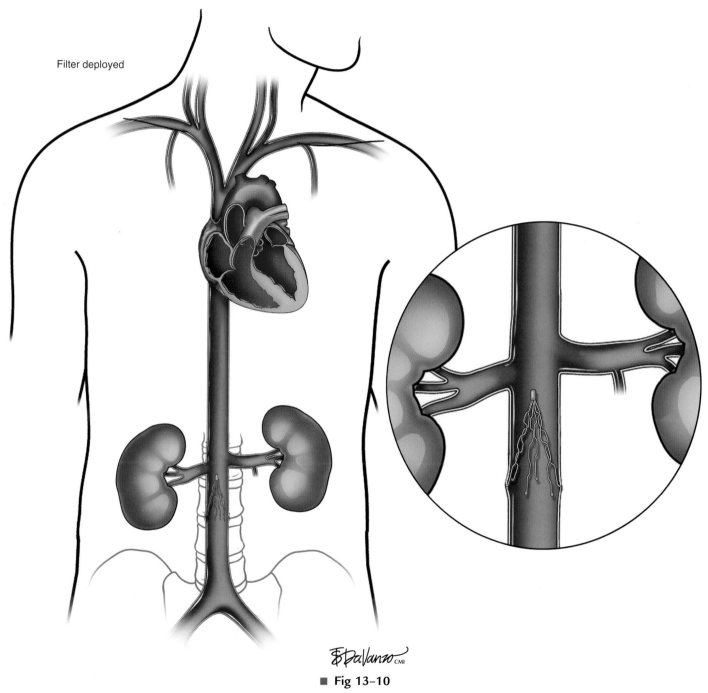

Filter deployed

■ **Fig 13–10**

Common Femoral Vein Approach

The common femoral vein usually is accessed using anatomic landmarks alone. The femoral pulse is palpated laterally. Ultrasound guidance may be easily applied in circumstances when the patient is obese or if the femoral pulse is absent. The common femoral vein cannulation techniques with an 18- or 21-gauge needle are similar to those that were described for internal jugular venous access (Figs. 13-11 through 13-16).

Text continued on p. 330

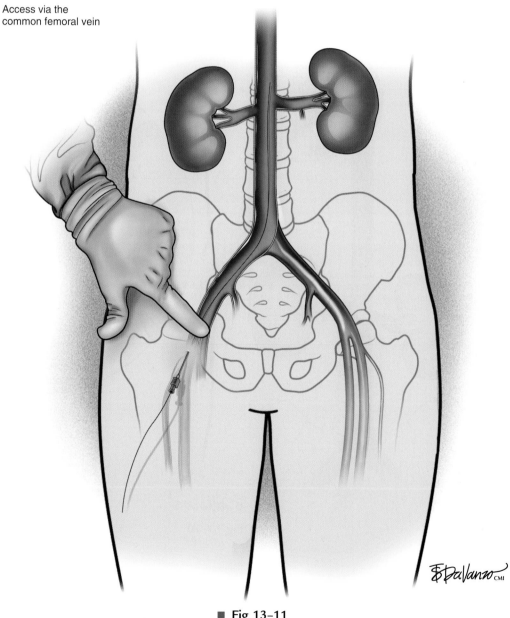

Access via the
common femoral vein

■ **Fig 13–11**

Sheath placed over
guidewire and advanced
into IVC

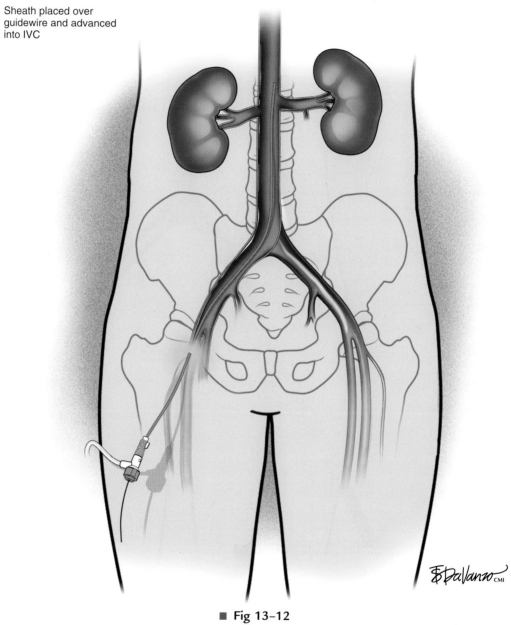

■ Fig 13–12

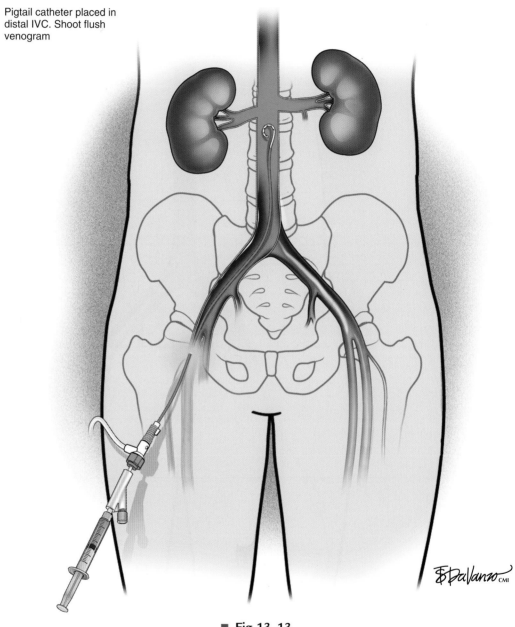

Pigtail catheter placed in distal IVC. Shoot flush venogram

■ **Fig 13–13**

If renal veins are not visualized
with flush venography,
exchange pigtail catheter (over
.035" guidewire) and place
Simmons catheter into left renal
vein. Shoot small puff (5-10 cc
of contrast) to confirm position.

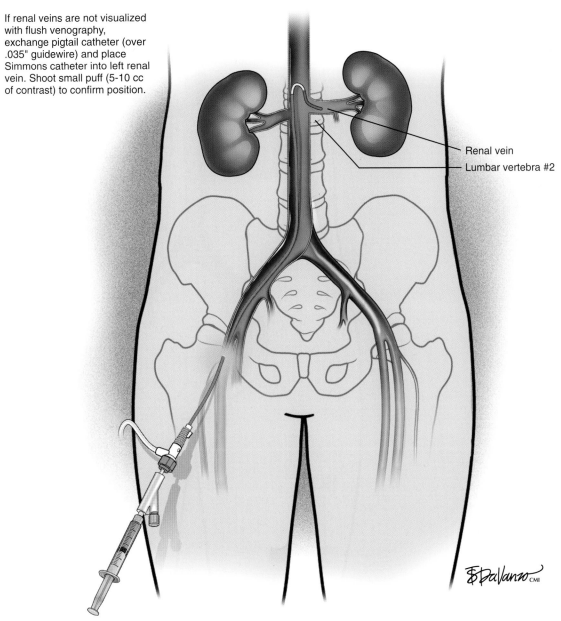

Renal vein

Lumbar vertebra #2

■ **Fig 13–14**

Filter is advanced within sheath

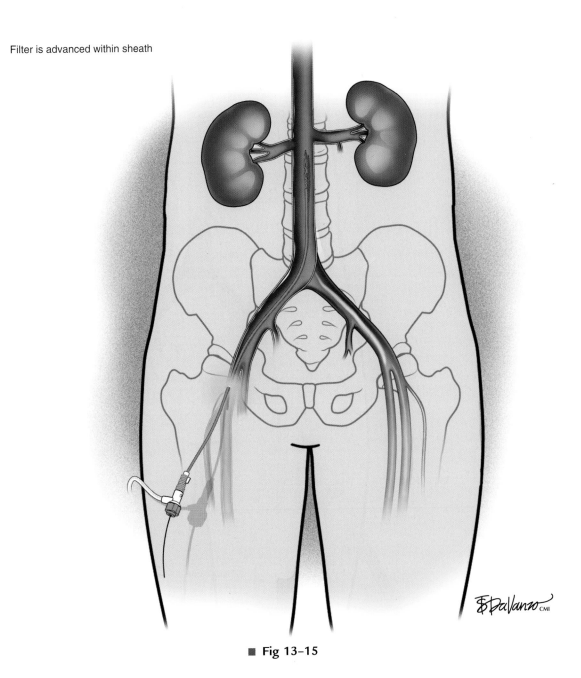

■ **Fig 13–15**

Filter deployed

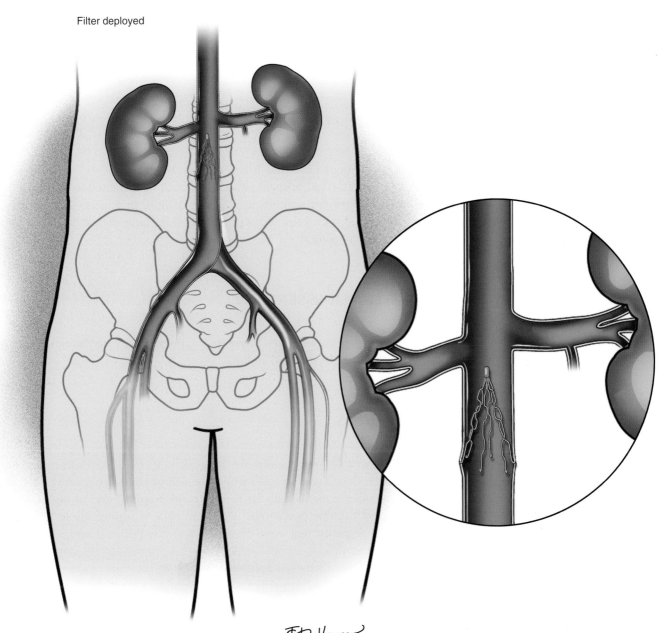

■ **Fig 13–16**

ANTICOAGULATION MANAGEMENT

The management of anticoagulation around the time of IVC filter insertion will depend on the indication for the filter. If the filter is to be inserted because of a contraindication to anticoagulation (e.g., active internal bleeding, recent major surgery, trauma, anticoagulation-related bleeding), then the IVC filter can be placed without periprocedural anticoagulation. However, if the indication was venous thromboembolism recurrence despite adequate anticoagulation, then the anticoagulation should not be discontinued around the time of the procedure.[3]

PEARLS AND PITFALLS

Once the filter is placed, remember to continually reassess anticoagulation.

If the plan is to remove an IVC filter, hospital programs should be instituted to track patients, ensure follow-up, and arrange for filter retrieval in a timely fashion. In patients who receive a permanent filter, yearly follow-up with plain kidney-ureter-bladder films should be obtained to assess for filter fracture or filter migration.

COMPLICATIONS OF IVC FILTER INSERTION

Complications include pneumothorax, access site thrombosis, pulmonary embolism, filter migration, filter infection, caval thrombosis, and IVC trauma.

COMPARATIVE EFFECTIVENESS

Success achieved with vena cava filters expanded the indications in some series to prophylaxis for free-floating thrombi longer than 5 cm,[4] in cases where the risk of anticoagulation was thought to be prohibitive such as in older patients with DVT, after major trauma,[5] and in high-risk situations such as orthopedic and bariatric operations.[6] Statistical data to support these indications are lacking, and enthusiasm for permanent vena caval filtration has declined with case reports of caval occlusion and filter fractures.

The development of retrievable filters has rekindled interest in their use, particularly during mechanical or thrombolytic treatment of large iliofemoral thrombi.[7] Unfortunately, data to date show equivalent complications, less secure fixation, and the added expense of multiple procedures. Improvements in techniques and devices should overcome some of these limitations but not the fundamental problem of knowing when embolic protection is no longer necessary.

REFERENCES

1. Krishnamurthy VN, Greenfield LJ, Proctor MC, Rectenwald JE. Indications, techniques, and results of interior vena cava filters. In: Gloviczki P, editor. Handbook of Venous Disorders. 3 ed. London: Hodder Arnold; 2009,299-313.
2. Kaufman JA, Waltman AC, Rivitz SM, Geller SC. Anatomical observations on the renal veins and inferior vena cava at magnetic resonance angiography. Cardiovasc Intervent Radiol 1995;18:153-157.
3. Kearon C, Kahn SR, Agnelli G, et al. Antithrombotic therapy for venous thromboembolic disease: American College of Chest Physicians Evidence-Based Clinical Practice Guidelines. Chest 2008;133:454-545.
4. Berry R, George J, Shaver W. Free-floating deep venous thrombosis. A retrospective analysis. Ann Surg 1990;211:719-723.
5. Langan EM 3rd, Miller RS, Casey WJ 3rd, et al. Prophylactic inferior vena cava filters in trauma patients at high risk: follow-up examination and risk/benefit assessment. J Vasc Surg 1999;30:484-488.
6. Sugerman HJ, Sugerman EL, Wolfe L, et al. Risks and benefits of gastric bypass in morbidly obese patients with severe venous stasis disease. Ann Surg 2001;234:41-46.
7. Thery C, Bauchart JJ, Lesenne M, et al. Predictive factors of effectiveness of streptokinase in deep venous thrombosis. Am J Cardiol 1992;69:117-122.

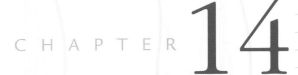

CHAPTER 14

Endovenous Thrombectomy and Thrombolysis

Rafael D. Malgor, Antonios P. Gasparis, and Nicos Labropoulos

HISTORICAL BACKGROUND

After the first episode of deep venous thrombosis (DVT), affected patients may develop pulmonary embolism (PE), recurrent DVT, or postthrombotic syndrome (PTS), and all carry significant morbidity and negative socioeconomic impact.[1] Important concepts in the natural history of the disease are recurrence, propagation, and recanalization with anatomic and/or hemodynamic changes following an episode of DVT. Spontaneous resolution of the DVT leaving intact the affected segment is rarely found, occurring only in one-third of patients.[2] Frequently, the segment affected by thrombosis develops reflux due to venous valve injury or some degree of residual obstruction.[3] Patients who develop a combination of reflux and venous obstruction following an episode of DVT have the highest risk of developing PTS.[3,4] A combination of reflux and obstruction is found in up to 86% of the patients, while occlusion alone is found in less than 10%.[5]

Patients with extensive proximal DVT, such as iliocaval or iliofemoral occlusions, have a worse prognosis compared with patients with infrainguinal thrombosis.[6,7] The resolution of venous obstruction with iliac thrombosis is often incomplete, and the incidence of PTS is higher.[4] Recurrent DVT is a very important factor in the natural history of the disease because other than exposing the patient to PE, it also increases significantly the risk for developing PTS.[8] In fact, it has been shown that a recurrent ipsilateral DVT is the strongest predictor for developing skin damage.[9] The risk of recurrent DVT was 40% (95% confidence interval [CI], 35.4% to 44.4%) after 10 years, being 53% (95% CI, 45.6% to 59.5%) in patients with unprovoked DVT and 22% in those with secondary DVT (95% CI, 17.2% to 27.8%).[10] Other important risk factors to develop recurrent DVT are age older than 65 years, incomplete thrombus resolution, and iliofemoral thrombosis.[6,9,11-13]

TREATMENT OPTIONS

To improve the long-term natural history of DVT, it is important to preserve venous function and outflow. Overall, the first line of treatment for DVT remains anticoagulation using either low-weight-molecular heparin (LMWH) or unfractionated heparin (UFH). Nonetheless, a review of 13 studies of proximal DVT showed total and partial resolution in only 4% and 14% of patients, respectively, who were treated with anticoagulation.[14]

Venous thrombectomy was first attempted in extreme cases of extensive DVT with impending venous gangrene aiming for limb salvage.[15,16] Indications for surgical thrombectomy are extensive proximal (iliofemoral) DVT when thrombolytic agents are contraindicated.[17] Therefore surgical thrombectomy has still not gained popularity, being performed in only a few specialized centers.[18] More recently, local thrombolysis and venous thrombectomy have been used together with very good outcomes.[19] Conversely, development of dedicated devises and safer use of thrombolytic agents has expanded percutaneous procedures. The goal with thrombolysis is to provide early thrombus removal with a minimally invasive procedure and low complications. By restoring venous flow, the objective is to prevent valve damage, venous hypertension, and recurrent thrombosis in an attempt to prevent PTS.

PATIENT SELECTION

Recommendations and patient's eligibility criteria for endovenous thrombectomy and thrombolysis via catheter-directed thrombolysis (CDT) or pharmacomechanical thrombectomy (PMT) have been defined as follows[17,20]:

- Extensive acute proximal (ileofemoral) DVT
- Less than 14 days from onset of symptoms or acute findings on duplex ultrasound
- Life expectancy of more than 1 year with good functional status
- Low risk of bleeding

While these are the most common recommendations for thrombolysis, deviations have been successfully reported, such as treatment of femoropopliteal DVT, thrombus longer than 14 days, and use of PMT in patients with higher risk of bleeding.

MODALITIES OF THROMBOLYSIS AND THROMBECTOMY

Systemic Thrombolysis

Over the past 50 years, variable outcomes were reported with systemic thrombolysis. Analysis of 13 contemporary studies including 591 patients found that the success rate of anticoagulation with heparin only showed total dissolution, partial lysis, and no improvement of the thrombus in 4%, 14%, and 82%, respectively.[14] Improvement with systemic thrombolysis was found in 45% of the patients in the same review.

Advantages of systemic infusion of thrombolytic agents were faster resolution of the clot load and less venous valve dysfunction compared with anticoagulation alone.[14] Nonetheless, the disadvantages of the technique include variable outcomes with potential serious complications such as increased risk of intracranial hemorrhage due to higher doses required to dissolve a distant thrombus.[21] In light of the variable success rate, systemic complications, and current advances in minimally invasive endovenous techniques such as CDT and PMT, systemic thrombolysis has been abandoned and now belongs to historical reports.

Catheter-Directed Thrombolysis

The higher risk of bleeding complications of systemic thrombolysis secondary to administration of high doses of thrombolytic agents via peripheral veins led to studies on devices to deliver intrathrombus thrombolytic agents.[21-23] In general, the technique consists of a multi–side-hole catheter that is positioned in the thrombus and remains parked in position to deliver localized thrombolytics and lysing the thrombus over time (Fig. 14-1).

Initial experience using CDT was reported by Semba and Dake using urokinase in 21 consecutive patients with iliofemoral DVT.[24] Total thrombus lysis was achieved in 72% of the limbs with overall angioplasty or angioplasty with stents required in 64%.[24] Subsequently, several series were published comparing anticoagulation alone with CDT.[14,23,25] The impact on quality of life (QoL) in 68 patients who underwent CDT and 30 patients treated with anticoagulation alone was assessed by Comerota and colleagues.[22] Notably, patients who underwent CDT reported better overall physical functioning, less stigma, and less health distress. Furthermore, health distress and symptoms were reduced in patients who had a successful versus a failed CDT treatment.

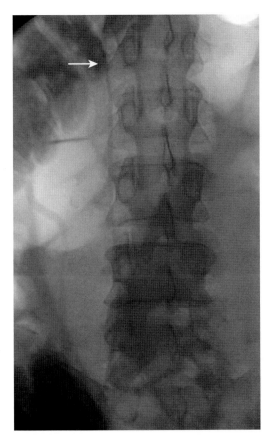

■ **Fig 14–1** Thrombolysis in a 49-year-old man who presented with right lower extremity swelling. He was found to have iliofemoral thrombosis extending to the hypoplastic segment of the perihepatic inferior vena cava. A 50-cm infusion catheter was placed via the popliteal vein. The tip of the catheter was positioned in the suprarenal portion of the interior vena cava (*arrow*). The infusion segment extended down to the common femoral vein.

The caveats of initial studies related to a small number of patients and single-center observation were addressed by a multicenter registry study with urokinase in 473 patients that showed complete lysis of the thrombus in 31% and partial lysis in 52% of the limbs with better results in patients with acute symptoms of DVT.[26] Patients with iliofemoral DVT had higher patency rates at 1-year follow-up than those patients treated for femoropopliteal DVT (64% versus 47%, $p < .01$), and the mean intensive care unit stay for monitoring thrombolytic therapy was 48 hours.[26] One patient had fatal intracranial bleeding and another required surgical evacuation of a subdural hematoma.

Two prospective randomized clinical trials (RCTs) have been reported. The first RCT enrolled 35 patients comparing CDT with streptokinase versus anticoagulation alone; it showed 72% of the limbs in the CDT group with no obstruction or reflux versus only 12% in the anticoagulant group at 6-month follow-up.[25] No major bleeding or mortality was reported. The second RCT, the CaVEnT (**Ca**theter-directed **Ve**nous **T**hrombolysis) trial, enrolled 118 patients to assess the long-term functional efficacy with frequency of PTS after 24 months and descriptive efficacy at 6 months' evaluation for patency rates.[23] Patency of the iliofemoral vein segment was 64% in the CDT group and 36% in the control group. In addition, lysis greater than50% was achieved in 88% of the patients who underwent CDT.[23]

The long interval of CDT treatment course remains problematic because of institutional requirements of an intensive care unit setting for monitoring. A longer infusion interval that is needed also raises concern of potential risk of major bleeding found in up to 11% of the patients.[26] In addition, the use of fluoroscopy for multiple follow-up venograms has directed efforts to accomplish thrombus removal in a more expeditious fashion than has currently been performed by PMT devices.[17,27]

Percutaneous Mechanical Thrombectomy

The advances of endovenous therapy are noticeable over the past two decades. The conception of PMT is a device that provides mechanical maceration of thrombus along with the ability to deliver local thrombolytics. This allows improved penetration of the thrombolytics into the thrombus by increasing the surface area, thereby theoretically decreasing treatment time and amount of thrombolytics delivered.

Two commercially available PMT devices are approved for treatment of DVT by the U.S. Food and Drug Administration (FDA): the Angiojet Thrombectomy system (Medrad/Possis Inc. Minneapolis, MN, and the Trellis-8 Peripheral Infusion System (Covidien, Mansfield, MA).[28] In addition, a brief discussion about the Ekos Endowave system (Ekos Medical, Bothell, WA) is pertinent due to distinct mechanism combining ultrasound waves to facilitate chemical thrombolysis.

The mechanisms of PMT elicited by the Angiojet and Trellis device system are distinct. The Angiojet system is based on the Bernoulli-Venturi principle that states that high speed of a flow decreases the fluid pressure and creates a zone of vacuum (Fig. 14-2). Therefore the high-speed saline injections cause dissolution of the thrombus into small particles that are aspirated and eliminated through an effluent port. Theoretically, the advantages of the system are less endothelial damage and valve dysfunction. The device can also be used in combination with thrombolytics. Drug is delivered into the thrombus with the catheter, allowed to immerse in the thrombus, and then aspirated with the effluent port opened.

Initial experience was reported by Kasijaran et al. in 17 patients showing 59% of overall (>50%) thrombus removal.[28] Bush et al. used the system in 23 limbs and reported complete and partial thrombus resolution in 65% and 35%, respectively.[29] A comparison between the Angiojet versus CDT using only urokinase showed reduced treatment duration and lower costs with the Angiojet pulse system.[30] Another study of 93 patients treated for symptomatic proximal DVT

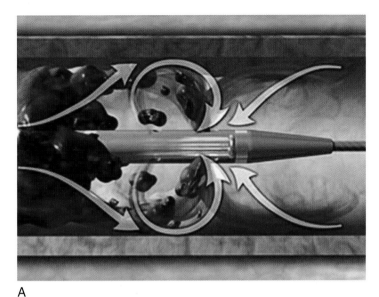
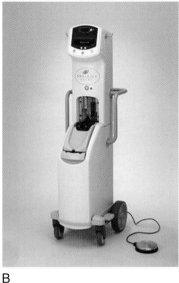

A   B

■ **Fig 14–2** Angiojet thrombectomy system. **A,** Catheter with saline infusion and aspiration port to retrieve thrombus. **B,** Pulse-suction Angiojet generator device.

showed lower mean intensive care unit stays and overall length of hospital stays and lower total hospital costs with Angiojet compared with CDT only.[27] One of the shortcomings of the system is a larger amount of fluid used to dissolve the thrombus, which can be impeditive in patients under fluid restriction, suggesting that precautions be used in cases of renal failure and decompensated congestive heart failure. Provoked hemolysis with increased bilirubin release in patients with liver failure may be another contraindication.

The Trellis-8 Peripheral Infusion System uses a dispersion spiral wire at higher spinning motion to macerated the thrombus in an isolated venous segment between a proximal and distal end balloon (Fig. 14-3). Initial experience with the device showed overall thrombus resolution in greater than 95% of limbs treated.[31,32] No major complications including PE or major bleeding were reported. Trabal et al. reported a series of 25 limbs treated with the Trellis system showing greater than 50% thrombus resolution in 92% of the limbs with significant shorter treatment time and reduced thrombolytic agent used compared with CDT.[33] In addition to thrombus burden resolution, the advantages of the Trellis system are its safety in patients with contraindications to thrombolytic agents and potentially less distal embolization due to isolation of a venous segment between two balloons.

The Ekos endowave functions by emitting high-frequency ultrasound waves that cause disaggregation of the fibrin in the thrombus, increasing permeability to the thrombolytic agents (Fig. 14-4).[34] The catheter consists of four lumens from 6 to 50 cm of functional area containing an ultrasound wire and three other ports for thrombolytic agents and saline infusion. Initial experience in a study of 53 limbs with acute, chronic, and acute-on-chronic DVT showed complete thrombus removal in 70% and overall (complete and partial) lyses rate of 91%.[35] There was no intracranial or retroperitoneal hematoma reported throughout the study. Further prospective, randomized studies on the use of the ultrasound-assisted thrombolysis are still expected.

An ongoing randomized multicenter trial, the ATTRACT trial, is designed to enroll 692 candidates to either PMT with anticoagulation versus anticoagulation alone in patients with symptomatic proximal DVT to assess the occurrence of PTS at 24-month follow-up.[36] The impacts on QoL, safety, and cost analysis are expected to be addressed.

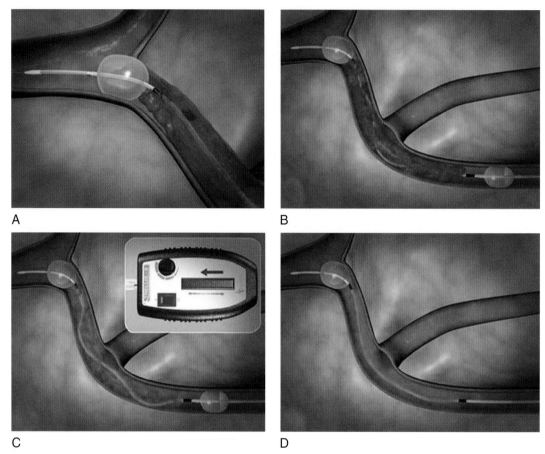

■ **Fig 14–3** The Trellis-8 Peripheral Infusion System. **A,** Catheter advanced through the thrombus in the right iliac vein with distal balloon inflation. **B,** Pulse-spray injection of thrombolytic (*purple strikes*) after inflation of the proximal balloon, isolating the segment of thrombosis. **C,** Initiation of the sinusoidal-shaped catheter macerating the thrombus (hand-held power generator showed in the uppermost portion of the picture). **D,** Dramatic reduction of the thrombus burden secondary to fragmentation caused by high-frequency wave shock. The distal balloon is deflated and the lysed thrombus is aspirated.

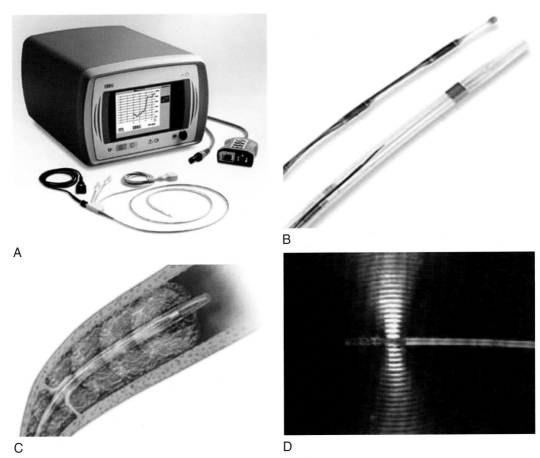

■ **Fig 14–4** Ekos Endowave system. **A,** Ultrasound (US) source generator with monitor. **B,** Ultrasonic catheter with emission probe. **C,** Disarrangement and lysis of the thrombus by ultrasonic waves and continuous lytic infusion. **D,** Detail of ultrasonic wave being emitted from distal probe.

ENDOVASCULAR SUPPLIES

- 21- or 22-Gauge micropuncture kit (0.014- or 0.018-inch platform)
- Angled and straight glidewire .035 inch (180 cm and 260 cm)
- 4- or 5-Fr angle glide catheter
- Multi–side-hole diagnostic catheter 60 and 90 cm
- 5-, 8-, and 9-Fr sheaths
- 4- or 5-Fr infusion catheters with 10-, 20-, 30-, 40-, and 50-cm lengths of infusion
- Trellis, Angiojet, and/or EkosSonic Devices Pack
- Inferior vena cava (IVC) filter as per operator's preferences if indicated
- Percutaneous transluminal angioplasty (PTA) balloons 6 to 18 mm
- Self-expanding stents 12 to 18 mm × 40 to 90 mm

IMAGING ASSESSMENT

- Ultrasound to guide percutaneous access
- C-arm or wall-mounted fluoroscopy for contrast venography
- Intravascular ultrasound (IVUS) in some cases if iliac vein stenting is indicated

OPERATIVE STEPS

Obtaining Access

The patient is taken to the angiography or dedicated operating room suite, prepped, and draped in the prone position. Please note that local anesthetic with 1% lidocaine is used to infiltrate the skin in the popliteal region. A direct popliteal vein stick under ultrasound guidance is performed with a micropuncture kit (Fig. 14-5). A 3- or 4-Fr micropuncture catheter is inserted and its position is checked with gentle hand injections of dilute contrast. Often, the injection reveals filling defects throughout the proximal popliteal, distal, and middle femoral vein. The 3-Fr catheter is exchanged over a wire to a 5-Fr sheath. One may choose access of posterior tibial vein for cases where extensive infrapopliteal involvement is of concern in providing adequate inflow, or for isolated iliac vein thrombosis the patient can be placed in the supine position and access can be obtained in the ipsilateral femoral vein. Other access sites described include the contralateral femoral vein and jugular vein. Our preferred access site is ipsilateral popliteal vein.

Inferior Vena Cava Filter Placement

A retrievable filter when considered is placed via the right internal jugular (Fig. 14-6). Use of an IVC filter during thrombolysis is controversial. The risks and benefits of the filter placement must

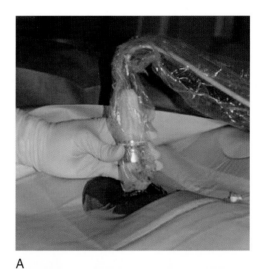

A

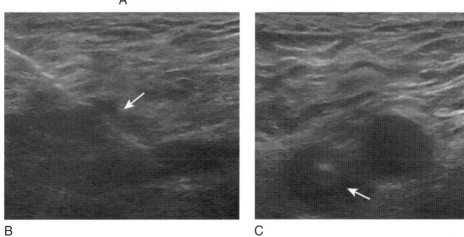

B   C

■ **Fig 14–5 A,** Ultrasound-guided popliteal vein access with the patient in the prone position. Access is obtained with a micropuncture set. The vein is accessed above or below the popliteal fossa. **B,** Needle being inserted in the popliteal vein (*arrow*). **C,** Transverse view confirming good position of the guidewire inside the popliteal vein (*arrow*).

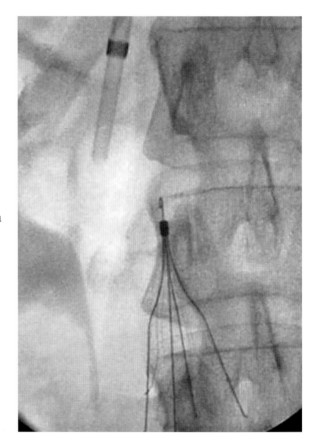

■ **Fig 14–6** Selective placement of inferior vena cava filter via a jugular approach.

be explained to the patient. The right side of the neck is prepped and draped in the usual sterile fashion. Under continuous ultrasound guidance the right internal jugular vein is cannulated with the 22-gauge needle using a micropuncture kit. Subsequently, the 3-Fr sheath is exchanged for a 5-Fr sheath over a wire, which is passed into the infrarenal vena cava. Through the sheath and over the wire a pigtail marking catheter is positioned in the distal IVC, its position is confirmed with gentle hand injections with dilute contrast media, and then a cavogram is obtained with a power injection. Measurements are taken and the IVC filter is chosen based on operator's preference. After IVC filter placement, hand injections through the sheath confirm the position of the filter and the opposition to the wall of the cava.

Catheter-Directed Thrombolysis

After access is obtained in the popliteal vein, a wire is advanced using a combination of an angled glidewire and glide catheter negotiating the iliofemoral segment to reach the IVC. Subsequently, the position of the catheter and patency of the IVC are confirmed with a venogram (Fig. 14-7, *A–D*).

A 5-Fr, 40- or 50-cm-long infusion catheter and the ball-tipped occluding wire are then placed through the catheter. This occludes the end-hole of the catheter and directs delivery of the thrombolytics through the infusion holes. In the case when a valved infusion catheter is used, the occlusion wire is not necessary because there is a occluding one-way valve at the end of the catheter. The infusion length of catheter is chosen based on the length of thrombus present that needs to be treated. The infusion portion of the multi–side-hole catheter is parked in the lowest part of the thrombus and positioned to cover the entire length of thrombus. The catheter is then connected to the infusion pump with an initial dose of 1 mg/hr of rt-PA, and 400 to 600 U of heparin runs through the sheath. Our preference is to use larger volumes of

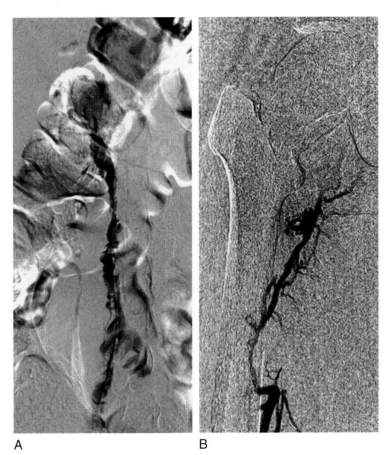

A   B

■ **Fig 14-7** A 49-year-old woman with bilateral lower extremity swelling and acute thrombosis of inferior vena cava (IVC), bilateral iliac, and right femoropopliteal veins. **A,** Initial venogram showing thrombosis extending from bilateral iliac veins into the IVC. **B,** Right femoral vein with proximal occlusion and patent deep femoral vein with collateral to the midportion of the femoral vein.

Continued

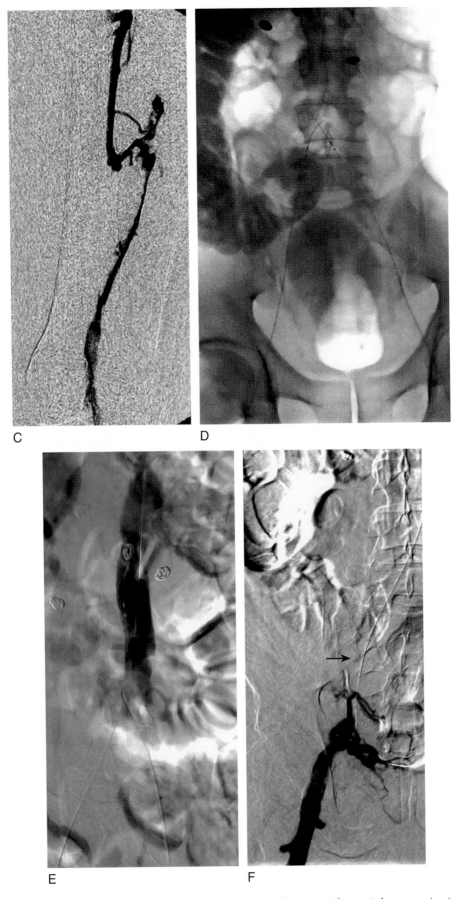

■ **Fig 14–7, cont'd C,** Distal third of the femoral vein with partial reconstitution via a collateral from the deep femoral vein. **D,** Placement of bilateral thrombolysis catheters positioned in the IVC confluence. **E,** Venogram 12 hours after CDT of the IVC with complete resolution of IVC thrombus. **F,** Residual thrombus in the right iliac vein (*arrow*).

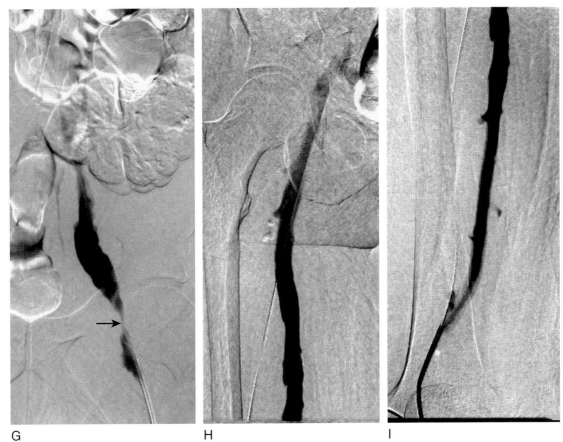

G   H   I

■ **Fig 14–7, cont'd   G,** Left iliofemoral veins partial resolution (*arrow*).
H, Completion venogram showing proximal resolution of thrombosis in the right
femoral vein after 24 hours of CDT. **I,** Patent distal portion of the femoral and
popliteal veins.

diluted rt-PA to improve lytic therapy if it is not contraindicated. This is theoretical and has never been studied. The catheter and sheath are both wrapped sterilely in the usual manner. The venogram of the more proximal iliac system is not necessarily performed if it is significant filling defect throughout the iliofemoral vein is present in a preprocedure imaging. At the end of the procedure, the patient is transferred to an intensive care unit for close monitoring throughout the thrombolysis course. A sequential treatment of an extensive iliofemoral and caval DVT using CDT is illustrated in Figure 14-7, *E–I*.

We advocate checking the complete blood cell count, serum chemistry, activated prothrombin time, and fibrinogen level every 4 to 6 hours while the thrombolytic agent is infused. The thrombolytic recheck is done every 12 hours to evaluate improvement.

Pharmacomechanical Thrombectomy

Trellis-8 Peripheral Infusion System. Access is obtained via popliteal vein as described earlier. An initial venogram is obtained as shown in Figure 14-8, *A*.

- The 5-Fr sheath is exchanged for an 8-Fr sheath to accommodate the Trellis catheter.
- The Trellis catheter is then advanced over a glidewire and parked in the segment of interest. Treatment is initiated in the most proximal segment (the segment closest to the heart) involved with the thrombus.
- The most common Trellis treatment length zone used is 30 cm. Specification of the sizes of the catheter is shown in Table 14-1. The specific length of the catheter encompasses the entire segment that is expected to be mechanically thrombectomized. If the treatment zone is longer than 30 cm, the venous segment is treated in serial segments starting from proximal to distal.
- The proximal end of the catheter is parked 1 to 2 cm above the proximal portion of the thrombus and the proximal balloon is inflated (Fig. 14-8, *B* and *C*). The glidewire is exchanged for the sinusoidal wire, and the distal balloon is inflated (Fig. 14-8, *D*).
- The motor is turned on at the highest rpm, and the direction of rotation is changed every 2 minute time interval. The combination of 5 mg of rt-PA mixed in 5 mL of heparinized saline is also infused at a rate of 1 mL/2 minutes (for a treatment time of about 20 minutes). This protocol of direction of rotation and drug infusion can be altered as per operator's preference.
- After 20 minutes of treatment, the distal end balloon is deflated, and fragments of thrombus, residual rt-PA, and blood are aspirated via the aspiration port while flushing the infusion port.
- The proximal balloon is deflated and the catheter is pulled back to a more distal segment with residual thrombus and the previous steps are repeated (Fig. 14-8, *E* and *F*).
- Thus, the response is gauged with repeat hand injections of contrast after device removal (Fig. 14-8, *G* and *H*). If residual thrombus is present, several options exist:
  - The Trellis catheter may be reinserted and additional PMT is performed in areas of residual thrombus.
  - If iliac vein stenosis and/or residual thrombus is present preventing adequate outflow, angioplasty and/or stenting may be required (Fig. 14-8, *I*).
  - Placement of the infusion catheter in areas of residual thrombus for CDT.

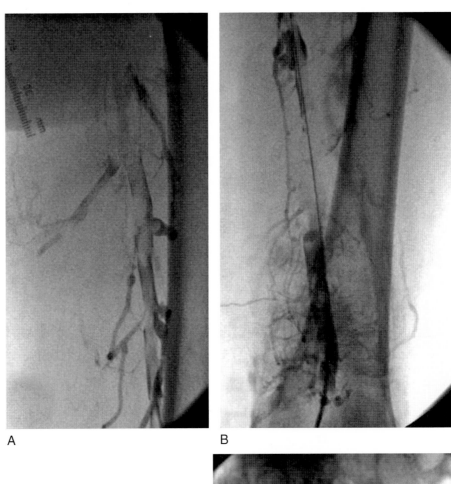

A

B

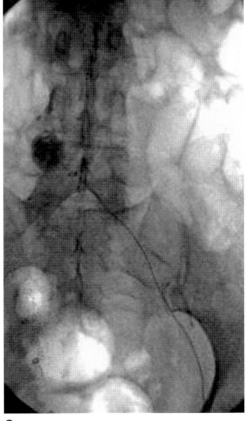

C

■ **Fig 14–8** A 54-year-old man presented with a new onset of left lower extremity swelling and pain due to extensive iliofemoral and popliteal vein thrombosis. **A,** Initial venogram confirming femoropopliteal deep venous thrombolysis. **B,** Subsequently, a wire is advanced through the thrombus. **C,** A 30-cm Trellis catheter is parked proximally to the thrombus and the proximal balloon is inflated.

Continued

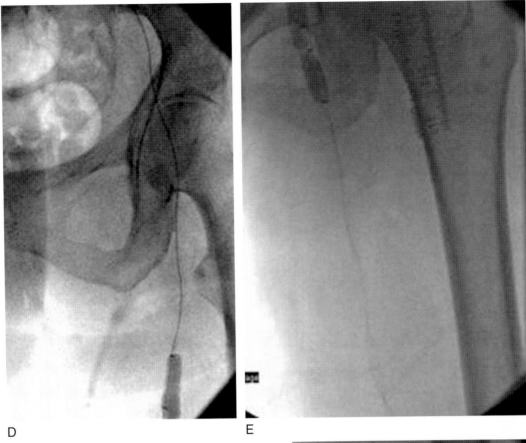

D

E

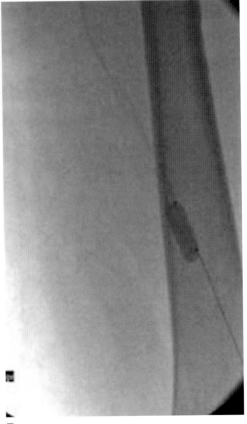

■ **Fig 14–8, cont'd D,** Subsequently, the distal balloon is inflated into the femoral vein, isolating the segment to be treated. **E,** Upon treatment completion of the proximal segment, the catheter is positioned for treatment of the femoropopliteal segment. **F,** The distal balloon is again inflated, isolating the new segment to be treated.

F

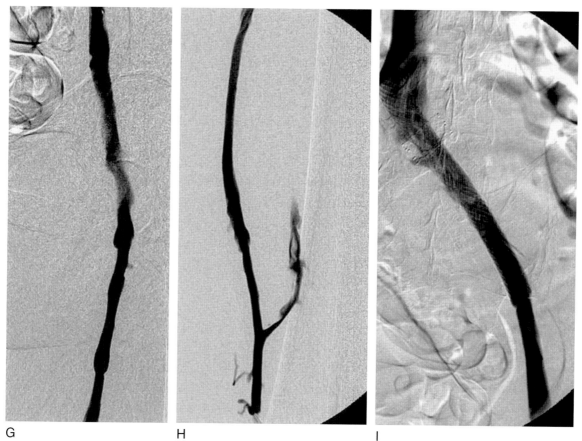

■ **Fig 14–8, cont'd G,** Venogram following PMT with most thrombi lysed in the femoropopliteal portion. **H,** Distal part of the treated segment. **I,** A 16 × 80-mm self-expanding stent was placed in the iliac vein to treat residual disease.

TABLE 14–1 FDA-Approved Commercially Available PMT Systems for Treatment of DVT

Trellis-8 Peripheral Infusion System		Angiojet Rheolytic System				
Length, cm	Treatment Zone, cm	Catheter	Length, cm	Sheath, Fr	Guidewire, in	Vessel diameter, mm
80	10	XMI RX+	135	4	.014	2-5
80	15	Spiroflex	135	4	.014	2-5
80	30	XVG	140	5	.014	3-8
120	15	Xpeedior	120	6	.035	4-12
120	30	DVX	90	6	.035	4-12

DVT, Deep venous thrombosis; *FDA,* Food and Drug Administration; *PMT,* pharmacomechanical thrombectomy.

Angiojet Rheolytic System (MedRad; Warrendale, PA). After micropuncture access is obtained in the popliteal vein and changed to a 6-Fr sheath, a glidewire is advanced with an angled glide catheter crossing the thrombosed area into the IVC. A preintervention venogram is obtained. Fig. 14-9, *A–C*, depicts an extensive ileofemoropopliteal DVT.

- The catheter is removed over the wire and the Angiojet DVX catheter is advanced.
- The DVX catheter is connected to the drive unit and the machine is tuned on to initiate the high pressure (10,000 psi) saline jets; the debris generated is aspirated to the effluent port (see Fig. 14-2, *A*). The catheter is positioned at the most proximal vein segment involved with thrombus.
- The catheter is pulled back slowly 1 cm for every pump cycle, treating the entire length. Often, two or three passes are necessary to achieve maximal thrombus resolution.
- If "power-pulse" technique is performed, the effluent port is closed to allow delivery of drug and no aspiration.
- Drug is delivered from proximal to distal at a pullback rate of 1 cm every pump cycle. Once drug is delivered into the thrombus, it is allowed to bathe for 15 to 20 minutes.
- The effluent port is then opened and the Angiojet catheter is passed from proximal to distal to aspirate thrombus and excess thrombolytics.
- Following treatment, a venogram is performed, and the decision is made to complete treatment, continue further treatment with pharmacomechanical thrombolysis, or place an infusion catheter (Fig. 14-9, *D* and *E*, illustrates the results after pulse-spray and Angiojet thrombectomy).
- If an underlying iliac vein stenosis is uncovered, it should be treated with PTA and stenting (Fig. 14-9, *F* and *G*).

EkoSonic Endovascular System (Ekos Medical, Bothell, WA). When the EkoSonic system is contemplated, a catheter must cross the thrombus over a .035-inch guidewire that is then exchanged with the ultrasonic (US) wire. The tip of the US wire exits the catheter, being parked at least 1 cm distal to the end of the catheter. Thrombolytic agent is delivered from the multi–side-hole catheter, and a mobile unit provides the temperature and US energy delivered. The patient is transferred to the unit and lytic re-recheck is performed every 4 to 6 hours or as per specific local protocols.

Venous Stenting and Angioplasty

The absolute indications for venous angioplasty and stenting are debatable. Angioplasty alone has not shown to be efficient to alleviate obstruction because of recoiling or persistent external compression. We advocate primary stenting whenever a significant residual stenosis is revealed. The presence of residual stenosis can be evaluated with venography or IVUS. Indirect signs of residual stenosis on venography include the presence of collaterals, intraluminal filling defects, or poor venous outflow. A direct evaluation of the residual obstruction can be obtained with IVUS. This also allows evaluation of the length needed to be treated and selection of the stent size. Most of the stents used are self-expandable and are 60 to 90 mm in length. The stent diameter for the common iliac should be 16 to 18 mm; for the external iliac, 14 to 16 mm; and for the common femoral vein, 12 to 14 mm. The key to venous stenting is to cover all diseased segments and obtain good inflow and good outflow. To achieve this, one may need to extend

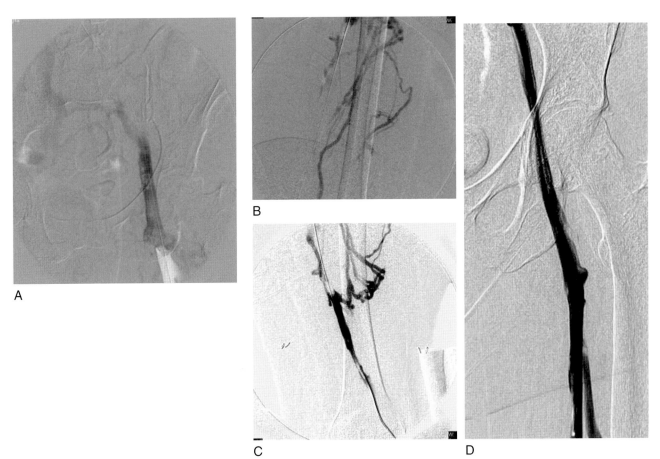

A

B

C

D

■ **Fig 14–9** A 62-year-old female patient who presented with left lower extremity swelling associated with thigh and calf pain. **A–C,** She was found to have extensive iliofemoral and popliteal deep venous thrombosis as shown in the diagnostic venogram. **D,** Venogram of proximal femoropopliteal segment following "pulse-spray" thrombolysis with 10 mg of t-PA using the Angiojet.

Continued

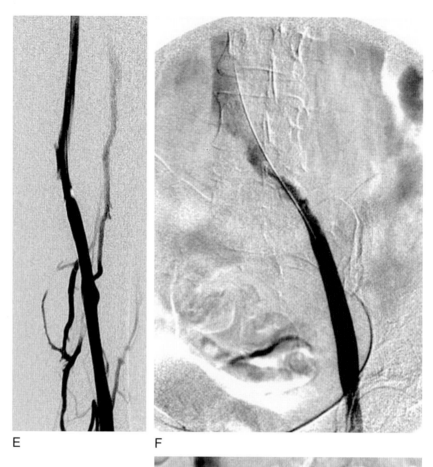

E   F

■ **Fig 14–9, cont'd** **E,** The distal femoropopliteal segment was successfully lysed as well. **F,** Completion venogram showing residual left iliac vein stenosis. **G,** Repeat venogram following deployment of 16 × 60-mm Wallstent.

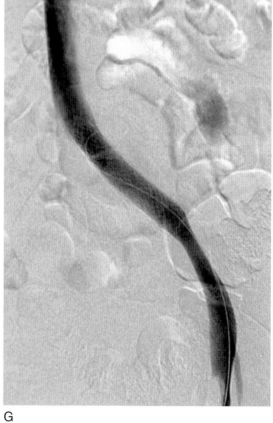

G

the stent into the IVC or below the inguinal ligament. Poststenting angioplasty with appropriately sized balloons is required to fully expand the stent. Completion venogram or IVUS is performed to evaluate flow and look for filling defects or residual stenosis.

HEMOSTASIS AND ANTICOAGULATION

During thrombolysis, low-dose anticoagulation is achieved with UFH. Following completion of thrombolysis, therapeutic anticoagulation is accomplished with UFH or LMWH. The patient is subsequently bridged to warfarin sodium that is continued and tailored to the patient's DVT presentation based on current guidelines.[17]

Puncture site hemostasis is effectively accomplished with manual compression or mechanical devices following completion of venography in the last lytic recheck.[37] In our experience, manual compression is appropriate with no need to use external mechanical compression devices.

Internal jugular and femoral vein access. Pressure is held manually for 10 to 15 minutes and a sterile dressing is applied to the puncture site. Application of heavy packs such as sandbags is not necessary.

Popliteal vein access. Manual compression for 10 to 15 minutes is applied, followed by the application of a mild to moderately tight Ace bandage wrapped around the venous puncture site right above and below the knee to confer hemostasis. A Coban bandage is then applied from foot to midthigh over a loose cotton layer to protect the skin. The patient is turned to the supine position after removal of the catheters, and the dressing is removed after 4 hours in the intensive care unit. Thereafter, the patient is encouraged to walk for 15 minutes.

COMPLICATIONS

Minor bleeding: Usually occurs from oozing and ecchymosis at the venous puncture site and does not require any treatment.

Major bleeding: Requires blood transfusion and usually occurs in the brain, retroperitoneum, muscles and gastrointestinal/genitourinary tract.

Venous wall injury: Wall damage during manipulation of catheters or rupture during balloon angioplasty.

Pulmonary embolism: Thrombus dislodgement into the pulmonary arteries during the procedure.

COMPARATIVE EFFECTIVENESS OF EXISTING TREATMENTS

Surgical thrombectomy was the first intervention attempted for limb salvage in cases of phlegmasia in patients with severe ischemia with impending venous gangrene. Contemporary results in a specialized center showed long-term patency of 80% at 5 years with no mortality.[38] Meticulous and technical refined operations require considerable efforts with a long learning curve. In light of advances in catheter technology and very good initial results with PMT devices, the surgical treatment is limited to cases of rapidly evolving massive DVT in patients with contraindications to thrombolytic agents and with impending limb loss.

PEARLS AND PITFALLS

Choosing the Access

The right choice of access site for CDT or PMT is critical for an appropriate treatment. In the majority of the series, the popliteal vein is the most commonly used puncture site followed by the contralateral femoral vein.[39]

The advantages of the popliteal vein include a straight pathway for instrumentation in the iliofemoral segment via an antegrade approach, avoidance of crossing an IVC filter, and shorter catheters required. Conversely, thrombus involving the popliteal vein and reduced torque to negotiate catheters and stents for contralateral limb treatment are relative contraindications.

Some specialists advocate the use of the internal jugular vein for thrombectomy and thrombolysis. The rationale of using this access is to facilitate treatment of bilateral iliofemoral DVT. Disadvantages are longer catheters and limited approach to distal femoropopliteal DVT.

An additional access is often not necessary for CDT or PMT unless an intervention such as stenting is required in selected cases of bilateral iliac vein stenosis.[40] Regardless of the preference of access, the needs of each patient should be considered, tailoring the best approach to a specific scenario of DVT.

Angioplasty and Stenting Post-CDT and PMT Therapy

Often, an iliac vein stenosis is found after CDT or PMT, compromising venous outflow. Angioplasty and stenting are always recommended when underlying venous lesions are present following a successful thrombolysis and thrombectomy.[17] We advocate the use of self-expanding stents over balloon-expandable stents. The stent diameter for the common iliac should be 16 to 18 mm; for the external iliac, 14 to 16 mm; and for the common femoral vein, 12 to 14 mm. Covering all venous segments with residual disease with stents and achieving good inflow and good outflow are very important to maintain patency. To accomplish this, one may need to use longer stents (60 to 90 mm) and extend the stents into the IVC or below the inguinal ligament. When stents are extended into the common femoral vein, patency of the femoral or deep femoral veins is essential. The use of IVUS appears attractive to better define anatomy and size the stents to attain precise apposition to the venous wall. However, the role of IVUS in procedures to treat acute DVT is not well defined.

Inferior Vena Cava Filter

The use of devices for thrombectomy ultimately may cause distal embolization that eventually dissolves through the use of thrombolytics or the intrinsic fibrinolytic system. Up to now, no fatal PE has been reported following CDT or PMT. However, five patients presented with symptomatic PE in a multicenter registry after CDT.[21] In our unreported experience, 30% of patients undergoing thrombolysis (PMT or CDT) experienced distal embolization (either PE or thrombus entrapped in the filter). Kolbel and colleagues analyzed data on 40 patients and found visible emboli within the filter in 45%.[41]

The role of IVC placement during CDT and PMT is not clear. Those who advocate the IVC filter placement based their decision on low morbidity and mortality of IVC placement, availability of temporary/retrievable filters, and potential complications such as PE.[41,42] The drawbacks of the IVC filter include the additional costs of the device, risks related to the procedure, and the need for IVC filter retrieval in the future. Some specialists suggest selective use of filters in patients with free-floating thrombus in the IVC.[43] Current guidelines recommend against routinely placed IVC filters aiming at prophylaxis[17] but do not specify the use during CDT or PMT.[31]

FIVE SALIENT REFERENCES

1. Kearon C, Kahn SR, Agnelli G, et al. Antithrombotic therapy for venous thromboembolic disease: American College of Chest Physicians Evidence-Based Clinical Practice Guidelines (8th Edition). Chest 2008;133(6 Suppl):454S-545S.
2. Mewissen MW, Seabrook GR, Meissner MH, et al. Catheter-directed thrombolysis for lower extremity deep venous thrombosis: report of a national multicenter registry. Radiology 1999;211:39-49.
3. Comerota AJ, Throm RC, Mathias SD, et al. Catheter-directed thrombolysis for iliofemoral deep venous thrombosis improves health-related quality of life. J Vasc Surg 2000;32:130-137.
4. Lin PH, Zhou W, Dardik A, et al. Catheter-direct thrombolysis versus pharmacomechanical thrombectomy for treatment of symptomatic lower extremity deep venous thrombosis. Am J Surg 2006;192:782-788.
5. Vedantham S, Vesely TM, Sicard GA, et al. Pharmacomechanical thrombolysis and early stent placement for iliofemoral deep vein thrombosis. J Vasc Interv Radiol 2004;15:565-574.

REFERENCES

1. Heit JA. The epidemiology of venous thromboembolism in the community. Arterioscler Thromb Vasc Biol 2008;28:370-372.
2. Meissner MH, Zierler BK, Bergelin RO, et al. Coagulation, fibrinolysis, and recanalization after acute deep venous thrombosis. J Vasc Surg 2002;35:278-285.
3. Labropoulos N, Patel PJ, Tiongson JE, et al. Patterns of venous reflux and obstruction in patients with skin damage due to chronic venous disease. Vasc Endovasc Surg 2007;41:33-40.
4. Prandoni P. Long-term clinical course of proximal deep venous thrombosis and detection of recurrent thrombosis. Semin Thromb Hemost 2001;27:9-13.
5. Labropoulos N, Gasparis AP, Pefanis D, et al. Secondary chronic venous disease progresses faster than primary. J Vasc Surg 2009;49:704-710.
6. Prandoni P, Villalta S, Bagatella P, et al. The clinical course of deep-vein thrombosis. Prospective long-term follow-up of 528 symptomatic patients. Haematologica 1997;82:423-428.
7. Labropoulos N, Waggoner T, Sammis W, et al. The effect of venous thrombus location and extent on the development of post-thrombotic signs and symptoms. J Vasc Surg 2008;48:407-412.
8. Agnelli G, Becattini C, Prandoni P. Recurrent venous thromboembolism in men and women. N Engl J Med 2004;351:2015-2018; author reply 2015-2018.
9. Labropoulos N, Jen J, Jen H, et al. Recurrent deep vein thrombosis: long-term incidence and natural history. Ann Surg 2010;251:749-753.
10. Prandoni P, Noventa F, Ghirarduzzi A, et al. The risk of recurrent venous thromboembolism after discontinuing anticoagulation in patients with acute proximal deep vein thrombosis or pulmonary embolism. A prospective cohort study in 1,626 patients. Haematologica 2007;92:199-205.
11. Labropoulos N, Spentzouris G, Gasparis AP, et al. Impact and clinical significance of recurrent venous thromboembolism. Br J Surg 2010;97:989-999.

12. Prandoni P, Kahn SR. Post-thrombotic syndrome: prevalence, prognostication and need for progress. Br J Haematol 2009;145:286-295.

13. Douketis JD, Crowther MA, Foster GA, et al. Does the location of thrombosis determine the risk of disease recurrence in patients with proximal deep vein thrombosis? Am J Med 2001;110:515-519.

14. Comerota AJ, Aldridge SC. Thrombolytic therapy for deep venous thrombosis: a clinical review. Can J Surg 1993;36:359-364.

15. Mahorner H. A new method of management for thrombosis of deep veins of the extremities: thrombectomy, restoration of the lumen and heparinization. Am Surg 1954;20:487-498.

16. Fontaine R, Briot B, Vujadinovic B, et al. [Results, after five months, of bilateral thrombectomy in the legs for alterating venous thrombosis of a type called blue phlebitis (phlebitis with arteriospasm).]. Strasbourg Med 1955;6:172-178.

17. Kearon C, Kahn SR, Agnelli G, et al. Antithrombotic therapy for venous thromboembolic disease: American College of Chest Physicians Evidence-Based Clinical Practice Guidelines (8th Edition). Chest 2008;133(Suppl):454S-545S.

18. Juhan C, Alimi Y, Di Mauro P, et al. Surgical venous thrombectomy. Cardiovasc Surg (Lond Engl) 1999;7:586-590.

19. Blattler W, Heller G, Largiader J, et al. Combined regional thrombolysis and surgical thrombectomy for treatment of iliofemoral vein thrombosis. J Vasc Surg 2004;40:620-625.

20. Klein SJ, Gasparis AP, Virvilis D, et al. Prospective determination of candidates for thrombolysis in patients with acute proximal deep vein thrombosis. J Vasc Surg 2010;51:908-912.

21. Mewissen MW. Catheter-directed thrombolysis for lower extremity deep vein thrombosis. Techniques in vascular and interventional radiology. 2001;4:111-114.

22. Comerota AJ, Throm RC, Mathias SD, et al. Catheter-directed thrombolysis for iliofemoral deep venous thrombosis improves health-related quality of life. J Vasc Surg 2000;32:130-137.

23. Enden T, Klow NE, Sandvik L, et al. Catheter-directed thrombolysis vs. anticoagulant therapy alone in deep vein thrombosis: results of an open randomized, controlled trial reporting on short-term patency. J Thromb Haemost 2009;7:1268-1275.

24. Semba CP, Dake MD. Iliofemoral deep venous thrombosis: aggressive therapy with catheter-directed thrombolysis. Radiology 1994;191:487-494.

25. Elsharawy M, Elzayat E. Early results of thrombolysis vs anticoagulation in iliofemoral venous thrombosis. A randomised clinical trial. Eur J Vasc Endovasc Surg 2002;24:209-214.

26. Mewissen MW, Seabrook GR, Meissner MH, et al. Catheter-directed thrombolysis for lower extremity deep venous thrombosis: report of a national multicenter registry. Radiology 1999;211:39-49.

27. Lin PH, Zhou W, Dardik A, et al. Catheter-direct thrombolysis versus pharmacomechanical thrombectomy for treatment of symptomatic lower extremity deep venous thrombosis. Am J Surg 2006;192:782-788.

28. Kasirajan K, Gray B, Ouriel K. Percutaneous AngioJet thrombectomy in the management of extensive deep venous thrombosis. J Vasc Interv Radiol 2001;12:179-185.

29. Bush RL, Lin PH, Bates JT, et al. Pharmacomechanical thrombectomy for treatment of symptomatic lower extremity deep venous thrombosis: safety and feasibility study. J Vasc Surg 2004;40:965-970.

30. Kim HS, Patra A, Paxton BE, et al. Adjunctive percutaneous mechanical thrombectomy for lower-extremity deep vein thrombosis: clinical and economic outcomes. J Vasc Interv Radiol 2006;17:1099-1104.

31. Rao AS, Konig G, Leers SA, et al. Pharmacomechanical thrombectomy for iliofemoral deep vein thrombosis: an alternative in patients with contraindications to thrombolysis. J Vasc Surg 2009;50:1092-1098.

32. O'Sullivan GJ, Lohan DG, Gough N, et al. Pharmacomechanical thrombectomy of acute deep vein thrombosis with the Trellis-8 isolated thrombolysis catheter. J Vasc Interv Radiol 2007;18:715-724.

33. Martinez Trabal JL, Comerota AJ, et al. The quantitative benefit of isolated, segmental, pharmacomechanical thrombolysis (ISPMT) for iliofemoral venous thrombosis. J Vasc Surg 2008;48:1532-1537.

34. Braaten JV, Goss RA, Francis CW. Ultrasound reversibly disaggregates fibrin fibers. Thromb Haemost 1997;78:1063-1068.

35. Parikh S, Motarjeme A, McNamara T, et al. Ultrasound-accelerated thrombolysis for the treatment of deep vein thrombosis: initial clinical experience. J Vasc Interv Radiol 2008;19: 521-528.

36. Comerota AJ. The ATTRACT trial: rationale for early intervention for iliofemoral DVT. Perspect Vasc Surg Endovasc Ther 2009;21:221-224; quiz 224-225.

37. Coto HA. Closure of the femoral vein puncture site after transcatheter procedures using Angio-Seal. Catheter Cardiovasc Interv 2002;55:16-19.

38. Hartung O, Benmiloud F, Barthelemy P, et al. Late results of surgical venous thrombectomy with iliocaval stenting. J Vasc Surg 2008;47:381-387.

39. Comerota AJ, Aldridge SC, Cohen G, et al. A strategy of aggressive regional therapy for acute iliofemoral venous thrombosis with contemporary venous thrombectomy or catheter-directed thrombolysis. J Vasc Surg 1994;20:244-254.

40. Vedantham S, Vesely TM, Sicard GA, et al. Pharmacomechanical thrombolysis and early stent placement for iliofemoral deep vein thrombosis. J Vasc Interv Radiol 2004;15:565-574.

41. Kolbel T, Alhadad A, Acosta S, et al. Thrombus embolization into IVC filters during catheter-directed thrombolysis for proximal deep venous thrombosis. J Endovasc Ther 2008;15: 605-613.

42. Kwon SH, Oh JH, Seo TS, et al. Percutaneous aspiration thrombectomy for the treatment of acute lower extremity deep vein thrombosis: is thrombolysis needed? Clin Radiol 2009;64: 484-490.

43. Comerota AJ, Gravett MH. Iliofemoral venous thrombosis. J Vasc Surg 2007;46:1065-1076.

CHAPTER 15

Postthrombotic Syndrome

Rafael D. Malgor, Antonios P. Gasparis,
and Nicos Labropoulos

HISTORICAL BACKGROUND

Postthrombotic syndrome (PTS) remains an important health care problem in United States. A population-based study showed that the incidence of venous ulcers currently approaches 18 per 100,000 habitants per year.[1] The same study identified that PTS is responsible for economic expenses estimated at least $200 million.[1]

Diagnosis of PTS is based on history and clinical presentation. The syndrome consists of signs and symptoms of heaviness, intolerance to exercises, pain, leg edema, paresthesia, cramps, pruritus that may evolve to skin damage such as hyperpigmentation, lipodermatosclerosis, and ulcers (Fig. 15-1). The severity of PTS is measured by different scales and scores assigning points for the presence of each sign and symptom. Although there is a good association with PTS severity, further refinement and validation are necessary.[2-5]

Attention to differential diagnosis should be outlined. Trauma, congenital venous disease (i.e., venous malformations, valve aplasia) and other causes of ulcerative disease such as rheumatologic (lupus, scleroderma, rheumatoid arthritis), oncologic (squamous and basal cell carcinoma), or infectious disorders (syphilis, lymphangitis) are potential causes of misdiagnosis and inappropriate treatment.[6,7] Table 15-1 shows the location and cause of non–venous-related ulcers.

Not all patients who have had a documented episode of DVT sustain PTS. Recovery with no signs or symptoms of PTS occurs in two-thirds of the patients, and only the rest will eventually develop PTS with variable spectrum and severity.[8] It appears that other factors are involved in the disease process, rendering some patients more vulnerable than others to PTS changes. Predisposing factors for PTS are age, sex, hypercoagulable state, obesity, immobility, and, most important, ipsilateral recurrent DVT. The latter is deemed to be the strongest factor for PTS, as several prospective studies have shown high odds for skin damage.[9,10] Patients who had unprovoked DVT and are older than 65 years have a higher risk of recurrent DVT and therefore PTS.[11]

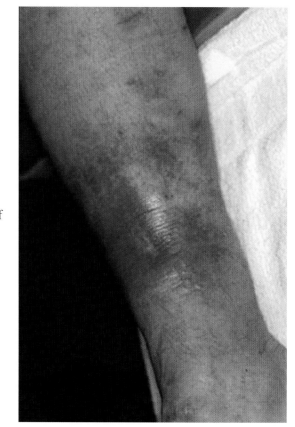

■ **Fig 15-1** Image of the right leg from a patient with previous venous thrombosis. Features of postthrombotic signs are seen in the medial aspect of the leg (CEAP classes 3, 4, and 5). This patient had also pain, itching, and burning sensation.

Residual thrombus was also reported as a cause of recurrent DVT[12] (Fig. 15-2). In addition, patients who had DVT in more than one site, popliteal valve insufficiency, or a calf DVT associated with a proximal DVT also have an increased risk of recurrent DVT.[13-15] Notably, the recurrence of DVT is likely to affect the proximal veins and is related to inadequate duration of anticoagulation.[9] In a recent review, the limitations of studies on recurrent DVT are discussed.[16] Most of the studies used a nonstandardized ultrasound analysis, giving limited or inaccurate information on the incidence of fatal pulmonary embolism (PE) as well as having poor documentation of anticoagulation and its monitoring. The effects of thrombolytic therapy and its socioeconomic and quality of life impact are also questions that remain unanswered.[16] These are important because ipsilateral recurrent DVT has a great impact on the development of PTS.

Biomarkers have been used to estimate the odds of developing PTS. In a recent study of 305 patients with PTS, persistent elevated levels of D-dimer in the course of DVT were investigated. Patients with elevated levels of D-dimer at 4 months following DVT after stopping anticoagulation showed a fourfold risk of PTS.[17]

Patients with asymptomatic DVT are also at risk of developing PTS. A systematic review including 364 patients with asymptomatic DVT showed that abdominal and orthopedic surgeries are major predictors for PTS. The drawbacks in the former study were different definitions of PTS according to each author's criteria, random use of anticoagulation upon diagnosis, and different diagnostic methods including venography, duplex ultrasound (DUS), and ^{125}I-fibrinogen uptake test. Regardless of distinct methodology found in the literature, if a poor DVT history is associated with marked PTS findings, it must prompt careful investigation with DUS first, especially following major abdominal or orthopedic surgery.

TABLE 15–1 Characteristics of the Ulcers Found on 21 Patients

Sex	Age (y)	Limb	Location on Calf	Duration (y)	Duplex	ABI	Medication	Pathology
M	63	L	u-1/med	3	nl	nl	abx	Undetermined
		R	u-1/med	3	nl	nl	abx	Undetermined
F	72	L	1/med	5	nl	nl		Vasculitis
		R	1/med	5	nl	nl		Vasculitis
F	52	L	m-l/med	4	nl	nl	abx	Chronic inflammation
M	73	R	1/med	8	nl	nl	abx	Chronic inflammation
M	54	R	1/ant-lt	2	nl	nl	abx	Chronic inflammation
M	68	L	m/post	1	nl	nl		Kaposi sarcoma
M	79	L	1/med	16		nl		Carcinoma
F	76	R	1/med	18	Venous reflux	nl		Squamous cell carcinoma
F	73	R	1/med	15	Venous reflux	nl		Squamous cell carcinoma
F	64	L	m-1/med	3	nl	nl		Undetermined
		R	m-1/med	3	nl	nl		Undetermined
M	71	L	1/med	4	nl	nl		No histology
F	82	R	m-1/med	7	nl	nl	abx	No histology
F	73	R	1/med	14	nl	nl		Basal cell carcinoma
M	78	L	m/med	2	nl	nl		Pyoderma gangrenosum
	59	L	1/med	0.17	nl	nl		Hydroxyurea
M	17	R	1/med	0.33	nl	nl		Sickle cell
M		L	1/med	0.25	nl	nl		Sickle cell
F	62	R	1/med	0.75	Mild reflux	0.7		Rheumatoid arthritis

Adapted from Labropoulous N, Manalo D, Patel NP, et al. Uncommon leg ulcers in the lower extremity. J Vasc Surg 2007;45:568-573.
ABI, Ankle-brachial index; *u,* upper calf; *m,* midcalf; *nl,* normal; *abx,* antibiotics; *post,* posterior; *ant-lt,* anterior lateral.

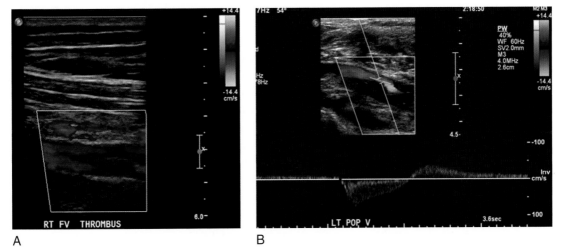

A   B

■ **Fig 15–2 A,** Chronic thrombus in a male patient who presented with swelling and pain of the right lower extremity. The femoral vein is partially recanalized as seen by the multiple channels and the intraluminal filling defects. **B,** A 55-year-old female patient sustaining leg edema, discoloration, and a venous ulcer. Reflux is seen in a partially recanalized popliteal vein thrombosis.

Progression of secondary cardiovascular disease (CVD) evolving to PTS has been demonstrated. A study of 73 limbs with secondary CVD showed overall progression in clinical CEAP classes in 31% of the limbs. Skin damage (C4-C6) rate strikingly rose from 4% at the first year to 25% in the 5-year follow-up. Other studies also investigated secondary CVD and clinical course of PTS.[12] In an Italian cohort of 355 patients, the incidence of PTS increased from 17% after the first year to 29% at 8 years of follow-up.[12] Development of reflux alone has been associated with PTS.[10-17] However, a combination of reflux and obstruction is associated with more severe PTS than reflux or obstruction alone.[10]

Patients with a hypercoagulable state such as carriers of factor V Lieden (FVL), prothrombin gene mutation, or proteins C and S have been investigated for occurrence of PTS. In a recent study, 667 patients with DVT who sustained hypercoagulable state demonstrated no association with increased risk of PTS. Furthermore, heterozygosis for FVL was even less associated with PTS than in noncarriers.[18] Another study of 387 patients tested for thrombophilia found no increased risk of PTS in carriers of FVL or prothrombin gene mutation.[15] The same study also showed that the intensity of persistent signs and symptoms in the first month after the episode of acute DVT predicted the incidence of PTS in a dose-dependent manner in the first 2 years.[15]

NONOPERATIVE TREATMENT

PTS generates high expenses for government and insurance companies due to disability premiums, loss of labor force, and need for rehabilitation and wound care. Thus, prevention should be always contemplated to minimize the socioeconomic impact of the disease. DVT prophylaxis is mandatory in different settings such as major surgeries, critically ill patients, and those with significant risk factors for DVT.[19]

Multiple reports have shown that elastic compression applied in patients with acute DVT may decrease the incidence of PTS by 50% at long term.[20,21] This was evident in two review papers that analyzed all the relevant prospective studies.[22,23] However, most of these trials had an inadequate sample size to resolve this conclusively. Currently, there is an ongoing randomized multicentre trial (SOX trial) that will provide data on the effectiveness of compression stockings on the prevention and severity of PTS, VTE recurrence, quality of life, and cost-effectiveness.[24] It will also prospectively evaluate the predictive role of biomarkers in the development of PTS.

In patients with established PTS, a few treatments are available. Initial treatment for all patients with PTS is nonoperative, with compression to the legs in different levels and intensity. The use of compression stockings in 387 patients could not predict the progression or lack of PTS. However, patients who did use compression stockings had a risk of 20% of developing PTS compared with 47% who did not use compression stockings.[12] The Cochrane collaboration review of 39 randomized control trials concluded that compression was more effective than no compression on ulcer healing.[25] It was also shown that multicomponent systems were more effective in ulcer healing compared with single-component systems.

The shortcoming of compression therapy is that up to 20% of patients are noncompliant, and compliance with stockings does not change regardless of the symptoms of PTS.[26] Complementary to the compression therapy, wound care is important to improve ulcer healing rates and patients' quality of life. Many techniques have been applied in different settings varying from local care to more extensive surgical debridement.

More recently, in a small prospective randomized study of patients with PTS, exercise training for 6 months was associated with improvement in quality of life and improvement in scores on the Villalta scale.[27] The authors concluded that these results should be confirmed in a large prospective randomized trial.

INTERVENTIONAL TREATMENT

Surgical and endovascular procedures are indicated when deep venous reflux or obstruction is present with or without superficial vein involvement in patients with skin damage or disabling symptoms. Prior to the endovenous techniques, obstruction used to be treated with bypass grafts. More recently, chronic venous obstruction is treated with balloon angioplasty and stenting. Bypass grafting is reserved for cases in which the endovenous approach is unsuccessful. However, the endovenous treatment for chronic venous obstruction is discussed extensively in Chapter 14. This chapter concentrates on the bypass grafting.

The treatment of proximal occlusion, including iliocaval segment, differs from that for femoropopliteal thrombotic occlusive disease. The higher velocity, significant blood volume, and better outflow of common femoral, iliac veins, and inferior vena cava (IVC) create a more amenable setting for treatment with either vein or prosthetic bypass grafts. A study of 44 venous reconstructions for nonmalignant iliofemoral and IVC occlusion was conducted at the Mayo Clinic.[28] A wide variety of possible options for IVC and iliofemoral segment reconstruction were used, including great saphenous vein (GSV) crossover grafts (Palma procedure), supported expanded polytetrafluoroethylene (ePTFE), spiral vein grafts, and femoral vein patch angioplasty (Fig. 15-3). The overall primary and secondary patency at 3 years was 54% and 62%, respectively. Conversely, lower primary and secondary patency rates were found for iliocaval and femorocaval bypasses when analyzed separately, reaching only 38% and 54% at 2-year follow-up. The lower patency found in those bypasses was deemed to be related to the ePTFE bypass grafts. A small number of procedures failed to show statistical significance, although a trend toward higher patency rates was shown for GSV bypass grafts. Highest patency was also achieved with GSV crossover grafts, reaching 77% in a 4-year period, similar to other reports in the literature.[28,29]

Several open surgical techniques have been used to correct venous reflux reconstructing the valves. The main procedures described are internal or external (transcommissural) valvuloplasty, axillary vein transfer, vein transplantation, or valve transplantation.[26,30,31] Overall, the results vary based on the technique used, the surgeon's expertise, and postprocedure care. A few specialized centers have been currently conducting open venous reconstruction or valvuloplasty.

The internal valve vein repair is carried out by performing a venotomy to expose the incompetent valve to reapproximate the valve leaflets (Fig. 15-4). In a study of 42 patients (52 limbs), Cheattle and Perrin reported an 85% valve competency and 9% ulcer recurrence rate at 1-year follow-up.[32] A long-term follow-up is provided in another study of 51 cases reported by Masuda and Kistner.[33] In the latter, the authors found better results in patients sustaining primary valve incompetency than secondary CVD and an overall clinical success of 60% in 10-year follow-up. The drawback is that the majority of patients sustained primary valve insufficiency and, therefore, the technique may rarely be used for patients with PTS due to possible chronic degenerative changes of the venous wall and valve system damage. In addition, the series comprises a small number of patients. A few other disadvantages of the internal technique include challenging limbs with small narrowed veins and multiple venotomies required in long diseased segments, increasing the operative time and complexity of the repair.

The external valve vein repair is another option that may expedite the operative procedure and simplify the repair (Fig. 15-5). The advantage of this technique is that multiple valves can be repaired in a single procedure. Despite the argument against blind suturing to tighten up the loose intercommissural space, the technique has shown decent results.[34,35] A large experience applying external or so-called transcommissural repair was reported in a study of 141 limbs. The ulcer-free rate when this technique was performed was 63% at 30-month follow-up.[34] Overall early complication rate was 9%, including a low early vein thrombosis rate of 3%. In contrast to

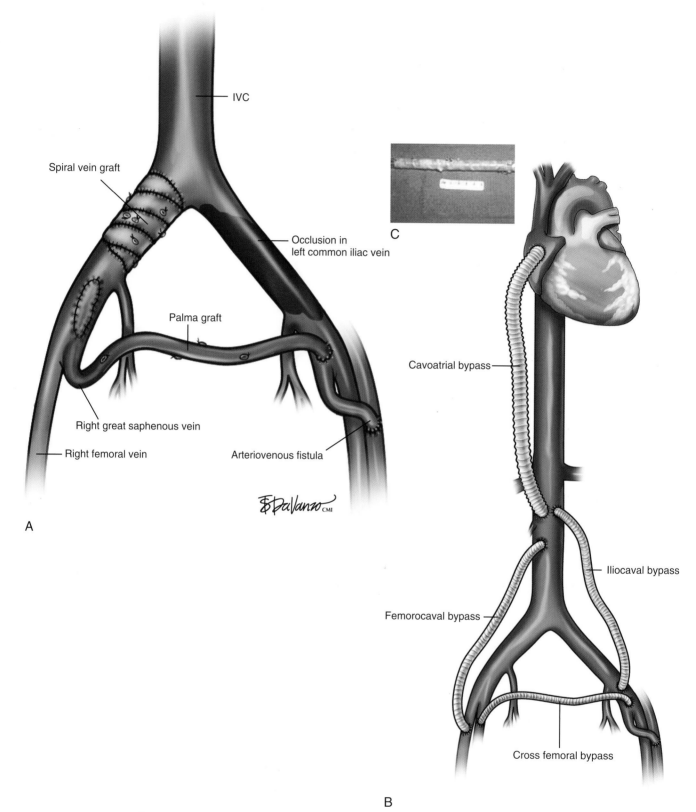

■ **Fig 15–3** Examples of venous repair and bypasses. **A,** A Palma procedure with an arteriovenous fistula, a common femoral vein venoplasty, and a spiral vein graft in the right common iliac vein. **B,** Different prosthetic bypasses. **C,** Spiral vein graft constructed over a chest tube. (*Modified from Jost CJ, Gloviczki P, Cherry KJ Jr, et al. Surgical reconstruction of iliofemoral veins and the inferior vena cava for nonmalignant occlusive disease. J Vasc Surg 2001;33:320-327.*)

Internal valve vein repair

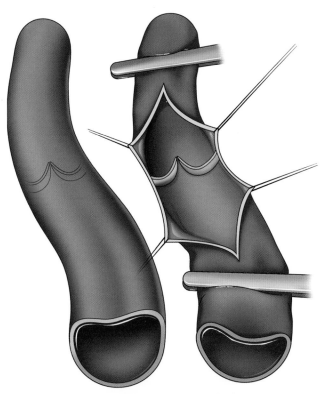

Venotomy with exposure of valve

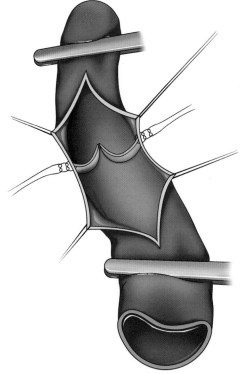

Edge repair with one interrupted suture

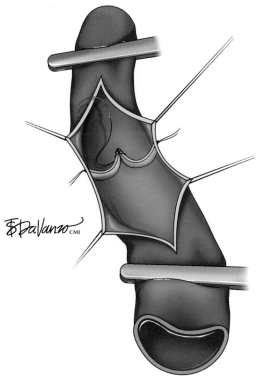

Intercommissural repair with running or interrupted sutures

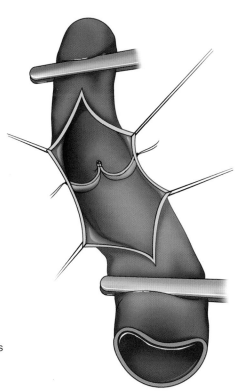

Competent valve showing good apposition of the leaflets

■ **Fig 15–4**

External valve vein repair

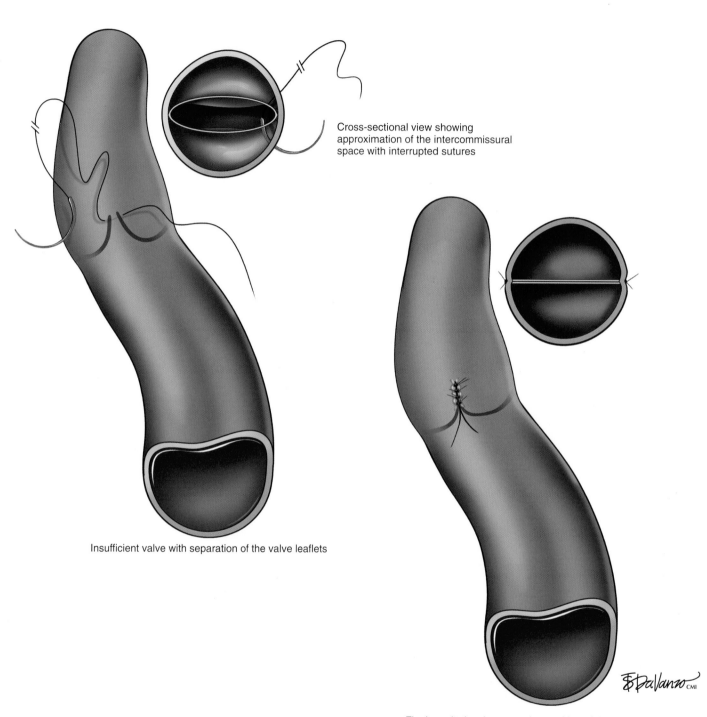

Cross-sectional view showing
approximation of the intercommissural
space with interrupted sutures

Insufficient valve with separation of the valve leaflets

Final result showing a good apposition of the valve leaflets
correcting the venous reflux

■ Fig 15–5

internal valve repair studies,[33,36] the durability achieved with transcommissural valve repair was found to be the same for patients with either "primary" or secondary CVD.[35]

The use of an external sleeve of Dacron or PTFE wrapped around the incompetent valve has been also applied to correct reflux.[37] It has also been used around axillary vein transplant procedures to prevent dilation of the valve and subsequent reflux.[38] Only a few reports exist with the external sleeve providing short-term data. In patients with PTS, this procedure will constrict the vein as there are no functioning valves; the reflux may be reduced but the effect of the obstruction is of concern.

The transfer or transplantation of venous segment with competent valves is a third alternative. The first autologous valved graft transplant used was the ipsilateral GSV.[39-41] The shortcomings of either in situ or transposition of a segment of GSV to the femoral vein are vein mismatch size, degenerative changes with vein incompetence secondary to vein wall dilatation, and the fact that isolated deep vein reflux with competent superficial vein is rare, limiting the use of GSV. Conversely, the axillary vein transfer (AVT) was proposed as another potential conduit to restore the directional venous outflow. The axillary vein is preferred instead of other deep veins because of the quality of the valves, good size match, and low degree of anatomic variation in that region (Fig. 15-6). Furthermore, the upper extremity blood return is mainly done by the superficial veins and therefore not being significantly impaired after axillary vein harvesting. However, a strip test is advocated to assess the axillary vein valve competency prior to transfer. Some authors reported up to 40% of axillary vein incompetency and advise in favor of valve repair in a bench or in situ procedure.[35] The spatial orientation of the anastomosis with precise trimming of the vein must also be accomplished in order to avoid reflux. Several authors have reported their experience with valved vein graft transfer.[31,36,42,43] Results are variable, ranging from 18% to up to 70% of recurrence of ulcers based upon follow-up time (1- to 5-year follow-up) and type of the conduit.[31,36,42,43] A more recent series of AVT reported long-term patency greater than 80% and ulcer-free recurrence greater than 60% at 10-year follow-up.[35]

Another technique of transfer was described by Ferris and Kistner in 1982.[44] It consists of ligation of the femoral vein below the level of valve incompetency and redirection of the flow to either the femoral or profunda vein (Fig. 15-7). Contraindications of the segmental femoral vein transfer are possible dilation of the recipient vein secondary to the increased rerouted flow and, subsequently, reflux involving the femoral and the target vein.

Allied to complex surgical reconstructions or vein transfer, a temporary or long-term arteriovenous fistula (AVF) is often necessary to increase the blood flow in order to keep the repair patent. The drawbacks of constructing a distal AVF are the potential risk of venous dilation and valve incompetency generating venous hypertension and ultimately skin damage. In addition, anticoagulation has been advocated in order to improve the patency rate. Mandatory life-long anticoagulation therapy is also a concern based on risks of bleeding and its morbidity and mortality. Other disadvantages of the open procedures are low patency rates and short-term and midterm follow-up with only few long-term retrospective series, frequently with small sample size.[28]

Experimental research has been carried out including neovalve construction, cryopreserved allograft, and prosthetic vein valve implants.[45-48] Some promising results of a multicenter phase I trial with cryopreserved allograft valves,[45] the "Maleti valve,"[47] and other neovalve implants[46] have been published. In preparation for neovalve reconstruction, endophlebectomy of trabeculated segments is recommended. The technique consists of longitudinal incision of the vein and resection of the fibrous septa with a microsurgery scissor or ophthalmic scalpel to the level of the intima layer. Relief of the obstruction in trabeculated veins is recommended and feasible prior to an axillary vein segment transfer or neovalve creation.[45,46]

A neovalve creation procedure has been developed.[49] The operation encompasses endophlebectomy of the venous segment and dissection of the intima layer, creating a flap that is positioned as a monocuspid or bicuspid valve with subsequent venorrhaphy in transverse fashion (Fig. 15-8). The largest experience reported is the Italian experience of 40 neovalve creations in

Axillary vein transposition

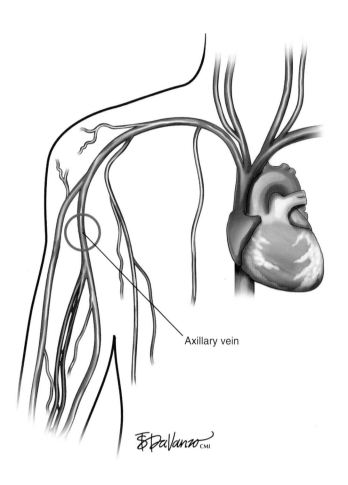

Axillary vein

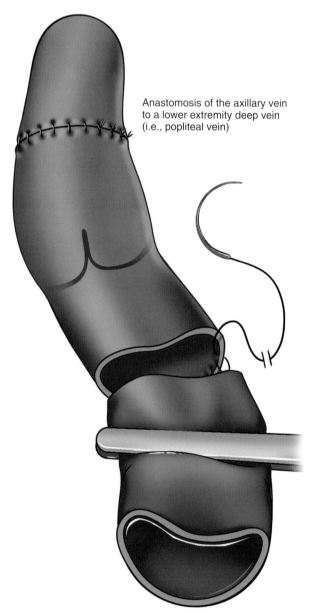

Anastomosis of the axillary vein to a lower extremity deep vein (i.e., popliteal vein)

■ **Fig 15–6**

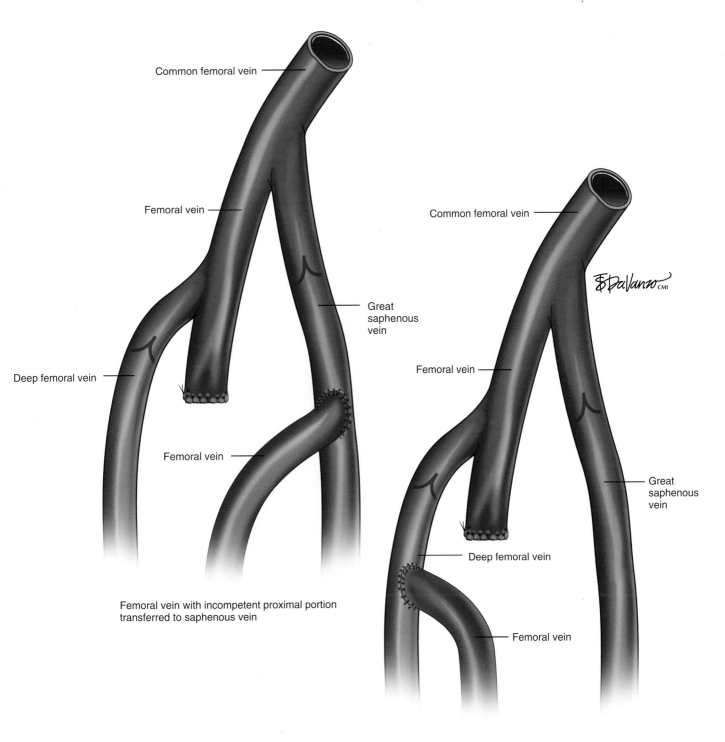

Femoral vein with incompetent proximal portion transferred to saphenous vein

Femoral vein with incompetent proximal portion transferred to deep femoral vein

■ **Fig 15–7**

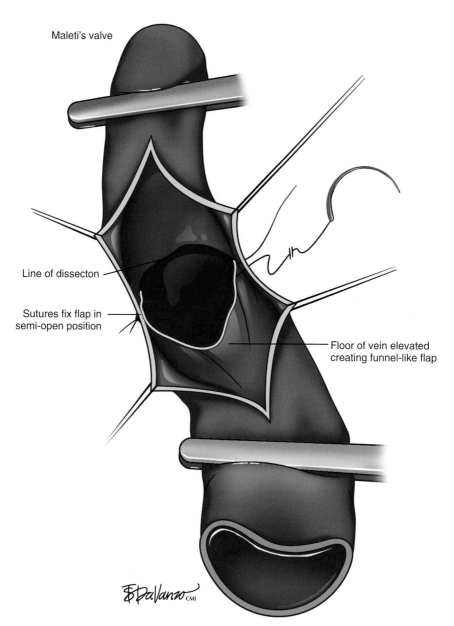

Maleti's valve

Line of dissecton

Sutures fix flap in
semi-open position

Floor of vein elevated
creating funnel-like flap

Creation of neovalve by parietal dissection and
fixing stitches to avoid readhesion

■ **Fig 15-8** The Maleti valve.

36 patients with recalcitrant ulcers.[46] Six valves failed in the first 19 procedures (phase I), but no failures were documented in the last 21 (phase II). No PE or major complications were reported, and overall recurrence of ulcers occurred in 8%. Mostly, the results were based on short-term and midterm follow-up (24 to 48 months for cumulative curves of competency rates). Nevertheless, to obtain good results of operative techniques for infrainguinal deep vein reflux, further investigation is necessary because of small number of patients, experience restricted to a very few centers, and scant long-term follow-up.

ENDOVASCULAR HORIZON

Endovenous therapy for PTS has emerged as the first option mainly for iliofemoral and IVC reconstruction because of its minimally invasive approach, lower morbidity, and promising results.[26,50] Indications and results of IVC, iliac, and femoral angioplasty and stenting are discussed in Chapter 16.

A few experimental implantable endovascular valves have been investigated. The idea of implanting valves via the endovascular approach was first done using an external jugular vein with a competent valve mounted in a Z-stent (Cook Medical, Bloomington, IN) that was deployed in either the external (n = 4) or common iliac vein (n = 1) in dogs.[51] One of five valves implanted was patent, competent, and with minimal inflammatory surrounding reaction. Interestingly, the normal-appearing valve was deployed in the common iliac vein, which has a higher flow pattern.[51] Different valve materials varying from glutaraldehyde-preserved bovine vein to a collagen tissue model of porcine small intestine submucosa (SIS) have been initially studied in animal models.[52,53] The former was made with thrombogenic material and leads to higher endothelial proliferation rate and therefore carries a higher risk of early occlusion of the valve.[54] The latter, which was built with SIS, has a nonthrombogenic and nonimmunogenic surface.[53] Both prototypes are mounted on Z-stents or, onto a nitinol-based stent.[52-56]

There were only two phase I trials reported with a total of five patients in the United States. The first enrolled two patients who underwent percutaneous insertion of a glutaraldehyde-fixed bovine venous valve via right internal jugular access.[57] Both patients were anticoagulated postprocedure, but the second patient had postimplant valve thrombosis. Despite catheter direct thrombolysis, the valve was incompetent but patent. The first patient had a patent and competent valve at 12-months follow-up. Clinical improvement was achieved in both patients, although aggressive compressing therapy and other superficial vein ablation or stripping procedures were required during the follow-up.[57]

The second phase I trial comprised three patients and was performed using the SIS bioprosthetic venous valve model.[58] The patients had percutaneous implantable valves in the proximal (n = 2) and distal (n = 1) portions of the femoral vein and were anticoagulated. All three implanted SIS valves were patent but with either some degree of valve leak in the first two cases or valve tilting in the third. At 12-month follow-up, all patients but one had clinical improvement.[58] A second generation of the SIS percutaneous venous valve stents with more precise spatial configuration to prevent tilting was already tested in animal model.[53]

Endovascular implantable bioprosthetic venous valves for agenesis or incompetent venous valve segments are feasible. However, further research is still warranted in order to improve patency and long-term valve competency.

FIVE SALIENT REFERENCES

1. Prandoni P, Villalta S, Polistena P, et al. Symptomatic deep-vein thrombosis and the postthrombotic syndrome. Haematologica 1995;80(2 Suppl):42-48.

2. Kahn SR, Kearon C, Julian JA, et al. Predictors of the post-thrombotic syndrome during long-term treatment of proximal deep vein thrombosis. J Thromb Haemost 2005;3:718-723.

3. Jost CJ, Gloviczki P, Cherry KJ Jr, et al. Surgical reconstruction of iliofemoral veins and the inferior vena cava for nonmalignant occlusive disease. J Vasc Surg 2001;33:320-327; discussion 27-28.

4. Raju S, Fredericks RK, Neglen PN, et al. Durability of venous valve reconstruction techniques for "primary" and postthrombotic reflux. J Vasc Surg 1996;23:357-366; discussion 366-367.

5. Maleti O. Venous valvular reconstruction in post-thrombotic syndrome. A new technique. J Mal Vasc 2002;27:218-221.

REFERENCES

1. Heit JA, Rooke TW, Silverstein MD, et al. Trends in the incidence of venous stasis syndrome and venous ulcer: a 25-year population-based study. J Vasc Surg 2001;33:1022-1027.

2. Prandoni P, Villalta S, Polistena P, et al. Symptomatic deep-vein thrombosis and the post-thrombotic syndrome. Haematologica 1995;80(2 Suppl):42-48.

3. Widmer LK, Zemp E, Widmer MT, et al. Late results in deep vein thrombosis of the lower extremity. VASA. Zeitschrift fur Gefasskrankheiten 1985;14:264-268.

4. Ashrani AA, Heit JA. Incidence and cost burden of post-thrombotic syndrome. J Thromb Thrombolysis 2009;28:465-476.

5. Ginsberg JS, Turkstra F, Buller HR, et al. Postthrombotic syndrome after hip or knee arthroplasty: a cross-sectional study. Arch Intern Med 2000;160:669-672.

6. Mekkes JR, Loots MA, Van Der Wal AC, et al. Causes, investigation and treatment of leg ulceration. Br J Dermatol 2003;148:388-401.

7. Labropoulos N, Manalo D, Patel NP, et al. Uncommon leg ulcers in the lower extremity. J Vasc Surg 2007;45:568-573.

8. Tran NT, Meissner MH. The epidemiology, pathophysiology, and natural history of chronic venous disease. Semin Vasc Surg 2002;15:5-12.

9. Kahn SR, Kearon C, Julian JA, et al. Predictors of the post-thrombotic syndrome during long-term treatment of proximal deep vein thrombosis. J Thromb Haemost 2005;3:718-723.

10. Labropoulos N, Gasparis AP, Tassiopoulos AK. Prospective evaluation of the clinical deterioration in post-thrombotic limbs. J Vasc Surg 2009;50:826-830.

11. Labropoulos N, Jen J, Jen H, et al. Recurrent deep vein thrombosis: long-term incidence and natural history. Ann Surg 2010;251:749-753.

12. Prandoni P, Lensing AW, Cogo A, et al. The long-term clinical course of acute deep venous thrombosis. Ann Intern Med 1996;125:1-7.

13. Fink AM, Mayer W, Steiner A. Extent of thrombus evaluated in patients with recurrent and first deep vein thrombosis. J Vasc Surg 2002;36:357-360.

14. Prandoni P, Frulla M, Sartor D, et al. Vein abnormalities and the post-thrombotic syndrome. J Thromb Haemost 2005;3:401-402.

15. Kahn SR, Shrier I, Julian JA, et al. Determinants and time course of the postthrombotic syndrome after acute deep venous thrombosis. Ann Intern Med 2008;149(10):698-707.

16. Labropoulos N, Spentzouris G, Gasparis AP, et al. Impact and clinical significance of recurrent venous thromboembolism. Br J Surg 2010;97:989-999.

17. Latella J, Desmarais S, Miron MJ, et al. Relation between D-dimer level, venous valvular reflux, and the development of the post-thrombotic syndrome after deep vein thrombosis. J Thromb Haemost 2010;8:2169-2175.

18. Spiezia L, Campello E, Giolo E, et al. Thrombophilia and the risk of post-thrombotic syndrome: retrospective cohort observation. J Thromb Haemost 2010;8:211-213.

19. Kearon C, Kahn SR, Agnelli G, et al. Antithrombotic therapy for venous thromboembolic disease: American College of Chest Physicians Evidence-Based Clinical Practice Guidelines (8th Edition). Chest 2008;133(Suppl):454S-545S.

20. Brandjes DP, Buller HR, Heijboer H, et al. Randomised trial of effect of compression stockings in patients with symptomatic proximal-vein thrombosis. Lancet 1997;349:759-762.
21. Prandoni P, Lensing AW, Prins MH, et al. Below-knee elastic compression stockings to prevent the post-thrombotic syndrome: a randomized, controlled trial. Ann Intern Med 2004;141:249-256.
22. Giannoukas AD, Labropoulos N, Michaels JA. Compression with or without early ambulation in the prevention of post-thrombotic syndrome: a systematic review. Eur J Vasc Endovasc Surg 2006;32:217-221.
23. Kakkos SK, Daskalopoulou SS, Daskalopoulos ME, et al. Review on the value of graduated elastic compression stockings after deep vein thrombosis. Thromb Haemost 2006;96: 441-445.
24. Kahn SR, Shbaklo H, Shapiro S, et al. Effectiveness of compression stockings to prevent the post-thrombotic syndrome (the SOX Trial and Bio-SOX biomarker substudy): a randomized controlled trial. BMC Cardiovasc Disord 2007;7:21.
25. O'Meara S, Cullum NA, Nelson EA. Compression for venous leg ulcers. Cochrane Database Syst Rev 2009:CD000265.
26. Meissner MH, Eklof B, Smith PC, et al. Secondary chronic venous disorders. J Vasc Surg 2007;46(Suppl S):68S-83S.
27. Kahn SR, Shrier I, Shapiro S, et al. Six-month exercise training program to treat post-thrombotic syndrome: a randomized controlled two-centre trial. CMAJ 2011;183:37-44.
28. Jost CJ, Gloviczki P, Cherry KJ Jr, et al. Surgical reconstruction of iliofemoral veins and the inferior vena cava for nonmalignant occlusive disease. J Vasc Surg 2001;33:320-327; discussion 327-328.
29. Harris JP, Kidd J, Burnett A, et al. Patency of femorofemoral venous crossover grafts assessed by duplex scanning and phlebography. J Vasc Surg 1988;8:679-682.
30. Neglen P, Raju S. Venous reflux repair with cryopreserved vein valves. J Vasc Surg 2003;37: 552-557.
31. Taheri SA, Elias SM, Yacobucci GN, et al. Indications and results of vein valve transplant. J Cardiovasc Surg 1986;27:163-168.
32. Cheatle TR, Perrin M. Venous valve repair: early results in fifty-two cases. J Vasc Surg 1994;19:404-413.
33. Masuda EM, Kistner RL. Long-term results of venous valve reconstruction: a four- to twenty-one-year follow-up. J Vasc Surg 1994;19:391-403.
34. Raju S, Berry MA, Neglen P. Transcommissural valvuloplasty: technique and results. J Vasc Surg 2000;32:969-976.
35. Raju S, Fredericks RK, Neglen PN, et al. Durability of venous valve reconstruction techniques for "primary" and postthrombotic reflux. J Vasc Surg 1996;23:357-366; discussion 366-367.
36. Eklof BG, Kistner RL, Masuda EM. Venous bypass and valve reconstruction: long-term efficacy. Vasc Med (Lond Engl) 1998;3:157-164.
37. Jessup G, Lane RJ. Repair of incompetent venous valves: a new technique. J Vasc Surg 1988;8:569-575.
38. Raju S, Fredericks R. Valve reconstruction procedures for nonobstructive venous insufficiency: rationale, techniques, and results in 107 procedures with two- to eight-year follow-up. J Vasc Surg 1988;7:301-310.
39. Cardon JM, Cardon A, Joyeux A, et al. Use of ipsilateral greater saphenous vein as a valved transplant in management of post-thrombotic deep venous insufficiency: long-term results. Ann Vasc Surg 1999;13:284-289.
40. Eriksson I, Almgren B. Surgical reconstruction of incompetent deep vein valves. Uppsala J Med Sci 1988;93:139-143.
41. Kistner RL, Ferris EB 3rd, Randhawa G, et al. The evolving management of varicose veins. Straub Clinic experience. Postgrad Med 1986;80:51-53, 56-59.
42. Sottiurai VS. Surgical correction of recurrent venous ulcer. J Cardiovasc Surg 1991;32: 104-109.

43. Nash T. Long term results of vein valve transplants placed in the popliteal vein for intractable post-phlebitic venous ulcers and pre-ulcer skin changes. J Cardiovasc Surg 1988;29: 712-716.

44. Ferris EB, Kistner RL. Femoral vein reconstruction in the management of chronic venous insufficiency. A 14-year experience. Arch Surg 1982;117(12):1571-1579.

45. Dalsing MC, Raju S, Wakefield TW, et al. A multicenter, phase I evaluation of cryopreserved venous valve allografts for the treatment of chronic deep venous insufficiency. J Vasc Surg 1999;30:854-864.

46. Lugli M, Guerzoni S, Garofalo M, et al. Neovalve construction in deep venous incompetence. J Vasc Surg 2009;49:156-162, 162 e1-2; discussion 162.

47. Maleti O, Lugli M. Neovalve construction in postthrombotic syndrome. J Vasc Surg 2006; 43:794-799.

48. Taheri SA, Schultz RO. Experimental prosthetic vein valve. Long-term results. Angiology 1995;46:299-303.

49. Maleti O. Venous valvular reconstruction in post-thrombotic syndrome. A new technique. J Mal Vasc 2002;27:218-221.

50. Raju S, Neglen P. Percutaneous recanalization of total occlusions of the iliac vein. J Vasc Surg 2009;50:360-368.

51. Dalsing MC, Sawchuk AP, Lalka SG, et al. An early experience with endovascular venous valve transplantation. J Vasc Surg 1996;24:903-905.

52. Gomez-Jorge J, Venbrux AC, Magee C. Percutaneous deployment of a valved bovine jugular vein in the swine venous system: a potential treatment for venous insufficiency. J Vasc Interv Radiol 2000;11:931-936.

53. Pavcnik D, Kaufman J, Uchida B, et al. Second-generation percutaneous bioprosthetic valve: a short-term study in sheep. J Vasc Surg 2004;40:1223-1227.

54. de Borst GJ, Teijink JA, Patterson M, et al. A percutaneous approach to deep venous valve insufficiency with a new self-expanding venous frame valve. J Endovasc Ther 2003;10: 341-349.

55. Pavcnik D, Uchida B, Timmermans H, et al. Square stent: a new self-expandable endoluminal device and its applications. Cardiovasc Interv Radiol 2001;24:207-217.

56. Pavcnik D, Uchida BT, Timmermans HA, et al. Percutaneous bioprosthetic venous valve: a long-term study in sheep. J Vasc Surg 2002;35:598-602.

57. Gale SS, Shuman S, Beebe HG, et al. Percutaneous venous valve bioprosthesis: initial observations. Vasc Endovasc Surg 2004;38:221-224.

58. Pavcnik D, Machan L, Uchida B, et al. Percutaneous prosthetic venous valves: current state and possible applications. Techn Vasc Interv Radiol 2003;6:137-142.

CHAPTER 16

Iliofemoral Venous Occlusive Disease

Jose I. Almeida

HISTORICAL BACKGROUND

In contrast to the right common iliac vein, which ascends almost vertically to the inferior vena cava (IVC), the left common iliac vein takes a more transverse course. Along this course, it underlies the right common iliac artery, which may compress it against the lumbar spine. This compression causes stasis of the blood, which is one element of the Virchow triad that precipitates deep venous thrombosis.

In approximately 40% of patients, the precursor to iliac vein obstruction is not thrombosis; rather, a nonthrombotic iliac vein lesion (NIVL), also known as May-Thurner syndrome[1] or iliac vein compression syndrome,[2] causes obstruction. A nonthrombotic blockage is defined as an absent clinical history of deep venous thrombosis coupled with absent findings on imaging studies such as contrast venography and ultrasound. Typically, an NIVL is caused by a stenosis of the left proximal common iliac vein by the right common iliac artery with secondary band or web formation.[3] This lesion is classically found in the left common iliac vein of younger females, but it is not uncommon in males or in elderly patients and it may involve the right limb. At least 15% of patients with limbs with primary disease have been shown to have stenosis of both common and external iliac veins.[4]

As depicted in Figure 16-1, the right common iliac artery always crosses the left common iliac vein at the confluence of the IVC and is where classic proximal left NIVL occurs. In 75% of cases (majority pattern), the right iliac artery continues its course to cross near the external iliac vein level, in which case it may induce right distal NIVL. In the minority pattern (22%), the right common iliac artery crosses the right common iliac vein; it then courses down over a longer length of the external iliac vein; it can thus induce either a proximal or distal right NIVL. The left distal lesion may be related to the crossing of the vein by the left hypogastric artery. These anatomic variations may explain why proximal NIVLs occur more frequently on the left side than

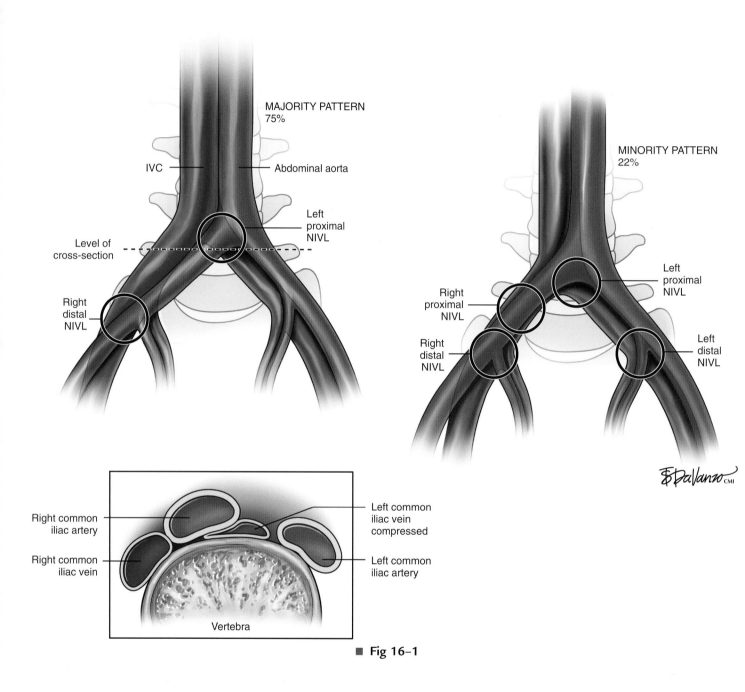

MAJORITY PATTERN
75%

IVC — Abdominal aorta

Left proximal NIVL

Level of cross-section

Right distal NIVL

MINORITY PATTERN
22%

Left proximal NIVL

Right proximal NIVL

Right distal NIVL

Left distal NIVL

Right common iliac artery

Right common iliac vein

Left common iliac vein compressed

Left common iliac artery

Vertebra

■ **Fig 16–1**

on the right side, why the left lesion is focal and the right is less so, and why the distal NIVL occurs equally on either side.

Although traditional venous corrective surgery concentrated on the correction of venous reflux below the inguinal ligament, the introduction of minimally invasive venous stenting with venography and intravenous ultrasonography (IVUS) provides the ability to treat the "obstructive" component of the disease above the inguinal ligament. The emphasis on IVUS as the key diagnostic tool was promulgated by Raju et al.,[5] who have shown that iliac venous stenting alone is sufficient to control symptoms in most patients with combined outflow obstruction and deep reflux.

ETIOLOGY AND NATURAL HISTORY OF DISEASE

The iliac vein is the common outflow tract of the lower extremity, and chronic obstruction of this segment can result in severe symptoms. The most frequent precursor to chronic pelvic venous outflow obstruction is iliofemoral deep venous thrombosis. Only 20% to 30% of iliac veins completely recanalize spontaneously after thrombosis, whereas the remaining veins recanalize partially and develop varying degrees of collaterals.[6] This may result in significant remaining obstruction to the venous outflow of the lower extremity. In the iliofemoral segment, collateral vein formation is relatively poor and thus results in more severe symptoms than does lower segmental blockage.[7] Distal obstructions are more readily compensated for because of robust femoropopliteal collaterals, profunda–popliteal vein connections, deep muscular tributaries in the thigh, and saphenosaphenous venous connections.

The high prevalence and pathologic role of NIVLs in patients with symptoms of chronic venous disease must be balanced with the frequent prevalence of NIVLs in the asymptomatic general population. These apparent contradictions can be resolved if the NIVL is viewed as a permissive condition predisposing to the development of chronic venous disease. Permissive conditions are diseases that may remain silent until additional insult or abnormality is superimposed. Symptom expression in many NIVL obstructions remains asymptomatic because it probably is a slowly progressive condition. Additional insult or pathologic conditions, such as trauma, cellulitis, distal thrombosis, secondary lymphatic exhaustion, or reflux, may render the extremity symptomatic.[8]

Other known permissive conditions that may remain variably silent but predispose to secondary disease and symptoms with additional insult include gastroesophageal reflux disease and asthma, ureteric reflux and pyelonephritis, cricopharyngeal spasm and Zenker diverticulum, esophageal reflux and cancer, diabetes and neuropathy, and middle lobe syndrome and pneumonia. The general principle in these complex diseases is to treat the permissive condition first, which alone may provide relief, and to prevent recurrence. Correction of secondary disease may be required only in recalcitrant and advanced cases.

In Raj and Neglen's series,[8] 75% of limbs with NIVLs and concurrent reflux experienced a good or excellent outcome with stent placement alone, even when the reflux component, severe in many, was uncorrected. These results support the concept that the NIVL plays a permissive role in the genesis of chronic venous disease symptoms. NIVLs are ubiquitous in chronic venous disease with severe symptoms, and liberal use of IVUS and stent correction when they are detected is recommended. Even patients with significant distal reflux are not precluded if the stents fail later, thus avoiding or postponing open reflux corrective procedures.

An alternative explanation for the observations presented here is to consider NIVLs and distal reflux as a continuum in progressive hemodynamic deterioration of the venous system; symptomatic decompensation occurs when the hemodynamics cross a certain critical threshold. However, no connection between NIVLs and distal reflux has yet been established. It should be emphasized that the hemodynamics of obstructive and reflux diseases are poorly understood, and their measurement even less so.

Of particular interest is the subset of patients with NIVLs with reflux who became symptom free with stent correction of the NIVL alone, even when the reflux component remains uncorrected. Notably, 67% of stasis ulcers in this subset also healed and remained healed at 2.5 years. Chronic venous disease symptoms, including stasis ulcers, are not due to reflux alone; the NIVL plays a role in ways yet to be understood. Ulcers also occur in NIVLs without reflux, although the incidence is higher with reflux.

When symptoms recur after initial remission following stent placement, stent malfunction is often found. Distal migration of the stent with recurrence of the lesion at the iliocaval junction, missed or incomplete treatment of the distal lesion, or, less commonly, in-stent stenoses were found in Raju and Neglen's series.[8] When corrected, the patient is usually returned to the status of symptom remission.

PATIENT SELECTION

When planning an invasive procedure on a patient, a surgeon preferably enters the operating room with an imaging study demonstrating a pathologic lesion. In the case of iliac vein occlusive disease, this is often not possible. The poor diagnostic sensitivity of venography was well documented by Negus et al.[3]; of practical importance is that up to half of the cases can be missed if frontal projection venograms alone are relied on for diagnosis.

Perhaps one of the major reasons why interest in iliac vein corrective surgery has lagged is the discomfort a surgeon feels when entering the operating room without a definitive diagnosis. Raju and Neglen[8] have one of the largest experiences in the world with iliac vein occlusive disease, and they have emphasized the value of intraoperative IVUS for diagnosis and treatment. Their vascular laboratory runs a battery of noninvasive tests on patients with signs and symptoms of venous disease, and their data demonstrate the insensitivity of these examinations to identify lesions[8] (Table 16-1). Magnetic resonance venography is operator dependent, and its routine use has not elevated this technique as the gold standard for diagnosis. Perhaps the most interesting phenomenon is the insensitivity of intravenous contrast venography. Although anteroposterior and oblique views may suggest some "pancaking" of the proximal iliac vein (Fig. 16-2), the common iliac vein often appears normal.

TABLE 16–1 Demographics, Intravascular Ultrasound Findings, and Preinterventional Hemodynamics in Stented Limbs with Nonthrombotic Iliac Vein Lesions with and Without Venous Reflux

Parameter	NIVLs With Reflux (n = 151)	NIVLs Without Reflux (n = 181)
Age, y	56 (20-85)	51 (18.90)*
Female-male ratio	110:36 (3.1:1)	146:31 (4.7:1)
Left-right limb ratio	105:46 (2.3:1)	136/45 (3:1)
IVUS degree of stenosis, %	70 (0-95)	70 (0-100)
Stenotic area, cm^2	0.66 (0.15-2.00)	0.53 (0.02-1.65)*
Ambulatory venous pressure, % drop	77 (0-97)	77 (0-99)
Venous filling time, sec	23 (2-132)	44 (0-165)
APG:VFI$_{90}$, mL/sec	2 (0-12.3)	0.9 (0.0-6.0)
Hand-foot pressure differential, mm Hg	1 (0-8)	1 (0-10)
Dorsal foot hyperemia pressure differential, mm Hg	6 (0-26)	5 (0-23)

Data are presented as ratio or median (range).
*p < .01, Not significant.
APG, Air plethysmograph; *NIVI,* Nonthrombotic iliac vein lesions; *IVUS,* intravascular ultrasound; *VFI$_{90}$,* venous filling index.

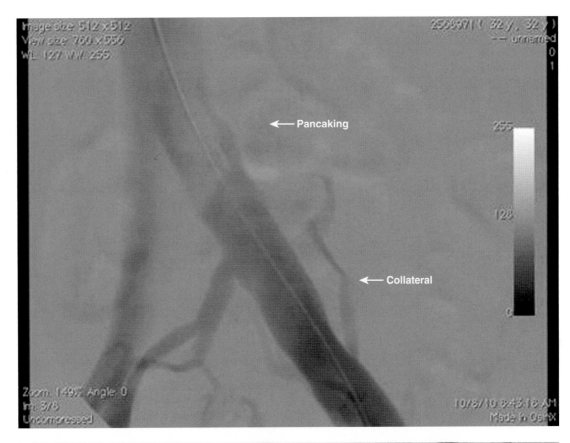

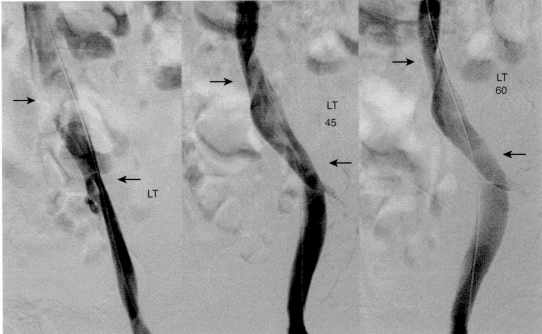

■ **Fig 16–2** Left iliocaval contrast venography with oblique views. "Pancaking" is seen at the iliocaval confluence.

IVUS is easy to use. Standard coaxial technique allows the operator to examine the target lesion by simply passing the device over a guidewire. It delivers no radiation and does not require the use of nephrotoxic contrast. The sound waves are emitted from the catheter tip transducer, usually in the 10- to 20-MHz range, and real-time ultrasound images of a thin section of the blood vessel are generated by computer. IVUS guidance has been used for the placement of IVC filters; it is a more accurate method than contrast venography of localizing the renal veins and measuring vena cava diameter.

ENDOVASCULAR INSTRUMENTATION

- 8-Fr to 11-Fr sheaths
- 5-Fr guide catheter
- Nonionic contrast
- High-pressure tubing for power injector
- .035-inch entry guidewire
- .035-inch stiff guidewire
- .035-inch angled hydrophilic glidewire
- 6- to 20-mm balloons
- 14- to 24-mm Wallstents (Boston Scientific, Natick, MA)

Imaging

- Standard ultrasound for percutaneous access
- IVUS
- C-arm or wall-mounted fluoroscopy for contrast venography

Access and Closure

- Micropuncture entry kit (0.018-inch platform)
- Angioseal closure kits

HEMOSTASIS AND ANTICOAGULATION

There is no standardization in this area. Most vascular surgeons feel comfortable providing anti-coagulation with standard unfractionated heparin. The decision of whether to add antiplatelet therapy is also physician preference.

OPERATIVE STEPS

The patient is taken to the endovascular suite and prepped and draped in the usual manner. The preferred approach is access to the femoral vein in the upper third of the thigh with the thigh slightly externally rotated and the knee slightly bent. The femoral vein lies inferior to the superficial femoral artery and slightly lateral in most cases. If access is planned via a popliteal approach, then the prone position is preferable, but for jugular or femoral vein access, the supine position is ideal (Fig. 16-3, *A*).

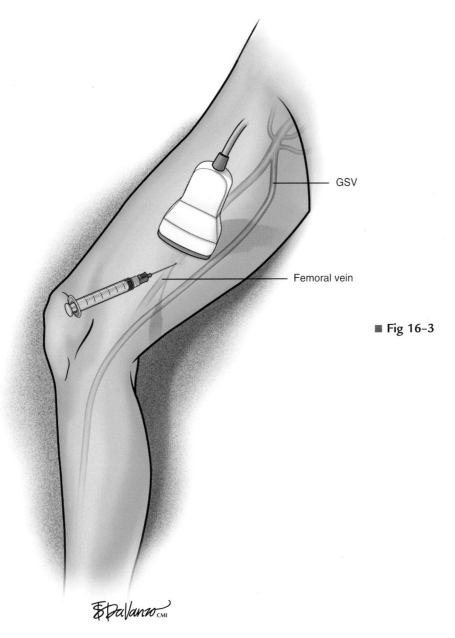

GSV

Femoral vein

■ **Fig 16–3**

A

Continued

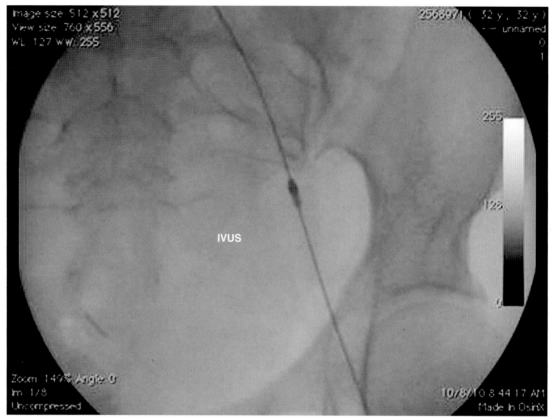

B

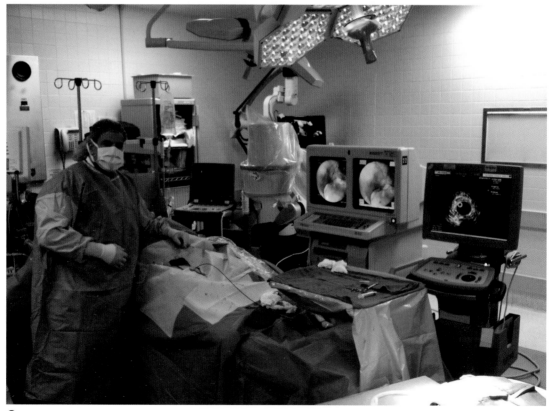

C

■ **Fig 16–3, cont'd**

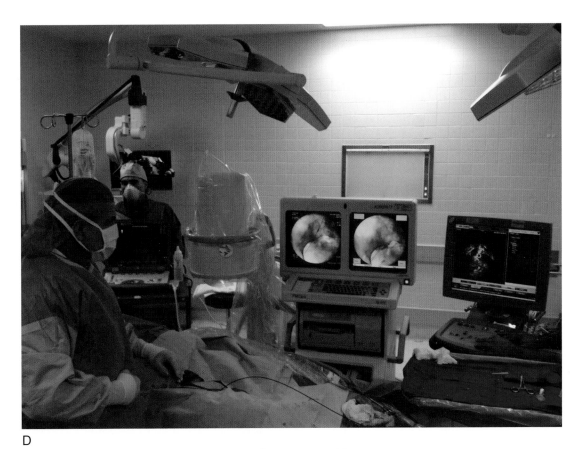

D

■ **Fig 16–3, cont'd**

Using ultrasound control, a 21-gauge needle is used for access and an .018-inch wire is placed with standard Seldinger technique. Using the 4-Fr microintroducer sheath, the .018-inch wire is exchanged for a .035-inch guidewire. Using fluoroscopic control, the .035-inch wire is navigated into the IVC. If the .035-inch wire meets resistance and there is difficulty entering the IVC, an intravenous contrast injection is performed to generate an anatomic roadmap. It is important never to force a wire that has met resistance. If resistance is met, the operator must stop and investigate the problem.

For contrast venography to be performed, a larger sheath is exchanged for the microintroducer over the existing .035-inch wire. A 6-Fr to 8-Fr sheath of 11 cm in length is ideal. The power injector is prepared and a digital subtraction contrast run is prepared by connecting high-pressure tubing from the injector to the side-arm of the sheath. Nonionic intravenous contrast (8 mL/sec for a total of 20 mL) is injected. The resulting image is examined for areas of stenosis, obstruction, and/or the presence of collaterals.

Nonthrombotic Iliac Vein Lesions

The most common lesion encountered for these cases is a stenosis at the confluence of the left common iliac vein with the IVC. Usually a standard .035-inch J-tipped guidewire will cross the lesion easily. In cases where the wire does not cross, a .035-inch hydrophilic angled glidewire is selected. In the majority of cases, the lesion will be successfully crossed with this wire. Hydrophilic glidewires are slippery by design; thus they are not ideal as working wires for tracking balloons, IVUS catheters, and stents. Therefore, the lesion is crossed; a 5-Fr guide catheter is used to exchange the angled glidewire for a .035-inch Amplatz super-stiff wire. The distal super-stiff wire is parked in the superior vena cava or subclavian or jugular vein. This maneuver is in anticipation of stent placement and will be explained later (Fig 16-3, *B–D*).

The IVUS catheter is brought into the field and mounted onto the .035-inch super-stiff guide-wire. IVUS imaging of the entire iliofemoral and caval outflow tract is performed. Particular attention is paid to the caliber of the veins as demonstrated by IVUS. The classic May-Thurner lesion is located at the left common iliac vein–IVC junction. This is the location where the right common iliac artery can be visualized as it crosses the left common iliac vein (Fig. 16-4, *A–D*). As mentioned earlier, distal NIVLs can be seen at the hypogastric artery crossing the external iliac vein, on either the right or left side (Fig. 16-4, *E* and *F*). Using the IVUS computerized software, the percent *area* reduction of the stenosis can be calculated by comparing the stenotic vein segment to an adjacent normal iliac vein segment (Fig. 16-4, *I*). There are no validated criteria to determine what percent area reduction constitutes a hemodynamically significant lesion; however, as a rule of thumb, a 50% area reduction is the treatment threshold.

Once the decision to treat is made, a larger sheath, usually 11-Fr, must be placed to accommodate the stent delivery system. In addition, stent delivery systems track more easily over .035-inch stiff wires; therefore, if needed, an exchange must be performed if a stiff wire is not in place. It is critical not to lose access once a lesion has been crossed with a wire, and an intermediate step is useful. A 5-Fr guide catheter will track over a glidewire into the IVC and can then be subsequently used for .035-inch stiff wire placement. After the .035-inch stiff wire is parked in the SVC, the 5-Fr guide catheter is removed and a balloon is brought into the field.

Iliac veins are compliant and fairly resistant to rupture; therefore a 14- to 18-mm-diameter balloon is usually chosen to dilate the lesion. The balloon is dilated to profile until the waist is obliterated. Sequential dilatations with larger balloons may be required to completely dilate the lesion. Since venous lesions almost always recoil after dilatation, stent deployment is required. Stent diameters of 16 to 18 mm are preferred since oversized stents are necessary. The most common stents used for iliac vein work are stainless-steel, self-expanding Wallstents (Figs. 16-5 through 16-9).

PEARLS AND PITFALLS

Intravenous Ultrasonography Findings

The proximal NIVL was three times more frequently observed on the left side, whereas the distal NIVL was equally distributed bilaterally. The proximal NIVL was typically very focal on the left side and was located at the iliocaval junction; the right proximal NIVL was less focal and was located 1 to 2 cm distal to the iliocaval junction.[8]

The median area of the more severe stenosis (proximal or distal), as measured by IVUS, was 0.58 cm^2 (normal, 1.5 cm^2) representing approximately 70% stenosis. Most NIVLs were "soft" compared with PTS or arterial lesions, with waisting of the balloon often relieved at less than 2 atm.[8]

Stent Deployment

The most dreaded complication is losing a stent and finding it in the heart. This phenomenon results when stents "jump" during deployment. Stents are packaged tightly in delivery sheaths

Text continued on p. 390

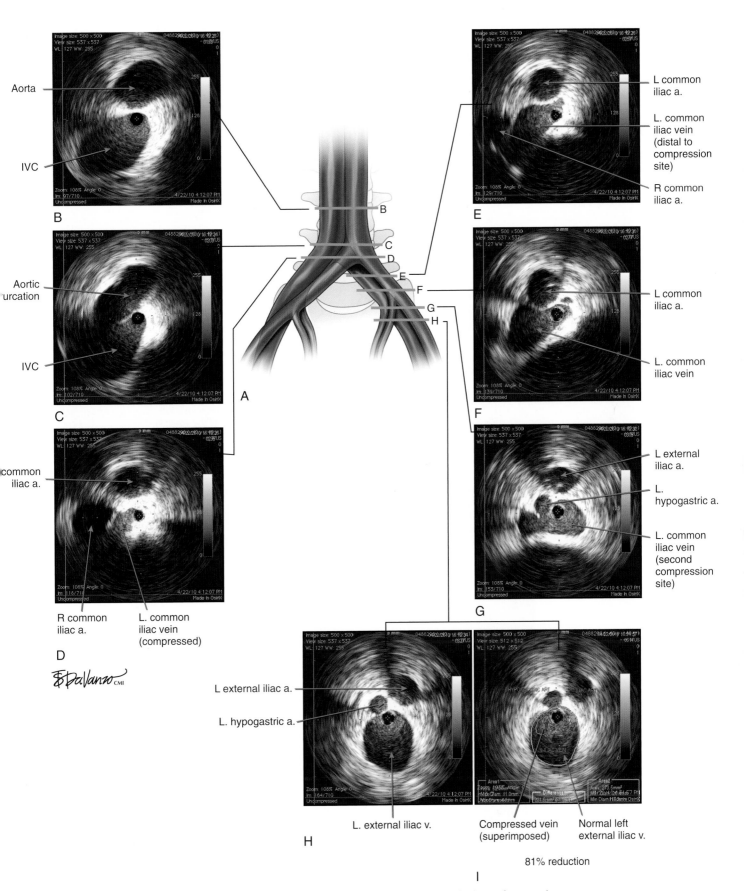

Aorta

IVC

B

Aortic
bifurcation

IVC

C

common
iliac a.

R common   L. common
iliac a.   iliac vein
                   (compressed)

D

$B.DaVanzo_{CMI}$

A

B   E   L common
                     iliac a.

                     L. common
                     iliac vein
                     (distal to
                     compression
                     site)

                     R common
                     iliac a.

C
D
E   F   L common
F   iliac a.
G
H

                     L. common
                     iliac vein

F

                     L external
                     iliac a.

                     L.
                     hypogastric a.

                     L. common
                     iliac vein
                     (second
                     compression
                     site)

G

L external iliac a.

L. hypogastric a.

                              Compressed vein   Normal left
                              (superimposed)   external iliac v.

L. external iliac v.

H   81% reduction

                                           I

■ **Fig 16–4** **A** to **H,** IVUS imaging depicting cross-sectional slices from pelvis to
just below inguinal ligament; notice the relationships between arterial and
venous anatomy. **I,** Computer-generated area measurements: left external iliac
vein (*blue*) used as normal-sized reference and superimposed image (*green*) of
left common iliac vein site of maximum compression. Calculated 81% area
reduction.

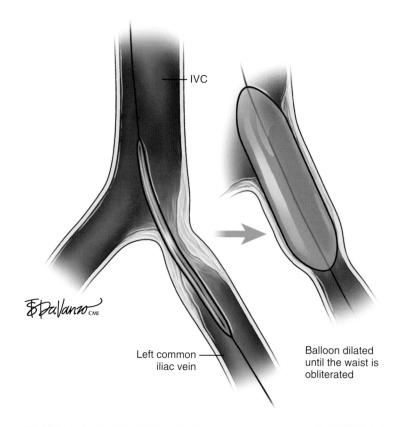

IVC

Left common
iliac vein

Balloon dilated
until the waist is
obliterated

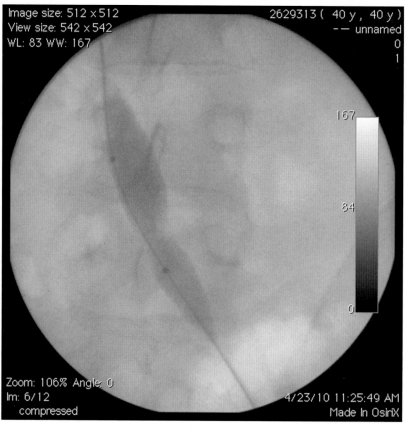

◼ **Fig 16–5**

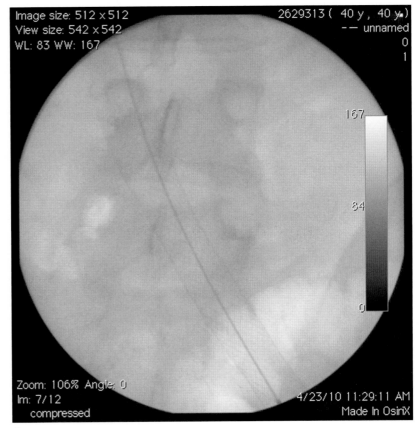

A

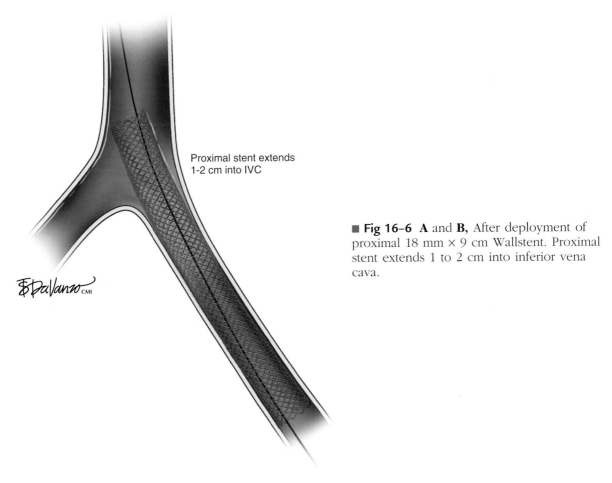

Proximal stent extends
1-2 cm into IVC

■ **Fig 16–6 A** and **B,** After deployment of
proximal 18 mm × 9 cm Wallstent. Proximal
stent extends 1 to 2 cm into inferior vena
cava.

B

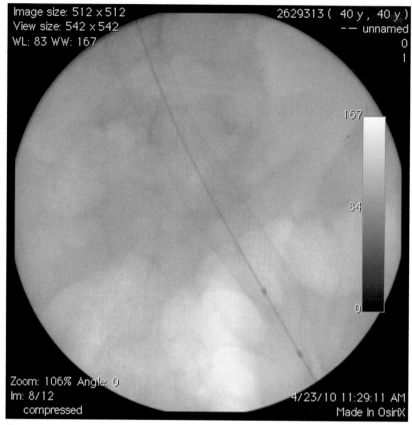

A

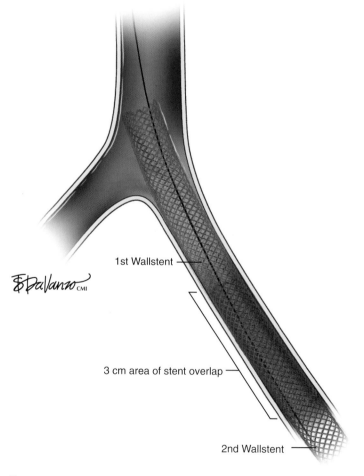

■ **Fig 16–7 A** and **B,** After deployment of second Wallstent (18 mm × 9 cm). Distal aspect of stent extends below inguinal ligament. There is a 3-cm area of stent overlap.

1st Wallstent

3 cm area of stent overlap

2nd Wallstent

B

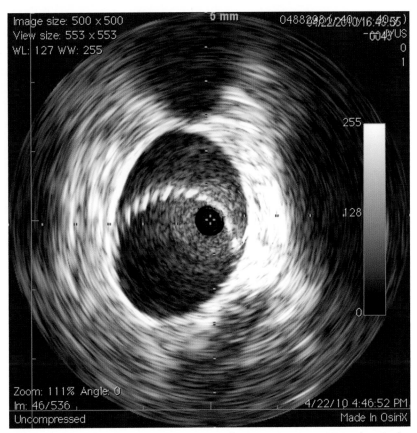

■ **Fig 16–8** Proximal stent extension into inferior vena cava. Note that it does not completely jail the outflow from the contralateral iliac vein.

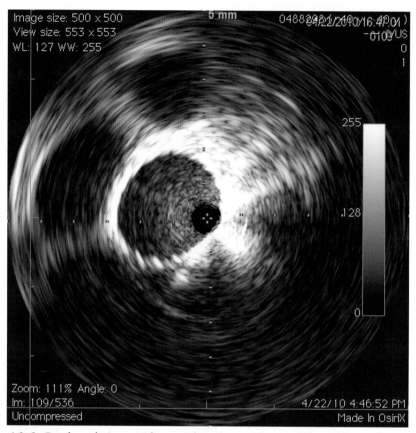

■ **Fig 16–9** Deployed stent with complete apposition to left common iliac vein wall. Complete obliteration of the stenosis at right common iliac artery compression site.

where their potential energy is stored. During deployment, the potential energy converts to kinetic energy as it expands and finds its resting place. The stent will then apply its outward radial force to the vessel wall and maintain an open vessel.

If the stent has the opportunity to find an open area to quickly release its energy, it will. Iliocaval stent deployment for NIVL routinely deploys across a tight iliocaval stenosis into the IVC. The IVC represents a large space where a stent may quickly, and uncontrollably, convert its potential energy into kinetic energy. Thus, the stent could "jump" into the IVC and float into the right ventricle if the operator is not careful.

Aside from careful deployment and stent oversizing, an important maneuver is parking the distal guidewire into the SVC or innominate vein prior to stent deployment. This technique will keep the stent "on a rail" and will not allow migration into the right atrium, the tricuspid valve, or, worse, the right ventricle. Stent retrieval with a snare, or capturing it with a balloon and redeploying it in another vessel is much easier when the stent is on a wire.

Advanced Techniques

Patients may require stenting of both limbs. Several techniques have been described by Neglen et al.,[9] but most noteworthy is the fenestration technique (Fig. 16-10).

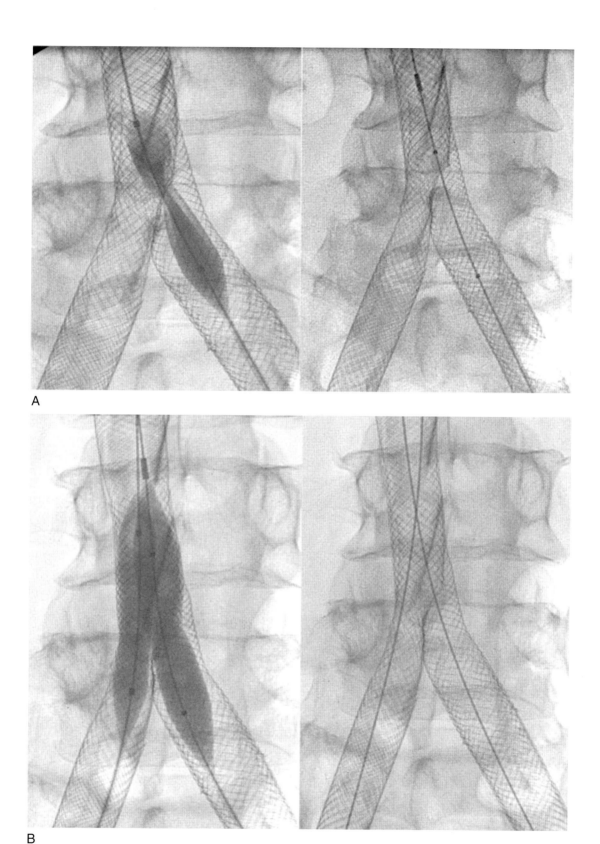

A

B

■ **Fig 16–10 A,** Fenestration of a stent, which is placed across the outflow of one stented limb after an inverted-Y fenestration. *Left,* A balloon is placed through the side of the stent and dilated (*right*), creating a fenestration and allowing unimpeded outflow. **B,** The unilateral dilation may sometimes infringe on the previous created window and result in stenosis. *Left,* It may be useful to perform balloon dilation at the stent confluence by the kissing-balloon technique to (*right*) ensure an uninterrupted outflow from both iliac veins. (*From Neglén P, Darcey R, Olivier J, et al. Bilateral stenting at the iliocaval confluence. J Vasc Surg 2010;51:1457-1466.*)

Postthrombotic Iliofemoral Venous Lesions

Patients presenting with iliac vein occlusive disease secondary to thrombosis are much more difficult to deal with technically, and stent patency is inferior to that of NIVL cases. Recanalization techniques are required (Fig. 16-11, *A–L*).[10]

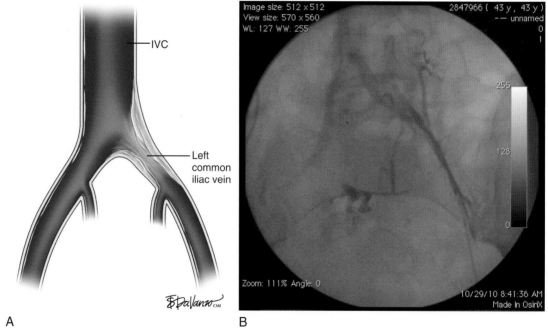

A   B

■ **Fig 16–11** Recanalization of a chronic left iliac vein occlusion secondary to previous iliofemoral deep vein thrombosis 20 years earlier. The left femoral vein was accessed percutaneously and an 8-Fr sheath was placed. With use of a .035-inch angled hydrophilic glidewire and a 4-Fr glide catheter, the lesion was crossed. Serial dilatation of the tract was performed with a 5-Fr balloon, 10-Fr balloon, 14-Fr balloon, and 16-Fr balloon. Intravenous ultrasonography confirmed intraluminal recanalization and left common iliac vein compression. The area was stented with a 16-mm Wallstent. The stent projected 2 cm into the inferior vena cava and was carried down to the confluence of the common femoral vein (CFV). Stent is carried below the inguinal ligament well into the CFV. The femoral vein is scarred from previous deep vein thrombosis, and the majority of drainage comes from the profunda femoris vein.

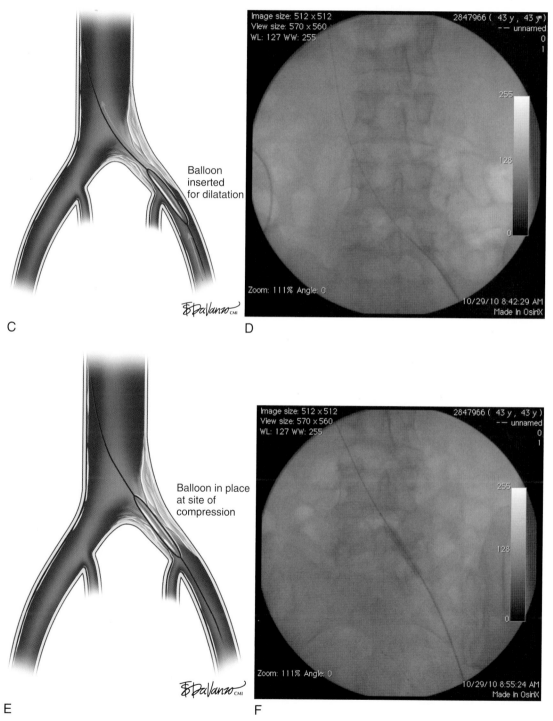

Balloon inserted for dilatation

C

D

Balloon in place at site of compression

E

F

■ **Fig 16–11, cont'd** For legend see the opposite page.

Continued

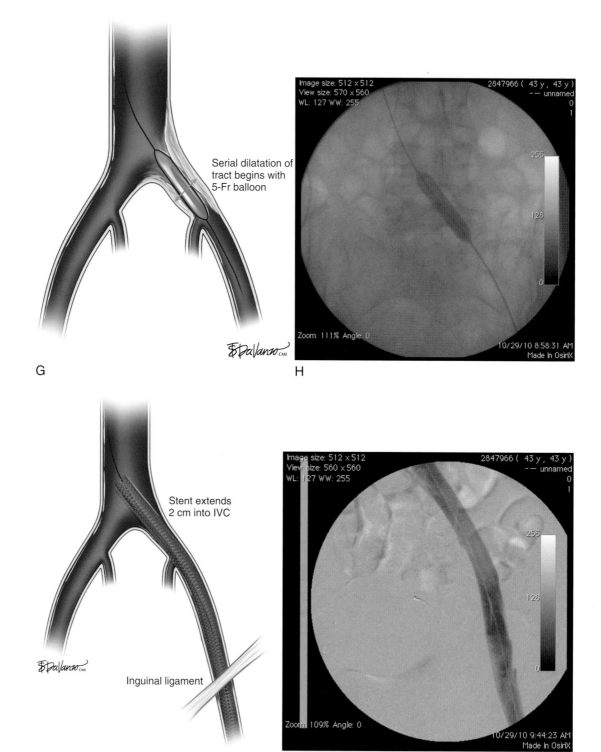

G

Serial dilatation of tract begins with 5-Fr balloon

H

I

Stent extends 2 cm into IVC

Inguinal ligament

J

■ **Fig 16–11, cont'd** For legend see page 392.

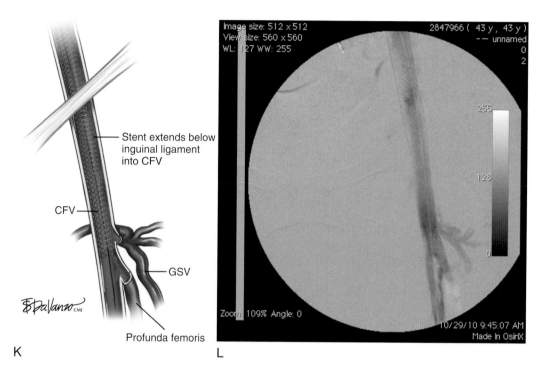

Stent extends below
inguinal ligament
into CFV

CFV

GSV

Profunda femoris

K

L

■ **Fig 16–11, cont'd** For legend see page 392.

COMPLICATIONS

- Stent thrombosis
- Stent fracture
- Stent migration

COMPARATIVE EFFECTIVENESS OF EXISTING TREATMENTS

Historically, the venous femoral-femoral bypass using great saphenous vein as a bypass conduit (Palma procedure) was the procedure of choice. Direct iliac vein surgery never gained much popularity. Iliac vein bypass using prosthetic grafts were alternatives. Anticoagulation, with or without adjunctive arteriovenous fistula support, was the norm to maintain primary patency of all venous reconstructions.

REFERENCES

1. May R, Thurner J. The cause of the predominantly sinistral occurrence of thrombosis of the pelvic veins. Angiology 1957;8:419-428.
2. Cockett FB, Thomas ML. The iliac compression syndrome. Br J Surg 1965;52:816-821.
3. Negus D, Fletcher EWL, Cockett FB, et al. Compression and band formation at the mouth of the left common iliac vein. Br J Surg 1968;55:369-374.
4. Neglen P, Berry MA, Raju S. Endovascular surgery in the treatment of chronic primary and post-thrombotic iliac vein obstruction. Eur J Vasc Endovasc Surg 2000;20:560-571.
5. Raju S, Darcey R, Neglén P. Unexpected major role for venous stenting in deep reflux disease. J Vasc Surg 2010;51:401-408.
6. Mavor GE, Galloway JMD. Iliofemoral venous thrombosis: Pathological considerations and surgical management. Br J Surg 1969;56:45-59.
7. Mavor GE, Galloway JMD. Collaterals of the deep venous circulation of the lower limb. Surg Gynaecol Obstet 1967;125:561-571.
8. Raju R, Neglen P. High prevalence of nonthrombotic iliac vein lesions in chronic venous disease: a permissive role in pathogenicity. J Vasc Surg 2006;44:136-144.
9. Neglén P, Darcey R, Olivier J, et al. Bilateral stenting at the iliocaval confluence. J Vasc Surg 2010;51:1457-1466.
10. Raju S, Neglen P. Percutaneous recanalization of total occlusions of the iliac vein. J Vasc Surg 2009;50:360-368.

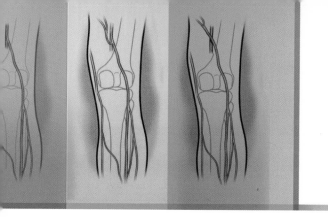

CHAPTER 17

Pelvic Congestion Syndrome and Ovarian Vein Reflux

Constantino S. Peña and James F. Benenati

BACKGROUND

Pelvic congestion syndrome (PCS) is an underdiagnosed condition causing chronic pelvic pain. PCS was first described by Taylor in 1948,[1] who described a number of specific patients suffering with pelvic pain; these patients had pelvic and ovarian varicosities from ovarian vein incompetence. Women with PCS are usually of menstruating age who report pelvic heaviness and pain that is aggravated by standing. They are typically multiparous and report that their symptoms worsen during the premenstrual period. These patients may also complain of dyspareunia.

CLASSIFICATION

As with many conditions there is a spectrum of pelvic venous syndromes that may affect patients. Scultetus et al.[2] classified these patients into four types. Type 1 includes patients with limited vulvar varices. Patients with hypogastric vein reflux (including internal pudendal and obturator branches), usually with vulvar varicosities and hemorrhoids, represent type 2. Type 3 patients are diagnosed with gonadal vein obstruction due to a mesenteric aortic compression of the left renal vein (nutcracker syndrome). Type 4 patients have gonadal vein insufficiency that is characteristic of PCS. These patients may have lower extremity varicosities that originate in the pelvis and may also have associated hypogastric vein reflux.

ETIOLOGY

The cause of PCS is unknown and poorly understood. However, autopsy studies have found that a percentage of patients may have congenital absence of valves in the left ovarian vein.[3] Interestingly, a significant number of patients (40%) with ovarian vein incompetence may remain asymptomatic. Additionally, the development of the incompetence and symptoms may be associated with mechanical stresses such as pregnancy as well as with certain hormonal effects.

DIAGNOSIS

The diagnosis of this condition requires a significant clinical suspicion because there are many disorders that present with pelvic pain. The diagnosis for many years relied on clinical suspicion that would be confirmed at the time of direct venography. Additionally, a number of cases have been diagnosed with the discovery of pelvic varicosities at the time of laparoscopy. The use of transabdominal and transvaginal ultrasound has been described as a manner to diagnose PCS in a patient with pelvic pain[4]; however, its accuracy in widespread practice is limited. At present, when there is a clinical suspicion, the diagnosis is confirmed with either computed tomography venography (CTV) or magnetic resonance venography (MRV).[5,6] MRV is the study of choice because of its lack of ionizing radiation and its ability to perform time-resolved imaging[7] (Fig. 17-1).

Interestingly, there are patients with unusual lower extremity varicose veins arising from the pelvis and vulvoperineal region without saphenofemoral insufficiency. These patients usually have anteromedial thigh varices but can be seen with many patterns. Although some of these patients have pelvic pain and associated PCS, up to 70% of the patients, in some series, did not have associated symptoms of pelvic pain and would not be consistent with PCS. Therefore the diagnosis hinges on the existence of ovarian vein incompetence along with the proper clinical symptoms of PCS. Because both MRV and CTV examinations are performed with the patient in the supine position, these imaging studies may be misleading. A normal imaging study does not exclude the diagnosis, especially with the proper clinical symptoms.

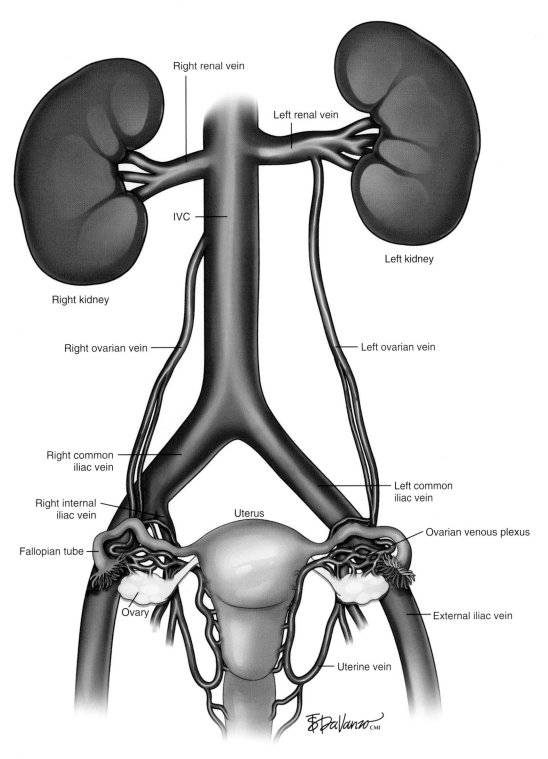

A

■ **Fig 17–1**

Continued

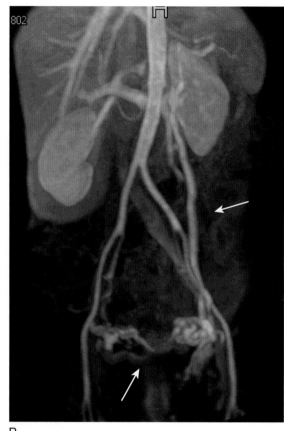

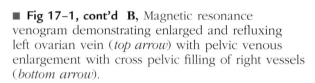

■ **Fig 17–1, cont'd B,** Magnetic resonance venogram demonstrating enlarged and refluxing left ovarian vein (*top arrow*) with pelvic venous enlargement with cross pelvic filling of right vessels (*bottom arrow*).

B

TREATMENT

In the early years of the condition, surgical treatment consisted of surgical ligation of the ovarian vein. Recently there have been reports of laparoscopic ligations. Most commonly, percutaneous transcatheter treatment is used. Transcatheter treatment was first reported by Edwards in 1993,[8] and these treatments have continued to adapt in technique over the years.

The percutaneous transcatheter treatment can be performed from either the femoral or jugular approach. We prefer the jugular technique as it allows a more natural angle into the left renal vein. Selection of the left as well as the right ovarian vein can be very difficult from the femoral approach because of the acute angle at the origin of the right ovarian vein with the inferior vena cava (Fig. 17-2). Injection of the left renal vein will usually depict the presence of a dilated (6 to 10 mm) left ovarian vein, which is incompetent (Fig. 17-3). There are usually cross pelvic collaterals filling the right ovarian venous system (Fig. 17-4). In a percentage of cases, the reflux causes filling of the internal iliac vein branches. Venography can be done during the Valsalva maneuver if the resting venogram does not demonstrate an enlarged ovarian vein.[9] Additionally, the venogram can be repeated in a semierect position if a tilt table is available.

It is important to exclude a compression of the distal left renal vein between the superior mesenteric artery and the aorta (nutcracker syndrome) as the cause of the left ovarian vein enlargement. This condition is diagnosed by an elevated pullback or simultaneously measured renocaval gradient. The gradient in this region should normally be 1 mm Hg or less and is typically greater than 5 mm Hg in patients with nutcracker syndrome.[10] This treatment for these patients involves relief of the compression using surgery or stent placement.

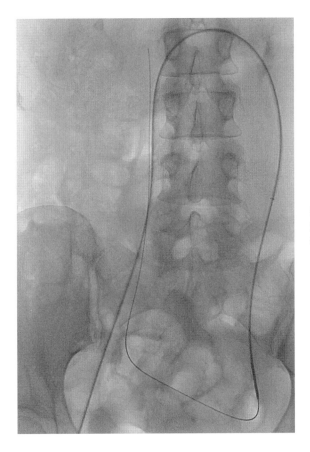

■ **Fig 17-2** Treatment of a patient from the femoral approach with subsequent catheterization of the right ovarian vein from the left ovarian vein.

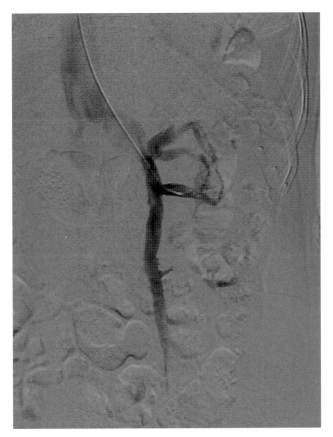

■ **Fig 17-3** Initial venogram after selecting the left ovarian vein with a multipurpose angiographic catheter confirming vein enlargement and reflux.

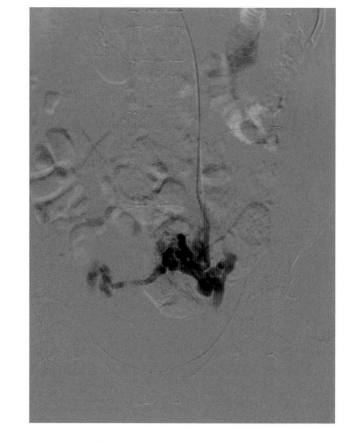

■ **Fig 17-4** Catheter venogram in the proximal left ovarian vein confirming reflux and cross filling of right pelvic veins.

The procedure begins with catheterization of the left renal vein and subsequently the left ovarian vein. The left ovarian vein is easily catheterized from a jugular approach with a multipurpose-shaped catheter and either a soft-tipped guidewire or a hydrophilic guidewire. The ovarian vein arises proximally from the left renal vein, usually around 1 cm lateral to the vertebral body. Once a catheter is engaged in the left ovarian vein, it is recommended to perform venography before navigating distally in the vein. This is to avoid spasm from the catheter manipulation. Imaging prior to the development of spasm is of great value to assess the vein and its branches and to plan treatment. Initial imaging may demonstrate a single, simple ovarian vein, or in many instances it may demonstrate numerous collaterals, which are of great importance because if left untreated they may provide collateral flow to the pelvis. On rare occasions, the ovarian vein may arise from a circumaortic renal vein or from the lower of two renal veins on the left side.

Once that the diagnosis has been established and the decision to treat the patient made, if the ovarian vein is large, a long 6-Fr sheath or guide catheter can be advanced into the vein for the purpose of using occluding devices and catheters in a coaxial fashion (Fig. 17-5). If a sheath or guiding catheter cannot be placed into the ovarian vein, a standard 5-Fr catheter can be used to negotiate the vein. It is important to place the catheter as proximal in the pelvis as possible. It is common to opacify small pelvic collaterals while the vulvovaginal varicosities can rarely be seen filling. We usually treat these small deep pelvic collaterals with the aid of a microcatheter and a combination of coils and liquid embolic agents and sclerosants (Figs. 17-6 and 17-7). However, care needs to be taken on superficial vulvovaginal varicosities. Treatment of the incompetence in the ovarian vein and deep pelvic vessels is usually sufficient to reduce the pressure load on these vessels. When transpelvic collaterals are identified, a microcatheter is used to catheterize these small transpelvic collaterals and gain access to the right ovarian system.

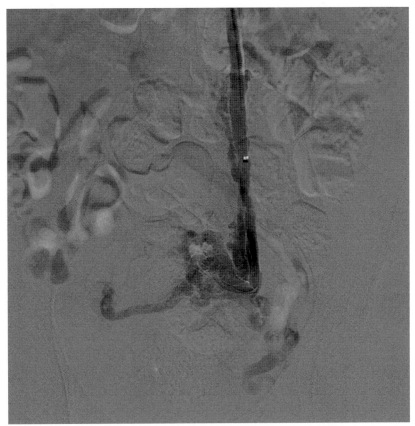

■ **Fig 17–5** Placement of a 45-cm 6-Fr sheath into the proximal ovarian vein. Venogram used as roadmap to cannulate dilated veins with coaxial catheter and microcatheter system.

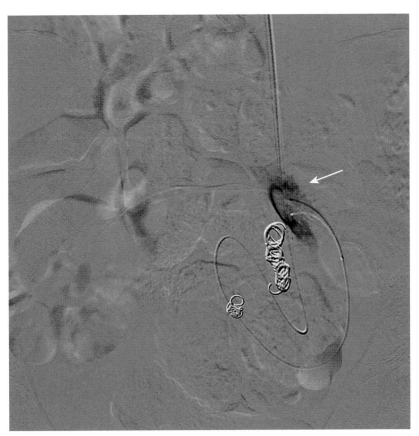

■ **Fig 17–6** After coil embolization of several large pelvic veins, a microcatheter was used to select internal iliac vein collaterals with subsequent filling into the common iliac vein (*arrow*).

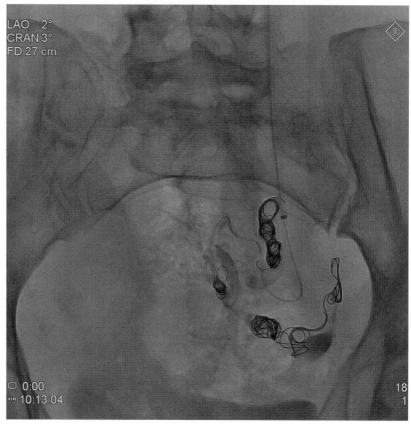

■ Fig 17–7 After embolization and sclerosis of the pelvic vessels as well as collaterals to the internal iliac branches.

In our practice, we traditionally treat the left ovarian vein and will study and then treat the right ovarian vein (Fig. 17-8). The right ovarian vein is usually more challenging to identify and catheterize. This vein usually arises from an acute angle slightly anterior and inferior to the right renal vein (Fig. 17-9). From the femoral approach, a reverse-curve catheter may be helpful, and from the jugular approach, a multipurpose- or cobra-shaped catheter often is ideal. Previous imaging can be extremely helpful to identify the origin of this vein prior to undertaking a search that may become prolonged. In less common instances, the right ovarian vein may arise farther below the renal vein than anticipated, from the right renal vein directly, or from a common trunk with lumbar veins.[11] Therefore, a detailed and methodical evaluation of the inferior vena cava must be conducted if the vein is not immediately obvious. At times in our practice, we have catheterized the left gonadal vein and passed a microcatheter across the transpelvic collaterals and up the right ovarian vein and then treated the patient working retrograde from the origin of the right ovarian vein back across the pelvic veins and up the left ovarian vein.

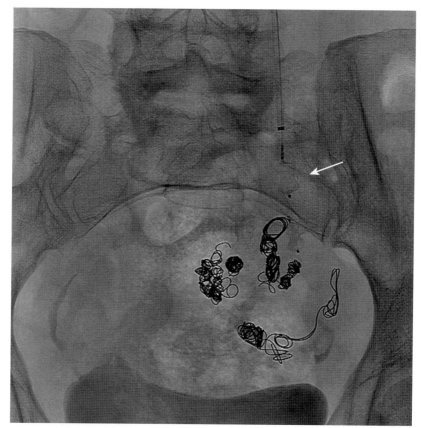

■ Fig 17–8 After treatment of the enlarged and refluxing vessels in the pelvis, the ovarian vein is embolized with coils or vascular plugs (*arrow*).

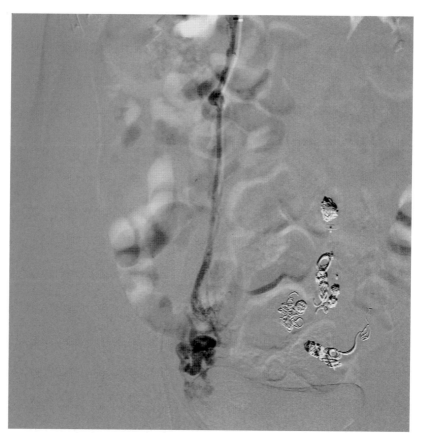

■ Fig 17–9 Catheter venogram of the right ovarian vein confirming enlarged right-sided pelvic veins, which were treated with sclerosis and several coils in the proximal ovarian vein.

Traditional treatment involves a combination of sclerotherapy of the small vessels and coil embolization of the ovarian vein and some of the larger collaterals (Fig. 17-10). With the catheters in the vessels below the pelvic brim, sclerosants and liquid embolic agents are used.[12] Specifically, sclerotherapeutic agents that are used are "off label" for this indication and include 3% STS (sodium tetradecyl sulfate) foam, 2% polidocanol (Aethoxysklerol), and 5% sodium morrhuate/Gelfoam slurry. Before the injection of any liquid sclerosant or embolic agent, it is advisable to determine the volume of agent needed as well as the rate at which the agent should be injected. This is achieved by testing with small contrast injections to determine how much contrast is needed to fill a group of collaterals and to evaluate the presence of reflux. Once this has been determined, the embolic agent is injected at the same rate. Care must be taken to avoid over-injection and refluxing into the inferior vena cava via collaterals. Other liquid embolic agents that have been used include glue (embucril), Onyx, and Gelfoam slurries. The ovarian vein may have a number of accessory veins requiring the packing of coils at several levels throughout the course of the left ovarian vein. Coils are oversized to prevent venous embolization of the coils.[13] Embolization plugs have also been used along with coils (Fig. 17-11).

Controversy exists as to the treatment of associated internal iliac and deep venous collaterals. Some authors will not treat internal iliac vein collaterals during the initial ovarian vein setting. If the symptoms continue, they will readdress these veins by selecting the internal iliac vein branches and embolizing them 3 to 8 weeks after the ovarian vein treatment.[14] Usually, if reflux into the internal iliac vein system can be identified at the time of initial venography, we treat these vessels to improve pelvic and lower extremity symptoms. The filling of thigh varicosities from the reflux is usually the cause of patients' extremity symptoms, especially in patients with no superimposed saphenofemoral incompetence. The size of the vessels may require coil embolization; however, in the proper setting, a controlled injection of sclerosants and liquid embolic agents can be used. In a significant percentage of patients, symptoms will not be relieved unless the internal iliac veins are treated. Again, great care must be taken to avoid reflux into the common iliac vein or inferior vena cava when treating these veins. Complications may include ovarian vein perforation, coil migration, and pain from nontarget sclerosant.

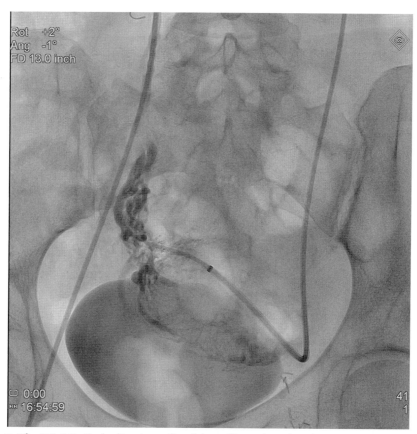

■ **Fig 17–10** Embolization of pelvic collateral with sclerosant and coils.

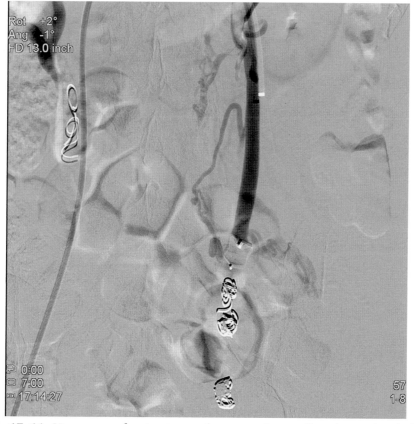

■ **Fig 17–11** Venogram after treatment demonstrating no flow into pelvis below vascular plug and coils.

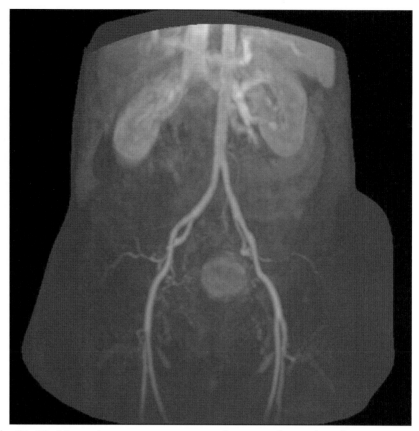

■ **Fig 17–12** Magnetic resonance venography several months after treatment demonstrating improvement in ovarian vein reflux.

TREATMENT EFFECTIVENESS

The published literature has demonstrated symptomatic response in more than 80% of patients treated.[14,15] In a series of 127 treated patients, there was an 83% improvement in symptoms with a 45-month follow-up (Fig. 17-12). It is common to have to re-treat to improve response, particularly in patients with associated internal iliac and deep pelvic collaterals, which may not be completely treated during the original procedure.

REFERENCES

1. Taylor HC. Vascular congestion and hyperemia; their effect on function in the female reproductive organs; clinical aspects of the congestion fibrosis syndrome. Am J Obstet Gynecol 1949;57:637-653.
2. Scultetus AH, Villavicencio JL, Gillespie DL, et al. The pelvic venous syndromes: analysis of our experience with 57 patients. J Vasc Surg 2002;36:881-888.
3. Ganeshan A, Upponi S, Hon LQ, et al. Chronic pelvic pain due to pelvic congestion syndrome: the role of diagnostic and interventional radiology. Cardiovasc Interv Radiol 2007; 30:1105-1111.

4. Park SJ, Lim JW, Ko YT, et al. Diagnosis of pelvic congestion syndrome using transabdominal and transvaginal sonography. AJR Am J Roentgenol 2004;182:683-688.
5. Hiromura T, Nishioka T, Nishioka S, et al. Reflux in the left ovarian vein: analysis of MDCT findings in asymptomatic women. AJR Am J Roentgenol 2004;183:1411-1415.
6. Jin KN, Lee W, Jae HJ, et al. Venous reflux from the pelvis and vulvoperineal region as possible cause of lower extremity varicose veins: diagnosis with computed tomographic and ultrasonographic findings. JCAT 2009;33:763-769.
7. Pandey T, Shaikh R, Viswamitra S, et al. Use of time resolved magnetic resonance imaging in the diagnosis of pelvic congestion syndrome. J Magn Reson Imag 2010;32:700-704.
8. Edwards RD, Robertson IR, MacLean AB, et al. Case report: pelvic pain syndrome: successful treatment of a case by ovarian vein embolization. Clin Radiol 1993;47:429-431.
9. Freedman J, Ganeshan A, Crowe PM. Pelvic congestion syndrome: the role of interventional radiology in the treatment of chronic pelvic pain. Postgrad Med J 2010;86:704-710.
10. Scultetus AH, Villavicencio L, Gillespie DL. The nutcracker syndrome: its role in the pelvic venous disorders. J Vasc Surg 2001;34:812-819.
11. Karaosmanoglu D, Karcaaltincaba M, Karcaaltincaba D, et al. MDCT of the ovarian vein: normal anatomy and pathology. AJR Am J Roentgenaol 2009;192:295-299.
12. Gandini R, Chiocchi M, Konda D, et al. Transcatheter foam sclerotherapy for symptomatic female varicocele with sodium tetradecyl sulfate foam. Cardiovasc Intervent Radiol 2008;31:778-784.
13. Liddle AD, Davies AH. Pelvic congestion syndrome: chronic pelvic pain caused by ovarian and internal iliac varices. Phebology 2007;22:100-104.
14. Kim HS, Malhorta AD, Rowe PC, et al. Embolotherapy for pelvic congestion syndrome: long-term results. J Vasc Interv Radiol 2006;17:289-297.
15. Maleux G, Stocks L, Wilms G, et al. Ovarian vein embolization for the treatment of pelvic congestion syndrome: long term technical and clinical results. J Vasc Interv Radiol 2000;11:859-864.

CHAPTER 18

Endovenous Management of Central and Upper Extremity Veins

Constantino S. Peña

In the era of central venous catheters and implantable pacemakers and defibrillators, upper extremity deep venous thrombosis (UEDVT) has become more frequent. Traditionally, upper extremity and central vein obstruction was associated with hypercoagulability, malignancy, and superior vena cava (SVC) syndrome. At present, central vein stenosis and thrombosis, usually from neointimal hyperplasia, are commonly seen in dialysis-dependent patients or in patients who have had placement of an indwelling central venous catheter. It is estimated that approximately 10% of all cases of deep venous thrombosis (DVT) occur in the upper extremity veins. Even though these cases are less likely to result in pulmonary embolism and postthrombotic syndrome than is lower extremity DVT, they are associated with a risk of pulmonary embolism (5.6%), venous gangrene, and disabling arm or neck swelling.

PRIMARY UPPER EXTREMITY DEEP VENOUS THROMBOSIS: PAGET SCHROETTER SYNDROME

UEDVT can be classified as primary, when it occurs without an inciting cause, and secondary, when it is related to an underlying catheter or previous catheter. Primary UEDVT, also known as effort thrombosis, usually occurs in healthy young individuals (third decade of life) who present with sudden, severe swelling of the upper extremity that may be associated with cyanosis and arm paresthesias. The condition is usually seen in patients after a repetitive activity and is known by the eponym Paget-Schroetter syndrome after a British and a German physician who simultaneously reported it. These patients usually have a compressive phenomenon at the thoracic outlet. It is traditionally seen at the level of the clavicular head and first rib. The scalenus anterior muscle and tendon, along with the bony structures, may compress the subclavian vein at this level, particularly at some stressed positions of the arm. The process can also be seen with the cervical ribs (Figs. 18-1 and 18-2). The combination of the compression of the costoclavicular portion of the axillosubclavian vein and repetitive stress leads to intimal damage and subsequent fibrotic reactions of the underlying vein. This intimal damage then promotes thrombosis. Patients with effort thrombosis must be identified because if this condition is not treated, it can progress and patients may experience chronic disability (25%-74%).

Treatment

As opposed to patients with secondary UEDVT, in these patients there is an extrinsic venous compression responsible for the thrombosis. The goal of treatment is to restore venous patency and relieve the compression. When effort thrombosis is suspected in a patient, we usually perform catheter-directed chemical thrombolysis (if the patient is a candidate) followed by limited angioplasty if needed to restore flow. The results of the angioplasty are variable depending on the underlying injury to the vein. The thought is that if the vein can be gently dilated to attempt to maintain patency, the patient can then undergo anticoagulation until decompression surgery. It is important to diagnose the compression during the thrombolysis procedure and understand that the long-term patency of angioplasty will be limited in the setting of external compression. Stents should never be placed in this compressive environment.

There is controversy about whether to operate immediately or several weeks after thrombolysis. Some surgeons will only operate in the setting of persistent symptoms. We typically treat these patients with immediate surgery shortly after thrombolysis to relieve the compression. Several weeks after surgery, the status of the vein can be reassessed with ultrasound and angioplasty can be performed as needed to maintain or reestablish flow.

Prior to treatment, it is common for patients to have a venous duplex ultrasound demonstrating thrombosis. A computed tomography scan or magnetic resonance image highlighting the venous phase may be helpful in demonstrating the compression and excluding other sources of central occlusion (Fig. 18-3). Ultrasound-guided vascular access is achieved traditionally into the basilic or brachial vein. It is important to establish that the vein being punctured is patent. A 4-Fr or 5-Fr mini-stick microcatheter system is used to perform an initial venogram and document the extent of thrombosis (Fig. 18-4). Once the entry vein is found to be satisfactory, a 5-Fr or 6-Fr vascular sheath is placed. The axillosubclavian thrombosis is crossed with a soft tip guidewire (Bentson wire; Cook Medical, Bloomington, IN) and an angled catheter (Kumpe or multipurpose). The catheter is exchanged for a thrombolysis catheter that is placed across the area of thrombosis (Fig. 18-5). The catheter infusion length is matched to the length of thrombosis, and the patient is treated overnight with thrombolytics. The choice and dose are usually dependent on the operator's choice, amount of thrombus, and patient risk factors. We usually coadminister peripheral low-dose heparin during the infusion, typically 300 units of heparin per hour (Fig. 18-6). In the setting of an acute decompensation requiring rapid thrombectomy or a patient who may not be a candidate for chemical thrombolysis, mechanical thrombectomy may be performed.

Text continued on p. 417

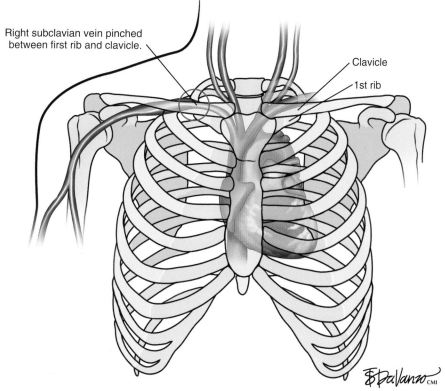

Right subclavian vein pinched between first rib and clavicle.

Clavicle

1st rib

■ **Fig 18–1** Diagram demonstrating the junction of both brachiocephalic veins into the superior vena cava.

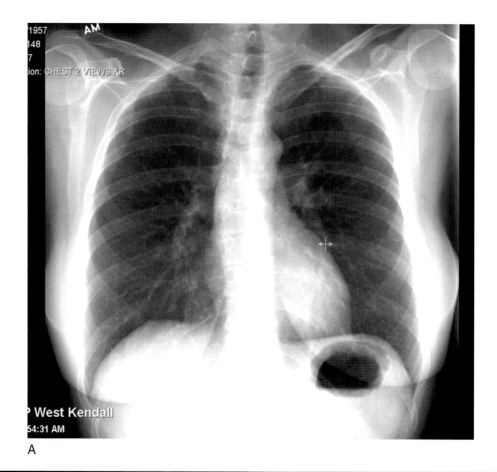

A

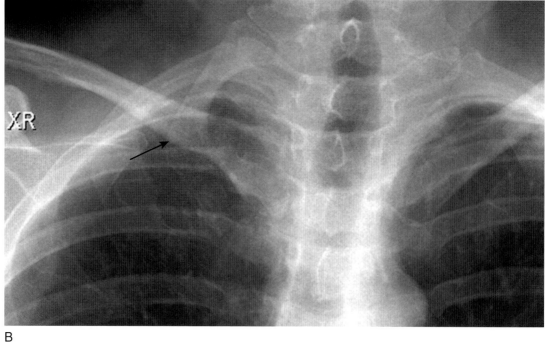

B

■ **Fig 18–2** A frontal chest radiograph (**A**) and magnified view (**B**) depict the presence of a right-sided cervical rib (*arrow*). This is just one of the possible causes of anatomic compression of the axillosubclavian vein.

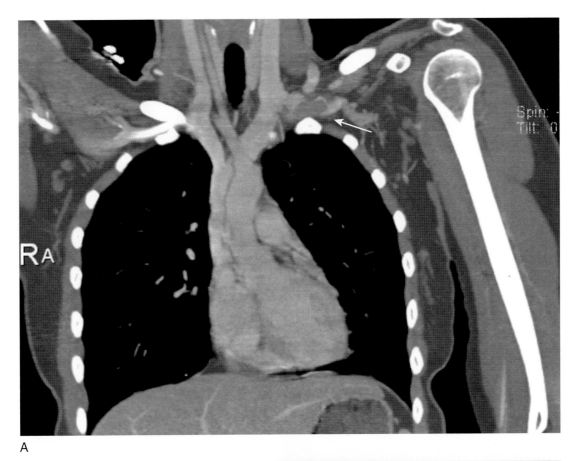

A

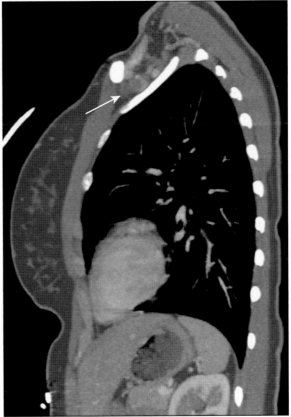

B

■ **Fig 18–3 A,** A coronal reformation of a computed tomography scan during the venous phase demonstrating a focal thrombosis of the left axillosubclavian vein (*arrow*). **B,** A sagittal reformation of a computed tomography scan during the venous phase demonstrating a focal thrombosis of the left axillosubclavian vein (*arrow*). Note location of the vein between the clavicle and the first in both reformations.

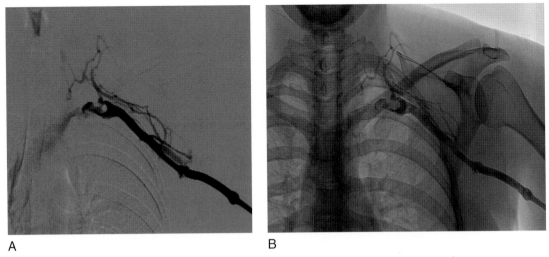

A   B

■ **Fig 18–4** A frontal left upper extremity venogram demonstrating occlusion with thrombosis of the left axillosubclavian vein in a subtracted (**A**) and unsubtracted (**B**) image.

■ **Fig 18–5** Frontal image demonstrating a wire across the occlusion and terminating in the inferior vena cava with a thrombolysis catheter (6-Fr EKOS ultrasound-aided infusion catheter [Bothell, WA]) positioned across the occlusion for overnight chemical thrombolysis.

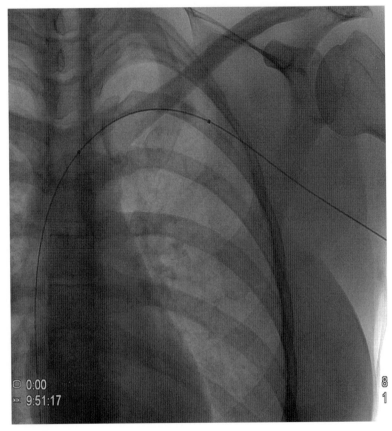

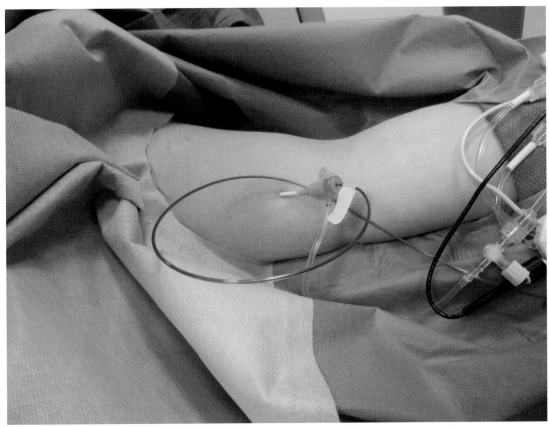

■ **Fig 18–6** Image demonstrating a 6-Fr sheath in the brachial vein with an EKOS infusion catheter through the sheath. This patient received 0.5 mg/hr of TPA (alteplase; Genentech, San Francisco, CA) infused via the EKOS catheter and 300 units/hr of heparin via the sheath.

After overnight catheter-directed thrombolysis, a venogram is performed to assess the patency of the axillosubclavian vein (Fig. 18-7). Usually, overnight thrombolysis is sufficient to clear the associated thrombus, but in certain patients a second day of thrombolysis may be necessary. As with any thrombolysis procedure, the patient is informed of the potential risk of bleeding and monitored carefully as well as with fibrinogen levels. A venogram is then performed in a provocative position to assess the amount of compression and secure the diagnosis. We usually abduct and externally rotate the arm over the patient's head. The area of compression on the vein is usually still present after thrombolysis (Figs. 18-8 and 18-9). Angioplasty can then be performed if there is a persistent high-grade stenosis (Fig. 18-10). A low-pressure balloon is used not solely to treat the venous obstruction but also to assess the amount of fibrosis and neointimal damage because a severely damaged vein may require a venous patch at the time of surgical decompression. The surgical decompression may be performed from a transaxillary or supraclavicular approach. A portion of the first rib along with the tendinous attachment of the transected anterior scalene muscle is usually removed (Fig. 18-11).

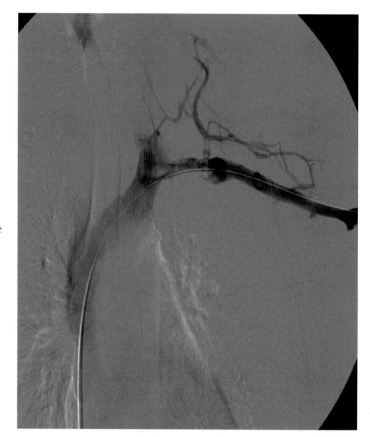

■ **Fig 18–7** Venogram after overnight thrombolysis demonstrating clearing of thrombus with minimal irregularity at the level of compression.

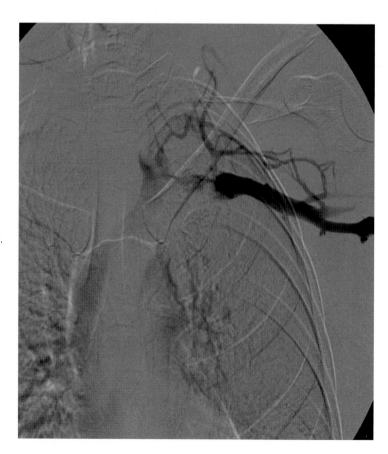

■ **Fig 18–8** Venogram performed with the patient in a stressed position.

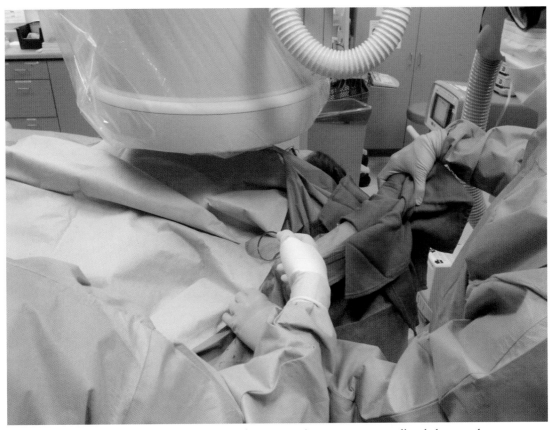

■ **Fig 18-9** Positioning of patient for stressed views. We usually abduct and externally rotate the arm.

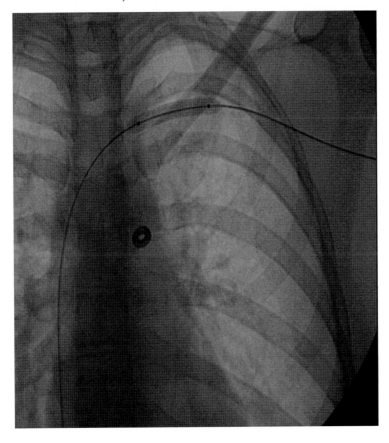

■ **Fig 18-10** Dilating the residual narrowing or venous thickening after lysis.

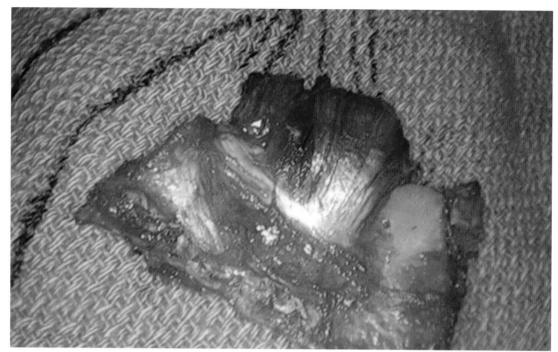

■ **Fig 18–11** Surgical specimen of the first rib with associated anterior scalene tendinous attachment. *(From Abilio Coello, MD, FACS, Miami Vascular Specialists.)*

SECONDARY PRIMARY UPPER EXTREMITY DEEP VENOUS THROMBOLYSIS

The frequent use of central and peripheral catheters has increased the incidence of upper extremity venous stenosis and DVT. These patients usually present with pain and/or arm swelling. Depending on the clinical situation, peripheral venous catheters are removed in favor of other access sites. Patient symptoms and extent of thrombosis determine if anticoagulation should be initiated for peripheral upper extremity venous thrombosis. Axillary, subclavian, and jugular thrombosis is usually treated with anticoagulation to improve symptoms and prevent pulmonary embolism. The placement of SVC filters in patients who are intolerant of anticoagulation is controversial, and usually only patients who have a suspected upper extremity thrombus pulmonary embolism or are at high risk of a life-threatening pulmonary embolism are treated with SVC filters. SVC filter placement is a higher risk procedure that should be carefully considered, especially because the incidence of life-threatening pulmonary embolism from an upper extremity source is unknown.

Patients with a central catheter–associated thrombosis are at slightly higher risk of pulmonary embolism. Pulmonary embolism has also been associated with the removal of these catheters in the acute setting of thrombosis. We will usually anticoagulate these patients and remove the tunneled central catheters only if the patient's symptoms persist or worsen on anticoagulation. Prevention of unnecessary subclavian punctures and catheter placement may limit the amount and extent of subclavian venous stenosis and thrombosis.

DIALYSIS ACCESS–RELATED CENTRAL VENOUS STENOSIS

Central venous stenosis occurs in a significant number (11% to 40%) of patients on hemodialysis. It is the leading cause of shunt dysfunction and is associated with venous hypertension and arm swelling. The cause of dialysis-associated central vein stenosis is unknown but is likely multifactorial. The neointimal fibrosis responsible for these central stenotic lesions may be associated with prior centrally placed catheters. The damage due to previous subclavian punctures has led the Kidney Disease Outcomes Quality Initiative (DOQI) guidelines to strongly discourage unnecessary subclavian punctures, but the presence of a central catheter, even from the jugular approach, may cause sufficient endothelial damage from the trauma associated with its continual motion within the body. The turbulent and high flow associated with upper extremity hemodialysis access may explain central venous stenosis in patients who have never received a central catheter.

The central venous stenosis not only can be symptomatic with severe arm swelling but also may limit the function of a hemodialysis access. The treatment of central vein stenosis associated with hemodialysis is traditionally angioplasty. Unfortunately, the 1-year patency of these treatments has been reported to be between 10% and 30%, and the use of multiple additional procedures to maintain secondary patency is the rule. The initial use of stents to treat central venous stenosis has been discouraged because of a similar patency rate to that of angioplasty and the possibility of stent compression in the thoracic outlet. In addition, there are no U.S. Food and Drug Administration (FDA)–approved uncovered stents for the venous system. Even though the results from angioplasty are limited, endovascular dilatation of these stenoses is preferred over surgical options because of its availability, noninvasiveness, low risk of morbidity, and ability to repeat as needed. DOQI guidelines recommend stent placement for central lesions that recur within 3 months after angioplasty and demonstrate immediate vessel recoil greater than 50% after angioplasty and vessel perforation. The patency of a stent in central venous stenosis is similar to that of angioplasty, but the ability of retreatment becomes limited (Figs. 18-12 and 18-13). The use of covered self-expandable stents has shown promise, particularly in the setting of peripheral dialysis graft anastomotic stenoses. Their use will likely increase in the central veins; however, the operator needs to be careful in not excluding other draining veins with a central covered stent.

Technically, angioplasty of central venous stenosis associated with hemodialysis is usually performed from the fistula and/or graft. In the setting of vessel occlusion, femoral access may also be needed. A sheath is placed in the access site, and a complete shunt study is performed with venography. The lesion is best treated over a working wire (Amplatz, Rosen, Torque). We usually begin with a low-pressure balloon (10- to 12-atm burst pressure). The sizing of the balloon is essential to prevent rupture. The dilatation of the stenosis is performed using a 3-minute inflation and a insufflator device to control the pressure administered. Care must be taken not to thrombose the access. If the stenosis is not dilated by the low-pressure balloon, a high-pressure balloon is used (Blue Max; Boston Scientific, Natick, MA, or Conquest; Bard, Tempe, AZ). If the stenosis was dilated by the low-pressure balloon inflation but demonstrated recoil, the decision can be made to stent the lesion, attempt a high-pressure balloon, or score the stenosis with a cutting balloon or similar product. It is important not to simply redilate with a larger-diameter balloon because this may risk rupturing the vein.

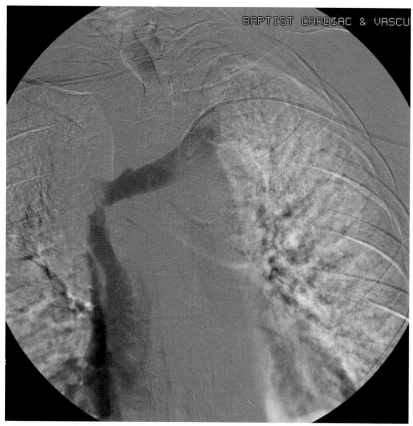

■ **Fig 18–12** A 57-year-old woman with end-stage renal disease and central stenosis at the junction of the left brachiocephalic vein and superior vena cava. The patient has an occluded right upper extremity system.

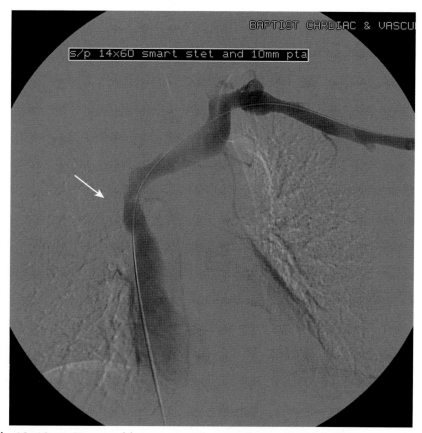

■ **Fig 18–13** A 57-year-old woman with central stenosis resistant to venoplasty and treated with a 14-mm × 60-mm Smart stent (self-expanding nitinol; Cordis Johnson & Johnson [Bridgewater, NJ]) dilated to 10 mm.

SUPERIOR VENA CAVA SYNDROME

Patients with SVC syndrome present with symptoms that include arm and neck swelling or pain as well as edema, erythema, orthopnea, and paresthesias. The symptoms may worsen with the patient in the recumbent position. SVC syndrome can develop progressively or acutely and is usually related to advanced oncologic disease such as lung cancer or mediastinal disease. However, SVC stenosis and its associated syndrome can also occur as a consequence of benign fibrosing conditions of the mediastinum such as sarcoidosis as well as previous radiation therapy and long-standing hemodialysis and the use of central venous catheters. The underlying condition consists of occlusion or severe stenosis of the central veins, preventing sufficient venous blood flow from returning into the right atrium. The jugular veins on each side of the neck join the subclavian vein to form the brachiocephalic vein in the chest. The right and left brachiocephalic veins then join to form the superior vena cava. The lesions may occur in the SVC or in a number of central extremity veins, creating the equivalent to an SVC lesion. Treatment for SVC syndrome can include chemotherapy or radiation therapy, especially for chemosensitive and radiosensitive masses, but the response may take a few days, which may be unacceptable to patients with severe symptoms.

Even though there are no FDA-approved stents for the venous system, stents are used "off-label" in patients with SVC syndrome with improvement in 70% to 90% of patients' symptoms. It is important to remember that the goal of treatment in patients with SVC syndrome is palliation. The long-term effects and patency of stents may not be relevant in patients with malignant obstruction or life-threatening symptoms. There is controversy surrounding stenting in the setting of SVC obstruction because a percentage of patients develop collateral pathways and may not become symptomatic. It is important to evaluate every patient individually, assessing symptoms and all available treatment options (Figs. 18-14 through 18-16). It is common for patients on hemodialysis to present with SVC syndrome due to central occlusions and stenosis (Figs. 18-17 through 18-19).

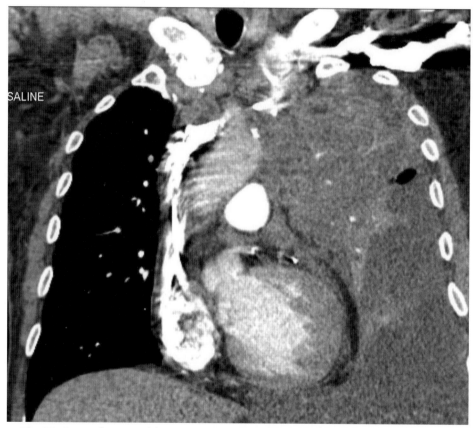

■ **Fig 18–14** A 61-year-old patient with left upper lobe lung cancer presents with left arm and face swelling. Computed tomography scan suggests brachiocephalic compression.

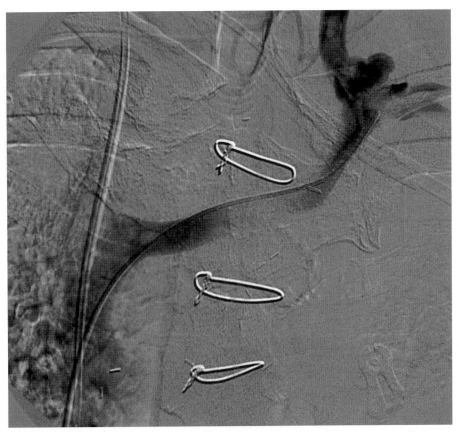

■ **Fig 18–15** Venogram confirms compression and severe stenosis.

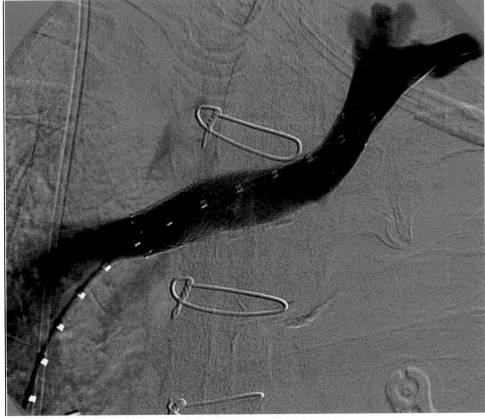

■ **Fig 18–16** Venogram after stent placement.

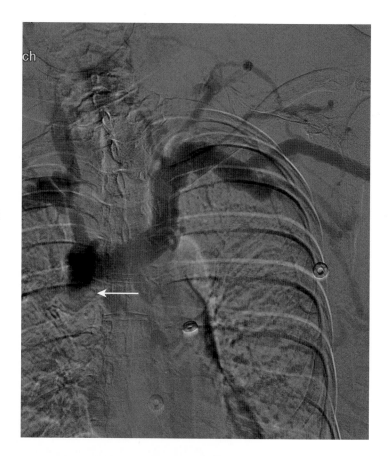

■ **Fig 18–17** A 48-year-old woman with end-stage renal disease presented with a swollen head and face and was found to have obstruction of the proximal superior vena cava (*arrow*).

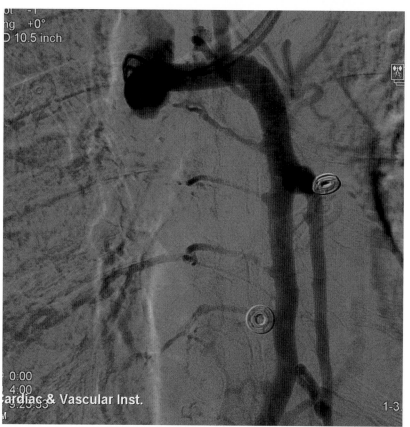

■ **Fig 18–18** Venogram demonstrates central outflow via dilated hemiazygous system.

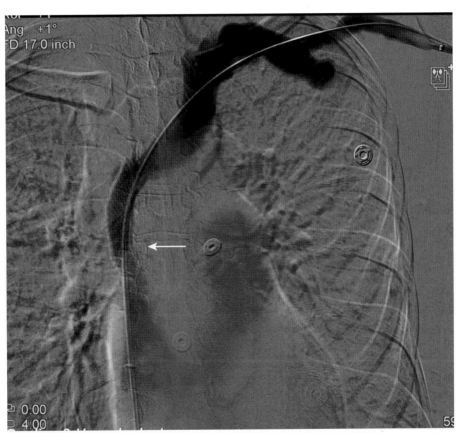

■ **Fig 18–19** After angioplasty and stent placement, there is restored inline flow into the right atrium with prompt symptom improvement (*arrow*).

Patients with SVC syndrome are initially studied using venography. A complete ultrasound examination including pulsed-wave Doppler and gray-scale imaging may be helpful to establish the number and degree of stenoses or occlusions prior to the venogram. If possible, a cross-sectional study such as a computed tomography angiogram or magnetic resonance angiogram with a venous phase may be obtained to confirm the level of stenosis and occlusion as well as highlight the amount of underlying mass effect or malignancy (Fig. 18-20).

Although it may not be necessary to treat both innominate veins to achieve a clinical outcome, bilateral central venous stenting may be needed to reestablish optimal flow. The goal is to restore flow into the right atrium (Figs. 18-21 through 18-23). The patency of the jugular veins is important because its intact drainage centrally is usually sufficient to relieve face and head symptoms. At the time of venography, brachial vein access is complemented by femoral and possibly jugular access. In the setting of acute thrombosis, chemical or mechanical thrombolysis may be necessary to uncover the underlying stenosis and minimize embolization. At our institution, we usually attempt to place the central stents first and then extend additional stents peripherally to help anchor the stents in place as needed. Stent migration is a complication and may be limited by the use of proper oversizing of the stents. The SVC is a thin vessel, and aggressive dilatation of stents should be avoided because caval perforation may occur, especially in patients after radiation therapy (Figs. 18-24 through 18-26).

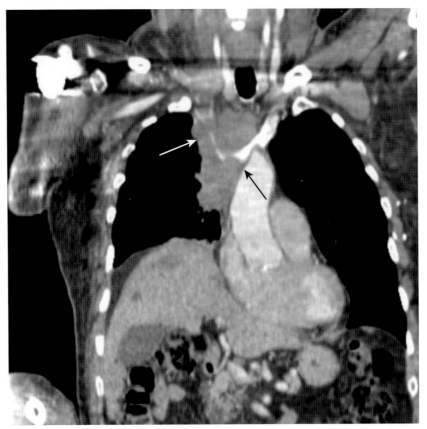

■ **Fig 18-20** A 76-year-old man presented with severe head pain and swelling. Computed tomography scan demonstrates known lung cancer, which is causing narrowing of both brachiocephalic veins. The right brachiocephalic vein appears occluded (*arrows*).

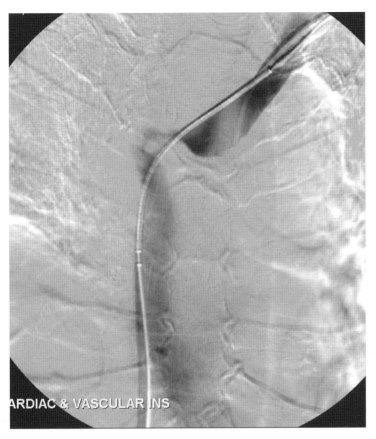

■ **Fig 18–21** A 76-year-old man with lung cancer and superior vena cava syndrome. Left upper extremity venogram demonstrates severe stenosis of the distal left brachiocephalic vein with a self-expandable stent being positioned for treatment.

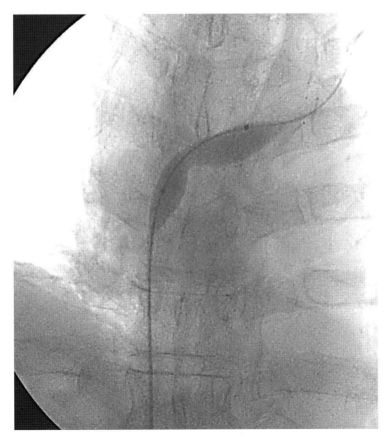

■ **Fig 18–22** Dilatation of the stent with a 12-mm balloon.

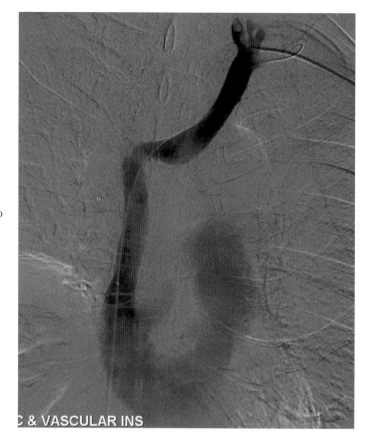

■ **Fig 18–23** Venogram poststent placement demonstrates prompt flow into the superior vena cava with dramatic improvement in the patient's symptoms.

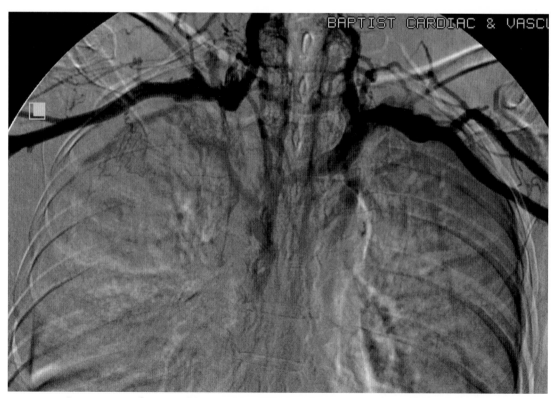

■ **Fig 18–24** A 61-year-old woman with superior vena cava syndrome whose bilateral upper extremity venogram demonstrates bilateral brachiocephalic vein occlusion.

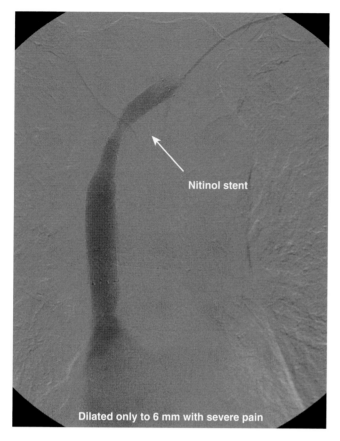

■ **Fig 18–25** Postrecanalization of left brachiocephalic vein; a 14-mm × 80-mm nitinol stent (SMART) was placed (*arrow*). Stent could be dilated only to 6 mm because of severe pain.

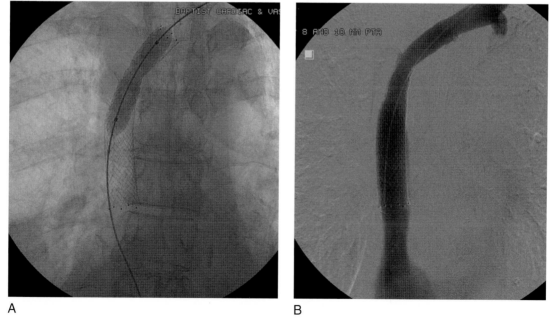

A   B

■ **Fig 18–26** Patient returned 6 days later, and the stent was dilated to 8 mm and 10 mm (**A**) with improved flow (**B**) with further improvement in symptoms.

NEW HORIZONS FOR MULTIPLE SCLEROSIS

Recent reports that patients with multiple sclerosis may have chronic cerebrospinal venous insufficiency have created renewed interested in the evaluation and treatment of central venous stenotic disease. Preliminary studies report that stenotic lesions in the azygous and jugular veins are more common in patients with a certain form of multiple sclerosis. These lesions may represent focal webs or traditional stenosis. Small studies have reported improvement in these patients' symptoms after treatment of these lesions with angioplasty. The assessment of these central lesions has included magnetic resonance venography, positional venous duplex ultrasound, and venography. Unfortunately, proper large-scale randomized studies are necessary to confirm these findings and prove the effectiveness of potential treatment options.

SUGGESTED READINGS

Bashit B, Parisi A, Frager DH, Suster B. Abdominal CT findings when the superior vena cava, brachiocephalic vein or subclavian vein is obstructed. AJR Am J Roentgenol 1996;167: 1457-1463.

Fassiadis N, Roidl M, South M. Are we managing primary upper limb deep venous thrombosis aggressively enough in the district? Int Angiol 2005;24:255-257.

Kapur S, Paik E, Rezaei A, Vu D. Where there is blood there is a way: Unusual collateral vessels in superior and inferior vena cava obstruction. Radiographics 2010;30:67-78.

Kucher N. Deep-vein thrombosis of the upper extremities. N Engl J Med 2011;364:861-869.

Lee WA, Hill BB, Harris EJ, et al. Surgical intervention is not required for all patients with subclavian vein thrombosis. J Vasc Surg 2000;32:57-67.

Lindblad B, Bornmyr S, Kullendorff B, Bergqvist D. Venous haemodynamics of the upper extremity after subclavian vein thrombosis. Vasa 1990;19:218-222.

Madan AK, Allmon JC, Harding M, et al. Dialysis access-induced superior vena cava syndrome. Am Surg 2002;68:904-906.

Owens CA, Bui JT, Knuttinen MG, et al. Pulmonary embolism from upper extremity deep vein thrombosis and the role of superior vena cava filters: a review of the literature. J Vasc Interv Radiol 2010;21:779-787.

Thomas IH, Zierler BK. An integrative review of outcomes in patients with acute primary upper extremity deep venous thrombosis following no treatment or treatment with anticoagulation, thrombolysis or surgical algorithms. Vasc Endovasc Surg 2005;39:163-174.

Tilney ML, Griffiths HJ, Edwards EA. Natural history of major venous thrombosis of the upper extremity. Arch Surg 1970;101:792-796.

Vendantham S, Benenati JF, Kundu S, et al. Interventional endovascular management of chronic cerebrospinal venous insufficiency in patients with multiple sclerosis: a position statement by the Society of Interventional Radiology, endorsed by the Canadian Interventional Radiology Association. J Vasc Interv Radiol 2010;21:1335-1337.

Zamboni P, Galeotti R, Menegatti E, et al. Chronic cerebrospinal venous insufficiency in patients with multiple sclerosis. J Neurol Neurosurg Psychiatry 2009;80:392-399.

Zamboni P, Galeotti R, Menegatti E, et al. A prospective open-label study of endovascular treatment of chronic cerebrospinal venous insufficiency. J Vasc Surg 2009;50:1348-1358.

CHAPTER 19

Venous Malformations

**Constantino S. Peña, Barry T. Katzen,
and Vittorio P. Antonacci**

Vascular malformations are probably the single most misdiagnosed entity in the vascular system. Essentially, vascular malformations are errors in vasculogenesis with the particular characteristics of the lesion determined by the vessel in the vascular system that is involved. As a result, these malformations can include arteries, veins, lymphatic vessels, or capillaries. These lesions occur in about 1.5% of the population and over 90% are present at birth. Venous malformations are the most common vascular anomalies.

While these lesions can have mass effect on adjacent structures, they are not tumors. A clearly organized classification system was presented by Mullikan, Glowacki, and colleagues in 1992, and this classification system was adopted in 1996 by the International Society for the Study of Vascular Anomalies (ISSVA). The classification system clearly separates tumors (e.g., hemangioma) from the vascular spaces that characterize a vascular malformation.[1]

WHAT ARE HEMANGIOMAS?

Hemangiomas are childhood masses characterized histologically by high endothelial cell turnover and are characterized by cell markers (GLUT-1, merosin, Lewis Y) that are otherwise found only in human placental tissue and that display phasicity characterized by a rapid proliferative phase, plateau phase, and slow involutional phase. The proper nomenclature for these lesions is infantile hemangioma. Infantile hemangiomas are benign vascular tumors that are not usually present at the time of birth but instead become evident within the first 2 to 3 weeks of life. They are the most common benign tumor of infancy. There is a subgroup of hemangiomas that present fully formed at birth known as congenital hemangiomas. These congenital hemangiomas (as opposed to infantile hemangiomas) do not exhibit the expected accelerated postnatal growth. Some congenital hemangiomas involve rapidly over the first year of life and are called rapidly involuting congenital hemangiomas (RICHs), while some may persist indefinitely without treatment and are called noninvoluting congenital hemangiomas (NICHs).[1]

The majority of infantile hemangiomas are localized and, although disconcerting to parents and care providers, are nonthreatening.[2] For these lesions, observation and routine monitoring by the pediatrician or dermatologist are acceptable treatment options. A minority of infantile hemangiomas can, however, cause significant morbidity. These require early recognition, timely referral to a specialist, and prompt intervention to minimize complications. Worrisome presentations include multiple hemangiomas and sensitive locations such as beard distribution, periocular, perioral, nasal tip, large regions of the face and neck, and the lumbosacral spine region. In general, larger hemangiomas located on the face are more likely to require treatment. One of the strongest indications for the use of the laser is the presence of ulceration. Other symptoms necessitating therapeutic intervention include congestive heart failure, airway obstruction, dysphagia, infection, failure to thrive, external auditory canal occlusion, visual axis impairment, and severe facial deformity.

Muscular skeletal hemangiomas are not hemangiomas. They are venous malformations that occur in the muscle. With the correct clinical history, a properly performed magnetic resonance imaging examination should be almost pathognomonic. Vertebral body hemangiomas are also not hemangiomas; they are venous malformations that occur in bone. Review of the literature demonstrates numerous studies demonstrating "increased vascularity" of these lesions. However, the increased vascularity is from the venous pooling in the lesion and not from arterial hypertrophy and neovascularity. Liver hemangiomas are not hemangiomas; they are venous malformations that occur in the liver.

Hemangiomas in adults are not hemangiomas; a hemangioma is a childhood-only birthmark. If a vascular birthmark was not present in the childhood stage, then it is not a hemangioma. Hemangiomas are NOT arteriovenous malformations (AVMs), and vice versa. While there is arterial inflow that identifies both these lesions, hemangiomas demonstrate typical tumor vascularity with a central arterial pedicle, and there is fairly minimal, if any, shunting identified in the outflow vessels. An AVM, on the other hand, may have significant venous shunting, with resultant low resistance arterial inflow and arterialized pulsatility in the venous outflow vessels. Venous enlargement is also common in AVMs, resulting from the pressurized shunted arterial flow into the nidus.

VASCULAR MALFORMATIONS

Vascular malformations are malformed or dysplastic embryologic spaces that are characterized by normal endothelial cell turnover and abnormal vascular anatomy characterized by the dysplastic vessels involved. All vascular malformations can be placed into one of three groups: low flow, high flow, and combined.

Low-Flow Vascular Malformations—Venous Malformations

Low-flow venous malformations are the most common form of vascular malformation—simplified, they are a number of tortuous vascular channels. They will be evident at birth and will grow with the child. These are common birthmarks present at birth, although they can be clinically occult if deep in location and usually do not become symptomatic until late childhood/early adolescence. Deep subcutaneous or intramuscular venous malformations often manifest with only local swelling and pain. The diagnosis can be difficult because extremity varicosities may be the only visible sign, especially in deep venous malformations. Superficial venous malformations can be seen with bluish-purple skin discoloration. Venous malformations can be divided into truncal and extratruncal lesions. On physical examination, these lesions are soft and easily compressible and will often demonstrate engorgement, especially when the affected extremity is placed in a dependent position. Extratruncal lesions occur from remnants of primitive vessels early in development and are usually dysplastic and diffusely infiltrative. They commonly involve the deep soft tissue structures but patients may have constant pain. Truncal venous malformations occur in differentiated and later-stage vascular structures and patients may have an impressive cutaneous manifestation with limb swelling and varicosities. Diffuse malformations involve multiple areas or regions and are usually part of a syndrome such as Klippel-Trenaunay syndrome. Diagnosis of a venous malformations can usually be made by clinical examination; however, imaging studies such as magnetic resonance imaging (MRI) are performed to evaluate the extent and guide treatment. On MRI, venous malformations are T1 isointense to muscle and T2 hyperintense and demonstrate late enhancement (Fig. 19-1).

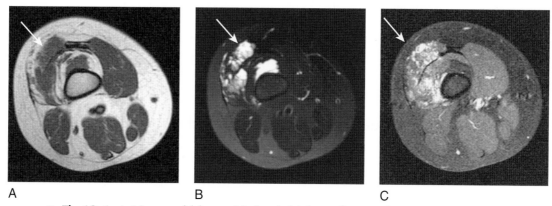

A   B   C

■ **Fig 19–1** A 10-year-old boy with focal thigh swelling and pain. Axial T1-weighted (**A**), T2-weighted (**B**), and T1-weighted after gadolinium (**C**) images demonstrating a T1 isointense and T2 hyperintense signal and enhancement after gadolinium in a venous malformation (*arrow*) in the lateral aspect of left lower extremity.

Low-Flow Vascular Malformations—Lymphatic Malformations

These lesions are abnormalities of lymphatic etiology that often appear in infancy or early childhood, with more than 90% of patients presenting by age 2. More than 75% of these lesions are seen in the craniocervical lesion. Patients with these lesions usually present for treatment earlier than those with venous malformations secondary to the cosmetic concerns of the localized mass effect or swelling caused by the lesions. Lymphatic malformations (LMs) will often fluctuate in size secondary to trauma, inflammation, or intralesional hemorrhage. Antibiotics are administered for fever or erythema. Unlike venous malformations, LMs are not usually painful. Larger LMs, however, can result in airway obstruction, speech abnormalities, and dysphagia. In the past, these lesions were called lymphangiomas or cystic hygromas. These outdated terms should no longer be used in clinical practice.

There are two subtypes of LMs: macrocystic LM and microcystic LM. Because the imaging characteristics and treatment options are different, it is important to recognize these subtypes. Macrocystic LMs appear similar to venous malformations on MRI except that they only demonstrate minimal, if any, peripheral enhancement. Macrocystic LMs are often easily accessible for sclerotherapy treatments. On the other hand, microcystic LMs are often only observed, with treatment options usually limited to surgical debulking and percutaneous management of cutaneous complications such as recurrent cellulitis or sclerotherapy treatment of bleeding superficial vesicles.

Low-Flow Vascular Malformations—Capillary Malformations

Capillary malformations (CMs) are capillary dilatations. They are characterized by ectatic papillary dermal capillaries and postcapillary venules in the upper reticular dermis and were commonly referred to as "port-wine" stains. CMs are present at birth and grow in size commensurate with the child as they have no tendency toward involution. At birth, CMs are usually pink or reddish and will usually darken with advancing age. They present as solitary lesions but can be associated with other vascular malformations. A typical worrisome location is the midline lower back region as CMs in this location may be associated with tethered spinal cord. Facial CMs may be associated with Sturge-Weber syndrome. Other conditions associated with CMs include Klippel-Trenaunay syndrome and Proteus syndrome.

High-Flow Vascular Malformations—Arteriovenous Fistulas

Arteriovenous fistulas (AVFs) are an abnormal connection between an artery and a vein. Although these high-flow lesions can be congenital, often they are acquired as the result of surgery, penetrating trauma, or erosion by adjacent disease processes. As blood follows the path of least resistance, flow in both the inflow artery and outflow vein increases. The resistance in the fistula can be low enough that the fistula tract causes a "steal phenomenon" to arterial supply distally and can actually cause a reversal of arterial flow in the distal arterial segment. This "parasitic circulation" can result in decreased arterial pressures in the distal capillary beds and cause tissue ischemia and pain. Treatment is usually from an endovascular approach, but this depends on the location of the AVF.

High-Flow Vascular Malformations—Arteriovenous Malformations

AVFs are abnormal connections between an artery and a vein that have a tortuous segment of dyplastic vessels (called the nidus) between the supplying artery or arteries and the draining vein or veins. Usually, these lesions are asymptomatic, but they can have varied symptoms, including heart failure, neuropathy, pain, or bleeding. Symptomatic small and superficial AVMs are occasionally treated with surgical resection; however, most AVMs are inoperable because they are large and diffuse in nature and involve important normal adjacent structures. With improvement of catheter technology, superselective techniques, and the use of liquid embolic agents, embolotherapy has emerged as the primary mode of treatment for the management of peripheral AVMs.

TREATMENT OF VENOUS MALFORMATIONS

Treatment of venous malformations has improved over the past decade as a result of advances in percutaneous and transcatheter embolotherapy and sclerotherapy. Localized and diffuse venous malformations have been treated with sclerotherapy, while some localized lesions may be resected. Sclerotherapy can be performed with ethanol, liquid, and foam detergents. In our practice, we treat venous malformations with ethyl alcohol embolization/sclerotherapy. In many ways it is similar to sclerotherapy performed for lower extremity varicosities, particularly when using agents such as sodium tetradecyl. When dehydrated ethyl alcohol is used, however, the potential for serious complications is increased by an order of magnitude. Local ethanol complications are related to the transmural necrosis of the agent and spread to the surrounding tissues.

Preprocedure evaluation of a malformation with either ultrasound or MRI is helpful not only in defining the extent of the abnormality but also in aiding to determine possible direct access into the lesion (Figs. 19-2 and 19-3). Access into the malformation is usually performed with ultrasound and fluoroscopic guidance (Fig. 19-4). Biplane fluoroscopy can be used if the location of the lesion allows. Direct comparison with the MR images can also be very helpful. Proper positioning on the angiographic table is critical to successfully access the malformation and to allow proper anesthesia monitoring. All alcohol embolization procedures are performed with the patient under general anesthesia to allow for proper sedation and pain management as well as to prepare should complications of treatment (such as cardiovascular collapse) occur. Additionally, a tourniquet for control with a calibrated cuff can be used if the location of the lesions allows. When using a tourniquet, we do not exceed diastolic blood pressure and often only use minimal pressures in the 20 to 40 mm Hg range.

The technique for the alcohol administration has evolved over the past 10 years. Previously, dehydrated ethanol was opacified with a small amount of ethiodized oil (Ethiodol) to increase the visualization of the administered alcohol under fluoroscopic control. Currently, we use a negative contrast technique. This consists of opacification of the malformation with contrast followed by administration of the ethyl alcohol that replaces the contrast on live fluoroscopic evaluation (Fig. 19-5). Once we have either treated the entire lesion or reached our sclerosant limits, the procedure is concluded (Fig. 19-6). The absolute maximum for ethyl alcohol is 1 mL/kg. In our practice, we rarely exceed 0.5 mL/kg in one procedure. A good working dose limit for ethyl alcohol is 0.25 mg/kg for the entire case. We also limit our total injected volume to 0.1 mL/kg/injection and allow at least 5 minutes between alcohol administrations. By adhering to these recommendations, we have completed safe treatment for many patients without the use of pulmonary arterial catheter monitoring.

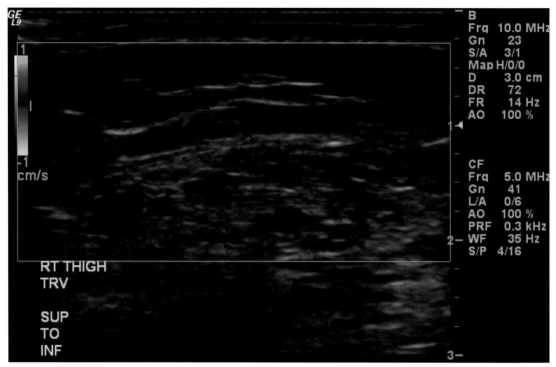

■ **Fig 19-2** Ultrasound Doppler examination demonstrates a heterogeneous lesion with no increased flow consistent with a low-flow vascular venous malformation.

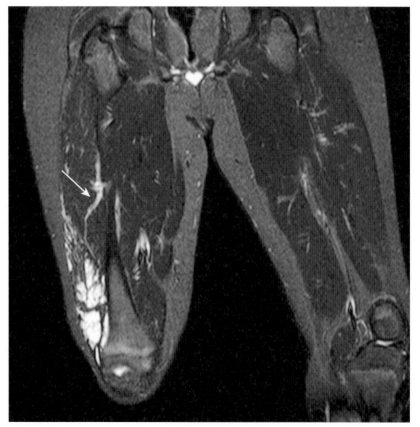

■ **Fig 19-3** Coronal fat-saturated T1-weighted image. After the addition of gadolinium, enhancement of the dysplastic draining vein is demonstrated (*arrow*).

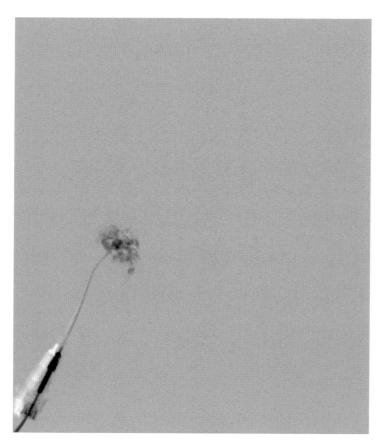

■ **Fig 19-4** Initial venogram with dilute contrast.

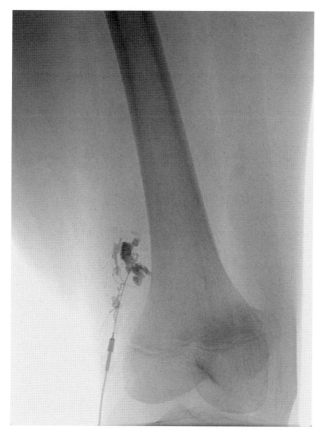

■ **Fig 19-5** Direct puncture venography using a small angiocatheter.

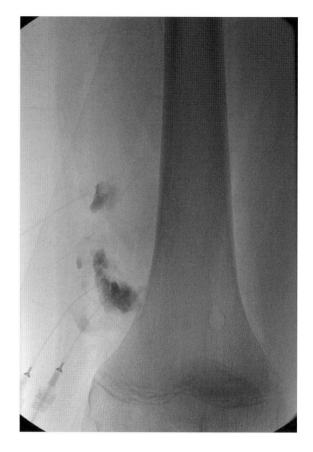

▪ **Fig 19-6** Posttreatment scout film demonstrating two separate treatment punctures.

Occasionally, a lesion can be treated in one session; however, most require several (two to four) treatments to reach our clinical endpoint of treating the pain associated with a symptomatic malformation. We do not treat asymptomatic lesions unless there is a significant cosmetic issue, which can occur with lesions on the face and neck. Treatments are usually spaced apart by 3 to 4 months to allow for postprocedural edema to resolve.

Our standard postprocedure orders include intravenous ketorolac, dexamethasone, and antibiotic coverage for the first 24 hours of treatment. Following overnight observation, patients are discharged home with an outpatient oral medication regimen of a methylprednisolone dose pack, ibuprofen therapy, and oral antibiotics.

Evaluation of the venous drainage of venous malformations is essential in their treatment. Malformations with no or limited venous drainage can be treated with embolic agents with higher effectiveness and less risk than malformations with normal draining vessels, while lesions with drainage into dysplastic veins or a venous ectasia can be most problematic to treat. Venous malformations may have a number of large-diameter connections to the deep venous system. It is important to control the injection to prevent the liquid embolics from entering these central veins. Burrows et al. have reported good result in 75% to 90% of their patient cohort treated with serial alcohol administration. However, many patients have chronic pain symptoms, and their clinical improvement may lag significantly behind a more technically successful treatment.

REFERENCES

1. Mulliken JB, Young AE. Vascular birthmarks: hemangiomas and malformations. Philadelphia: WB Saunders; 1988.
2. Bittles MA, Sidhu MK, Sze RW, et al. Multidetector CT angiography of pediatric vascular malformations and hemangiomas: utility of 3-D reformatting in differential diagnosis. Pediatr Radiol 2005;35:1100-1106.

OTHER SELECTED READINGS

Al-Adnani M, Williams S, Rampling D, et al. Histopathological reporting of paediatric cutaneous vascular anomalies in relation to proposed multidisciplinary classification system. J Clin Pathol 2006;59:1278-1282.

Bauman NM, Burke DK, Smith RJ. Treatment of massive or life-threatening hemangiomas with recombinant alpha (2a)-interferon. Otolaryngol Head Neck Surg 1997;117:99-110.

Cho SK, Do YS, Kim DI, et al. Peripheral arteriovenous malformations with a dominant outflow vein: results of ethanol embolization. Korean J Radiol 2008;9:258-267.

Rosenblatt M. Endovascular management of venous malformations. Phlebology 2007;22:264-275.

van der Linden E, Pattynama PMT, Heeres BC, et al. Long-term patient satisfaction after percutaneous treatment of peripheral vascular malformations. Radiology 2009;251:926-932.

van Rijswijk CSP, van der Linden E, van der Woude H-J, et al. Value of dynamic contrast-enhanced MR imaging in diagnosing and classifying peripheral vascular malformations. AJR Am J Roentgenol 2002;178:1181-1187.

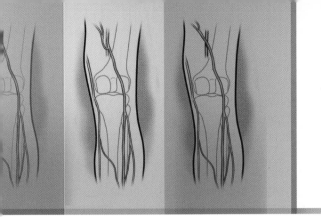

CHAPTER 20

Treatment of
Venous Ulcers

Ronald Bush

Venous ulcers affect 2% of the adult population. Millions of dollars are spent each year on the care of this difficult condition. There is as yet no consensus on the best therapy; the main treatment strategy has been compression therapy.

In this chapter, the etiology is examined from a hemodynamic and cellular aspect. Adjunctive treatments, both medical and surgical, are discussed. Finally, a new treatment option—terminal interruption of the reflux source (TIRS)—is introduced. First, all venous ulcers have a common denominator. The commonality is increased ambulatory venous pressure. A pressure above 45 mm Hg increases the risk of ulceration. The higher the pressure, the greater is the risk of eventual venous ulceration.[1] The increased pressure may be due solely to reflux at some point in the venous system or coexist with other factors.[2]

When evaluating a patient with a venous ulcer, an understanding of venous pathophysiology and the complex interaction at the cellular level must be understood. The etiology of the increased venous pressure should be documented. This may be from a superficial, deep, or perforating vessel or a combination of any of the three. There may be other contributing factors such as abdominal outflow compression or problems with venous or arterial capacity.

The eventual goal, if possible, is to provide relief of the increased venous pressure. This will ensure the best possible outcome and help reduce further ulcerations. Most therapy is directed at the local level when the patient is first seen. This is in the form of compression therapy.

Compression therapy with either elastic or inelastic dressings has been the historical treatment.[3,4] As compliance increases, so do the healing rates. However, with compression alone, there is still a high recurrence rate.[4,5]

Other adjuncts to improving ulcer healing have been described. Medical therapy has included rutosides, aspirin, and pentoxifylline.[6-8] Of course, local wound care is essential and irrigation and debridement of devitalized tissue are essential.

At the Midwest Vein and Laser Center, debridement is often carried out using a 3- to 10-mL syringe with saline connected to a 30-gauge needle. This technique in effect sends a high-pressure stream of saline that is directed at the ulcer base. This is very effective and better tolerated by the patient.

Many dressings have been advocated for the active ulcer. These range from simple gauze to impregnated foam dressings. Silver-impregnated dressings are used in our clinic when there is evidence of infection locally. However, there is no evidence of the superiority of one dressing over the other in promoting wound healing.

Skin grafts have been used as an adjunct in wound healing for venous ulcers. These grafts include full-thickness punch grafts, xenografts, or allografts. To date, in an updated review on skin grafting for venous ulcers, bilayer artificial skin used in association with compression dressings increased ulcer healing compared to compression alone.[9,10] In the study by Falanga et al.,[9] healing at 6 months was only 63% with allogenic human skin equivalent compared to 43% with compression alone.[9]

Surgical techniques such as stripping the great saphenous vein,[10,11] subfascial perforator ligation,[12,13] endoluminal thermal ablation,[14] and minimally invasive perforator therapy[15] have been used as adjuncts in the treatment of venous ulcers. Nontargeted foam sclerotherapy has also been mentioned as a treatment modality.[15-17] Except for foam sclerotherapy, none of these procedures has proved to increase the healing rate of venous ulcers. These adjunctive procedures are mostly directed at preventing future occurrences.

Recently, the TIRS technique was introduced.[18] The TIRS technique targets only those vessels in close proximity to the venous ulcer.

The basis of this theory is that venous ulceration is a local manifestation of a systemic problem. The high venous pressure in a vein or veins draining the ulcer bed, or in some instances a perforator directly in continuity with the ulcer, is responsible for the local phenomenon of ulceration. If the venous hypertension is relieved, then healing should accelerate.

When using the TIRS technique, patients at Midwest Vein and Laser Center had rapid healing of ulcers compared to compression alone or compression with other adjunctive procedures. In a series of 20 patients treated with the TIRS technique, healing occurred in 90% of patients within 8 weeks. All patients had been compliant with compression for 18 to 24 months prior to treatment.[18]

The exact mechanism of action at the microscopic level is as yet unknown in the TIRS technique. The genesis of ulceration at the microscopic level is generally believed to be an inflammatory response. According to this theory, continuous high-pressure leads to eventual necrosis. The necrosis is mediated by complex interaction at the cellular level. Rapid healing observed after occluding these high-pressure venous effluents with foam sclerotherapy must be related to a marked reduction in ambulatory venous pressure at the local level. Unfortunately, there is no reliable means to measure pressures in those smaller distal venous channels or, for that matter, at the tissue level. Hence, an assumption is made that healing is mediated through a local reduction of venous pressure at the ulcer site. The response has been rapid in most patients; however, there may be other mechanisms that are also contributing that are so far not known.

The TIRS technique requires good interpretive ultrasound skills and the ability to safely deliver the foamed sclerotherapy with the aid of ultrasound guidance. Only the most distal venous branches draining the area of the ulcer are identified. In some patients, especially those with anterior calf ulcers, a perforator leading directly to the ulcer bed may be identified (Figs. 20-1 and 20-2). The proximal source of reflux (i.e., saphenous vein, classic posterior tibial perforator, or other source proximally) is ignored. Only the distal vessel or vessels are targeted initially (Fig. 20-3 through 20-13). *Text continued on p. 454*

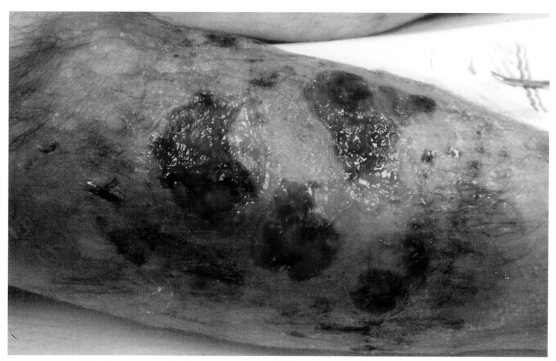

■ **Fig 20-1** Anterior leg ulcers secondary to chronic venous hypertension.

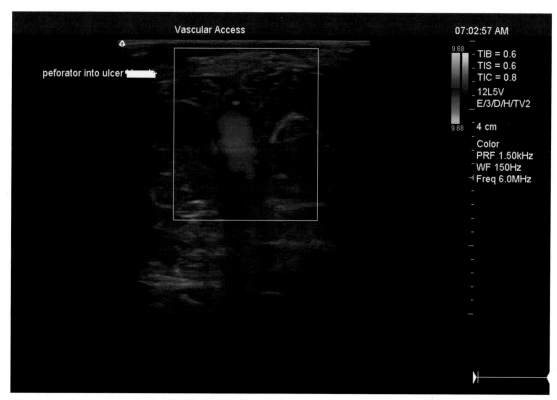

■ **Fig 20-2** Perforator into superior ulcer bed.

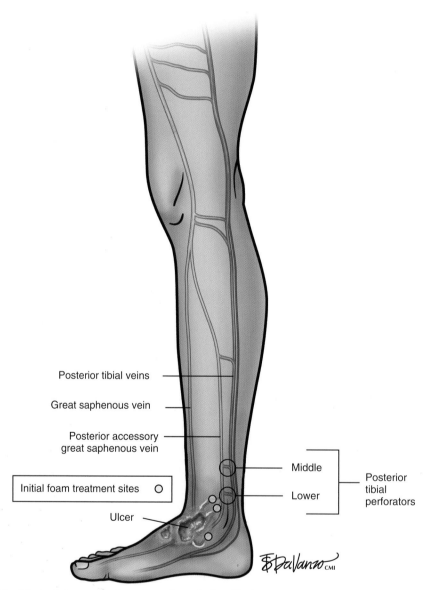

Posterior tibial veins

Great saphenous vein

Posterior accessory
great saphenous vein

Middle

Lower

Posterior
tibial
perforators

Initial foam treatment sites ○

Ulcer

■ **Fig 20–3** Schematic drawing of medial calf ulcer associated with posterior calf perforator.

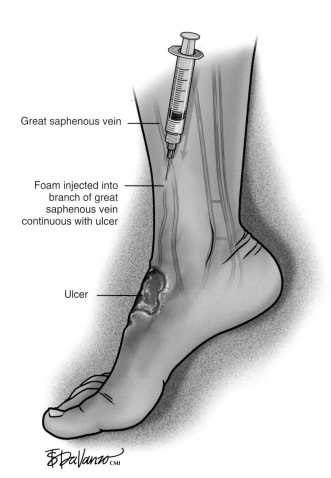

Great saphenous vein

Foam injected into
branch of great
saphenous vein
continuous with ulcer

Ulcer

■ **Fig 20–4** Schematic drawing of anterior
ulcer secondary to incompetent branch of
the saphenous vein with associated greater
saphenous insufficiency.

■ **Fig 20-5** Schematic drawing of anterior ulcer secondary to perforator associated with deep venous insufficiency.

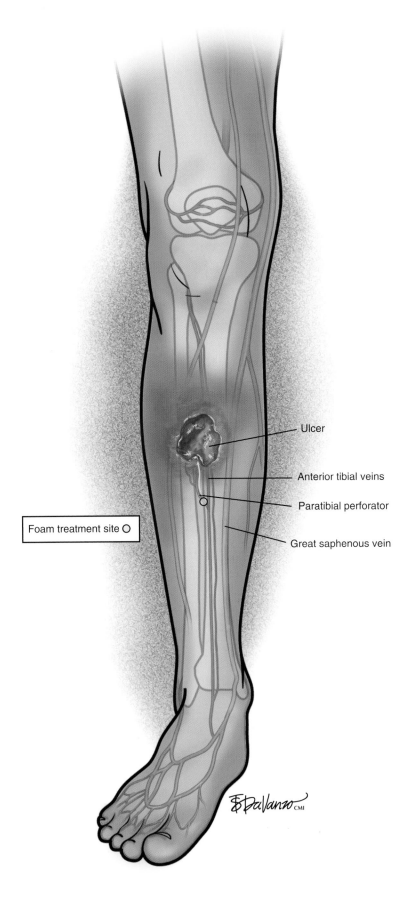

Ulcer

Anterior tibial veins

Paratibial perforator

Great saphenous vein

Foam treatment site O

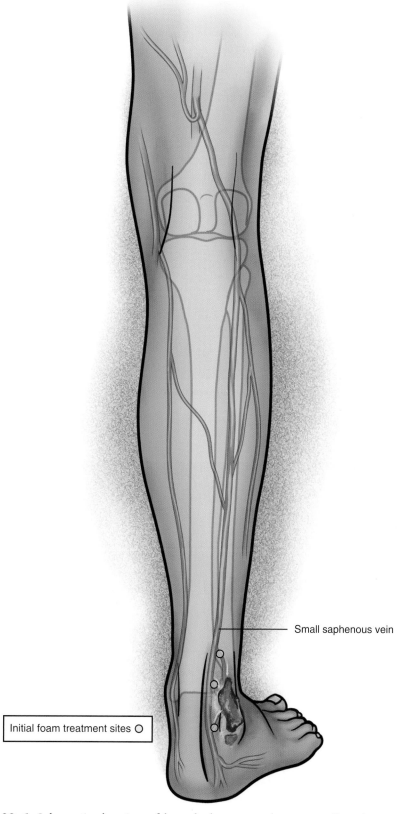

Small saphenous vein

Initial foam treatment sites ○

■ **Fig 20–6** Schematic drawing of lateral ulcer secondary to small saphenous vein insufficiency.

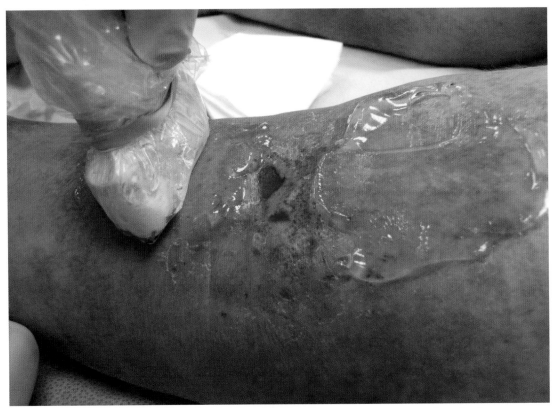

■ **Fig 20–7** Using ultrasound to demonstrate vessels draining ulcer bed.

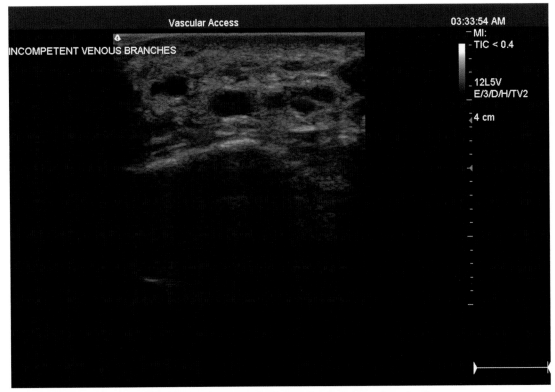

■ **Fig 20–8** Ultrasound of vessels draining ulcer bed.

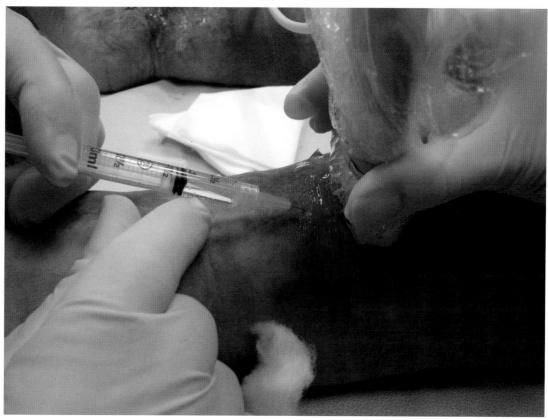

■ **Fig 20–9** Local anesthesia to skin delivered with a 30-gauge needle with tumescent solution.

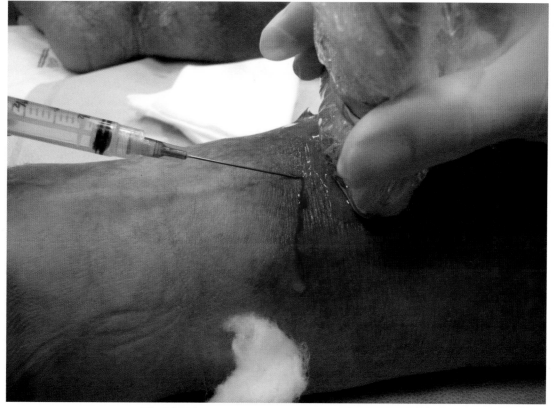

■ **Fig 20–10** Percutaneous puncture of target vessel.

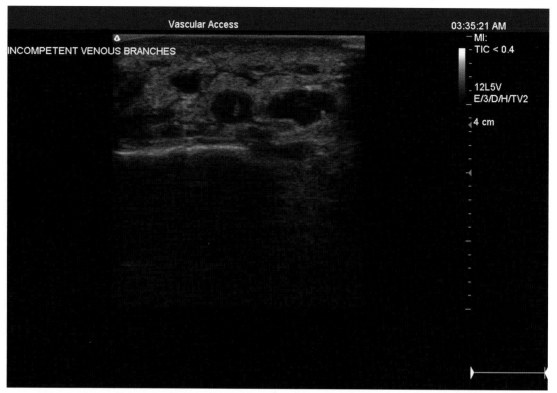

■ **Fig 20–11** Needle in target vessel.

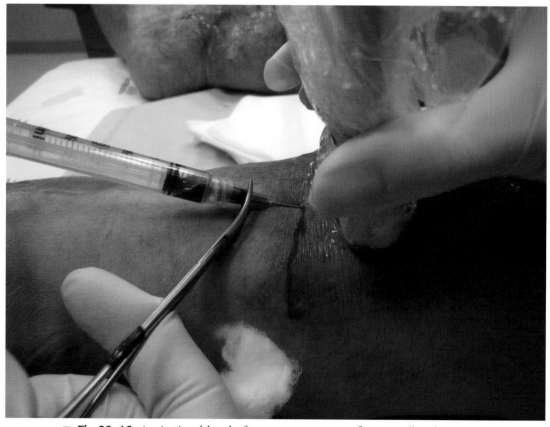

■ **Fig 20–12** Aspirating blood after puncture to confirm needle placement.

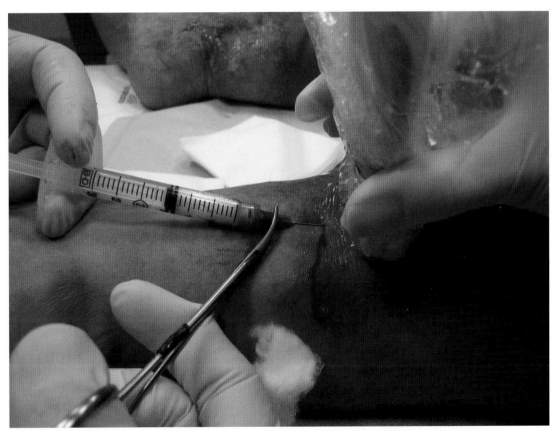

■ **Fig 20–13** Injecting sodium tetradecyl sulfate (Sotradecol) foam.

Using ultrasound guidance, these vessels are cannulated with needle penetration through normal skin, as far from the ulcer margin as possible. A 3-mL syringe and a 22-gauge needle are used in our clinic. Cannulation is performed superior to the ulcer if chronic skin change exists inferiorly. After penetrating the target vessel, the foam is slowly injected (Fig. 20-14). In our clinic, a 4:1 mixture of sodium tetradecyl sulfate (Sotradecol) and CO_2 is used. After injection of the foamed solution, compression is applied and local wound care is performed. The patient is re-scanned at weekly intervals and foam injections are repeated if necessary. A 1% concentration is used, unless extenuating circumstances such as concurrent anticoagulation or high flow exist. A 3% foamed solution of sodium tetradecyl sulfate is then used.

Definitive treatment of the proximal reflux source such as thermal ablation of the saphenous vein or perforator interruption is done at a later date, to help prevent future ulcer occurrences. In some cases, concurrent treatment can be done. However, many times insurance dictates must be addressed and the more definitive procedures are performed 6 to 8 weeks after the first ultrasound-guided treatment. Most patients have had rapid healing by this time, and local infection and pain have abated.

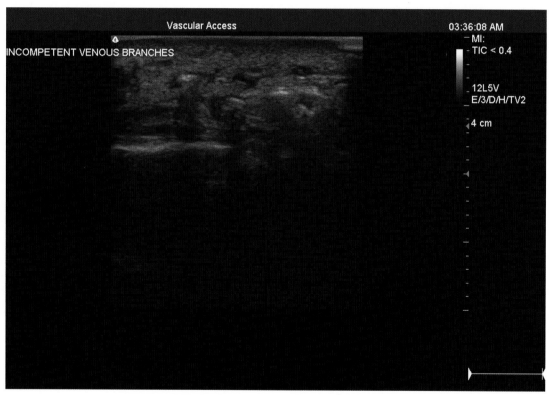

■ **Fig 20-14** Postprocedure ultrasound.

REFERENCES

1. Payne S, London N, Newland C, et al. Ambulatory venous pressure: Correlation with skin condition and role in identifying surgically correctible disease. Eur J Vasc Endovasc Surg 1996;11:195-200.
2. Raju S, Neglen P, Carr-White P, et al. Ambulatory venous hypertension: component analysis in 373 limbs. Vasc Endovascular Surg 1999;33:257-266.
3. Fletcher A, Cullum N, Sheldon T. A systematic review of compression treatment for venous leg ulcers. BMJ 1997;315:576-580.
4. Erickson C, Lanza D, Karp D, et al. Healing of venous ulcers in an ambulatory care program: the roles of chronic venous insufficiency and patient compliance. J Vasc Surg 1995;22: 629-636.
5. Scriven J, Taylor L, Wood A, et al. A prospective randomized trial of four-layer versus short stretch compression bandages for the treatment of venous leg ulcers. Ann R Coll Surg Engl 1998;80:215-220.
6. Falanga V, Fujitani R, Diaz C, et al. Systemic treatment of venous leg ulcers with high doses of pentoxifylline: efficacy in a randomized, placebo-controlled trial. Wound Repair Regen 1999;7:208-213.
7. Colgan M, Dormandy J, Jones, P, et al. Oxpentifylline treatment of venous ulcers of the leg. BMJ 1990;300:972-975.
8. Gohel M, Davies A. Pharmacological agents in the treatment of venous disease: an update of the available evidence. Curr Vasc Pharmacol 2009;7:303-308.
9. Falanga V, Margolis D, Alvarez O, et al. Rapid healing of venous ulcers and lack of clinical rejection with an allogeneic cultured human skin equivalent. Arch Dermatol 1998;134: 293-300.
10. Barwell J, Davies C, Deacon J, et al. Comparison of surgery and compression with compression alone in chronic venous ulceration (ESCHAR STUDY): randomized controlled trial. Lancet 2008;363:1854-1859.
11. Homans J. The operative treatment of varicose veins and ulcers, based on classification of these lesions. Surg Gynecol Obstet 1916;22:143-158.
12. Pierik E, Van Urk H, Hop W, Wittens C. Endoscopic versus open subfascial division of incompetent perforating veins in the treatment of venous leg ulceration: a randomized trial. J Vasc Surg 1997;26:1049-1054.
13. Glovicski P, Bergan J, Rhodes J, et al. Mid-term results of endoscopic perforator vein interruption for chronic venous insufficiency: lessons learned from the North American subfascial endoscopic perforator surgery registry. The North American Study Group. J Vasc Surg 1999; 29:489-502.
14. Rautio T, Ohinmaa A, Perala J, et al. Endovenous obliteration versus conventional stripping operation in the treatment of primary varicose veins: a randomized controlled trial with comparison of the costs. J Vasc Surg 2002;35:958-965.
15. Poblete H, Elias S. Venous ulcers: New options in treatment: minimally invasive vein surgery. J Am Coll Cert Wound Special 2009;1:12-19.
16. Hertzman P, Owens R. Rapid healing of chronic venous ulcers following ultrasound-guided foam sclerotherapy. Phlebology 2007;22:34-39.
17. Cabrera J, Redondo P, Becerra A, et al. Ultrasound-guided injection of polidocanol microfoam in the management of venous leg ulcers. Arch Dermatol 2004;140:667-673.
18. Bush R. New technique to heal venous ulcers: terminal interruption of the reflux source (TIRS). Perspect Vasc Surg Endovasc Ther 2010;22:194-199.

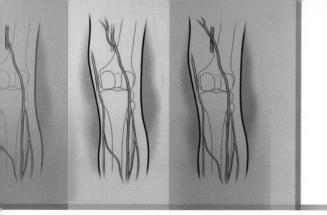

CHAPTER 21

Severity Scoring and Outcomes Measurement

Michael A. Vasquez and Carolyn E. Munschauer

HISTORICAL BACKGROUND

I have but one lamp by which my feet are
guided, and that is the lamp of experience. I
know no way of judging the future but the past.

—Patrick Henry

With these words from 1775, Patrick Henry set a standard for the role of progress. Moving forward demands a look back and a commitment not to abandon the lessons of the past to the lure of an untested future.[1]

The approach to accepting change and advancement in medicine and surgical technology is much the same. The promises of the new must meet the expectations built from the experience of the old. The responsibility of the physician is to rigorously evaluate new developments through analysis of data and to share those findings with his or her patients and other physicians.[1]

There is evidence of the recognition of varicose veins as early as ancient Egyptian and Greek periods, including a familiar tablet in Athens, Greece, of a man displaying a leg with visible varicosities.[2] Other writings have offered descriptive accounts of circulation, arteriography and venography, the introduction of heparin, and the embolectomy catheter. From Oribasius in the fourth century, who also wrote about surgical procedures for varicose veins, to Harvey in the 17th century, these writings described in detail the structure and function of the circulatory system.

By the 19th century, reports were emerging on interventions for arterial and venous disorders, which led to increased understanding of the course of disease and healing. Mott used arterial ligation to treat aneurysms and other disorders, while European physicians focused on the diagnosis and treatment of venous disease, with ligation, injection of varicosities, identification of reflux and its role in venous disease, and ulcer treatment with Unna paste among the significant advancements of this time. In 1803, von Loder provided a thorough description of the communicating and perforating veins in the legs.

The 20th century brought new advances in vascular diagnosis and therapy for arterial and venous disease. Homans made the direct association between ulcers and varicosities, leading to the use of surgical therapy involving excision of the saphenous vein, its branches, and perforators. This led to a focus on venous disease, including ambulatory venous ligation, injection of sclerosants, perforator ligation, diagnostic venography, venous bypass grafting, and the introduction of low-dose heparin. In 1938, Linton demonstrated a direct link between anatomy and pathophysiology in his description of the role of perforators in venous ulcers; by ligating the perforating veins, he decreased pressure in the superficial system and improved ulcer healing.

In an article about the discovery of venous valves, Scultetus et al. wrote: "With the formidable advances of the diagnostic methods and new therapeutic modalities, we will be able to make earlier diagnoses, begin treatment sooner, and increase life expectancy. However, we must not forget the origin of our knowledge—the past."[3]

The end of the 20th century and the first decade of the 21st century have marked a change of focus in venous disease and therapy. Although treatments were regularly being offered for many vascular conditions, the outcomes were only sporadically evaluated. After introducing several valvular reconstructive procedures, Kistner found that reporting methods were not standardized across facilities, preventing interinstitutional trials and confounding results reporting.[4] According to Mozes and Gloviczki, "The time has come to standardize the clinical classes of venous disease, to compare treatment and outcome, and to speak the same language when we talk about venous problems all around the world."[5]

This realization that the language of diagnostic and treatment information needs to be universal has shifted the focus of physicians to organize information to provide a framework for clinical practice and research.[4] Dayal and Kent[6] wrote about the need for reporting standards to address important elements of assessment, including clinical classification of disease, a grading system for risk factors, categorization of operations and interventions, complications encountered with grades for severity or outcomes, and criteria for improvement, deterioration, and failure.

Results should be evaluated alongside other options such as the natural course of the disease itself, nonsurgical therapies, additional surgical interventions, or alternative ways of performing an intervention.[7] Developing and using proper outcomes assessment tools should be paramount in the minds of those treating venous disease. The assessment of outcomes in chronic venous disease is multifactorial and is more complicated than in other vascular conditions.[8] The end points of comparison must be objective usable measures that reflect signs, symptoms, and patient quality of life.[9] Rutherford said, "Comparing results is not a simple matter, but if we develop a good, readily usable approach to outcomes comparisons, one by which the results of our labors can be properly judged, the results are great."[7]

ETIOLOGY AND NATURAL HISTORY

In the 1950s, life table analysis was used to examine and predict survival and success rates from many surgical procedures. When the concept was applied to cancer survival in the mid 1970s, it gained acceptance as a valid reporting method for outcomes assessment.[10] Reports of short- and long-term survival after procedures for lower extremity ischemia became more common in the 1970s and 1980s, culminating in the 1986 findings of an ad hoc committee of the Society for Vascular Surgery/North American Chapter, International Society for Cardiovascular Surgery.[11] This group was charged with standardizing reporting practices for lower extremity ischemia. It was one of several subcommittees that met to determine reporting standards for numerous vascular conditions and therapies. Around this same time, reports were being published on clinical outcomes and quality-of-life assessment. Many of the instruments used were able to be applied to the emerging field of venous disease.

The 36-Item Short Form Health Survey (SF-36) is a generic quality-of-life survey developed from components of multiple surveys used in the 1970s and 1980s. It was first used in a developmental form in 1988 and in a standard form in 1990. It is designed to assess physical health (the patient's level of functioning) and mental health (an indication of well-being) by breaking these categories into eight domains: physical and social functioning, role limitations because of physical or emotional problems, mental health, pain, vitality, and perception of health. This survey has been widely used and validated in small and large studies, most notably the Bonn Vein Study.[11a] This German study evaluated 3072 participants and was designed to determine the rate of occurrence and severity of chronic venous disease among the general public. The SF-36 was useful in this study because of its specific objectives. Patients were enrolled from the community without prior knowledge of their venous disease status. By using the reliability and validity of the SF-36 along with physical examinations, it was possible to determine the rate of occurrence of chronic venous disease and its effect on several quality-of-life variables. The International Quality of Life Assessment Project aims to translate and adapt the SF-36 into all major languages. If this undertaking is successful, the SF-36 will gain strength internationally as a measure of health-related quality of life.[12,13]

In addition to generic measures, patient-reported disease-specific instruments have been used extensively in reporting chronic venous disease and therapy. A patient-reported outcome (PRO) is any report of patient health condition made by the patient and reported as said, without physician interpretation. Such an instrument can be used during the diagnostic phase to measure symptoms or disease states and following therapy to evaluate changes and treatment effect. The U.S. Food and Drug Administration recommends the use of a PRO instrument when the element being measured is best known and expressed by the patient.[14]

These PRO surveys are noted to have increased sensitivity to the element being measured because of their focus on particular disease processes and treatments. Four instruments specific to venous disease have been used and validated in the past several years, and a new instrument is undergoing wider validation. These patient-reported surveys provide valuable information on the individual effect of venous disease. Understanding the elements that compel patients to seek treatment is important in planning therapy that will address their main concerns.

The Chronic Venous Insufficiency Questionnaire (CIVIQ) has had two versions. The first version, CIVIQ 1, was developed in French in 1994, and it was validated in English between 1997 and 1999 in the Reflux Assessment and Quality of Life Improvement with Micronized Flavonoids study.[15] The survey evaluated physical, psychological, social, and pain effects.

Different numbers of questions were asked in each category, rendering the instrument difficult to score. A revised version, CIVIQ 2, equally distributed the effects across 20 questions to provide a composite score. Both versions of the CIVIQ have been used and validated.[12]

The Venous Insufficiency Epidemiological and Economic Study (VEINES) instrument was validated in 2006. It consists of 35 items in two categories to generate two summary scores, one for quality of life and another for symptoms. The quality-of-life survey has 25 items that estimate the effect of disease on quality of life, and the symptom survey has 10 items that measure symptoms. The focus is on physical manifestations rather than psychological and social elements. Along with score division into categories of symptoms and disease effect, this makes the VEINES instrument useful for many clinical applications. The VEINES has been validated in four languages.[12]

The Aberdeen Varicose Vein Questionnaire is a 13-question survey developed in 1993 addressing all elements of varicose vein disease. Examined are physical and social issues, including pain, ankle edema, ulcers, and the use of compression therapy as well as the effect of varicose veins on daily life and as a result of cosmetic issues. It is scored from 0 (no effect) to 100 (maximum effect). Specifically addressing the effect of varicose veins on quality of life, including cosmetic impact, this questionnaire was designed to improve the sensitivity of response among all patients, even those with less severe physical symptoms. This survey has been validated and used for all types of venous disease.[12,16]

The Charing Cross Venous Ulceration Questionnaire was developed and validated in 2000 to provide a quality-of-life measure for patients with venous ulcers. Before the existence of this instrument, there was no standardized measure of the effects of treatment for venous ulcers. The survey contains 20 questions scored from 0 (no effect) to 5 (maximum effect). The instrument is scored from the sum of these individual question scores. It has been validated and used in patients with ulcers.[12,17]

The Specific Quality of Life and Outcome Response–Venous (SQOR-V) survey was initially validated in French in 2007 and was continuing to undergo validation in English in 2010. It differs from the other patient-reported surveys in its focus on the relationship between the patient's primary complaint and his or her venous disease. It groups questions regarding symptoms, cosmesis, effect on activities and habits, and worry about the health implications of venous disease. Most of its 15 questions are broken into specific subcategories to elucidate thorough information about each aspect of the patient's concerns.[12,18]

Physician-generated assessment instruments provide another perspective on the management of venous disease and are valuable tools in determining the level of disease and the efficacy of treatment. Two of these instruments now in use are the Clinical, Etiology, Anatomy, Pathophysiology (CEAP) classification and the Venous Clinical Severity Score (VCSS).

The CEAP classification was developed in 1994 as a common descriptive platform for the reporting of diagnostic information in chronic venous disease. The clinical component is scored for active disease severity from 0 (none) to 6 (active ulcers). The etiology section categorizes the venous disease as congenital, primary, or secondary. The anatomic classification identifies affected veins as superficial, deep, or perforating. The pathophysiologic section details the presence or absence of reflux in the superficial, communicating, or deep veins and any incidence of outflow obstruction. The revised CEAP classification, published in 2004, is widely used as the reporting standard in venous disease but is not without drawbacks. Although an excellent descriptive tool, the revised CEAP classification is static and is limited in its ability to reflect response to treatment, especially in the C4 and C5 categories.[12] This is most evident if the CEAP classification is used as a stand-alone instrument.

The VCSS was designed in 2000 by a committee of experts to include nine recognized features of venous disease. Each is scored from 0 to 3. The recently revised VCSS[19] updates terminology, clarifies application, and combines important language of PROs to reflect severity changes across the spectrum of symptomatic venous disease. The feature that sets the revised VCSS apart from other physician-assessed instruments is its ability to reflect status changes in response to therapy. This is owing to the nature of the categories, which are broken down into elemental aspects of venous disease. The clinical descriptors include vein size and location, the use of compression therapy, skin changes (including pigmentation, inflammation, induration, and ulcers), and edema and its distribution as noted by the patient at different points in the day and by the physician; pain is identified as being "aching, heaviness, fatigue, soreness, and burning." The revised VCSS is thought to have retained its sensitivity, while better identifying issues of patients with milder venous disease (Table 21-1). The course of outcomes assessment thus far has offered two choices for the type of assessment performed: physician assessed and patient reported. The data derived from physician-assessed instruments may not always be an indication of the effect of disease or the value to the patient of the changes following treatment, even seemingly slight improvements.[20,21] However, valuable data can be generated much more readily with little burden to the clinician. Input of these data into available online registries in the United States and in Europe is important to ensure that new therapies meet high standards of safety and reliability and that they address the variables considered important to the physician and the patient.[21,22]

Although physician- and patient-reported tools provide useful information on symptoms and sequelae, the primary difference between them is perspective. It has become evident that some combination of both types of instruments will provide the most comprehensive understanding of common elements. As shown in Figure 21-1, this concept combines the more scientific evidence-based approach of the physician instrument and the focus in the patient-reported assessment on disease elements that are of primary importance to the patient.[18,23-25]

Regardless of the instrument or approach chosen, the manner in which the data are interpreted and reported is important in evaluating the effect of treatment. It is a long and exacting process for a survey tool to become a valid standardized reporting practice and eventually to evolve into a comprehensive measure of results that is widely accepted in clinical practice and research.[4,7]   *Text continued on p. 466*

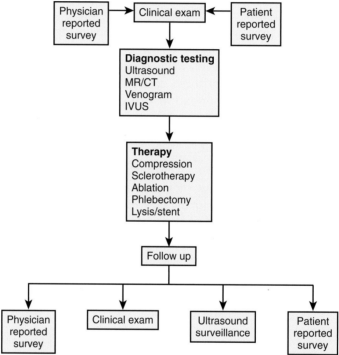

■ **Fig 21–1** Algorithm for decision making and outcomes assessment in chronic venous disease. The initial clinical exam determines the appropriate diagnostic studies. Patient- and physician-generated assessment tools are administered as part of the decision-making process to help determine the therapy option that will address the most relevant concerns of physician and patient. In the follow-up period, routine ultrasound surveillance and clinical examination confirm the outcome of the procedure, while serial use of patient- and physician-generated surveys follow clinical improvement and progress of patient concerns.

TABLE 21–1 Revised Venous Clinical Severity Score

	None: 0	Mild: 1	Moderate: 2	Severe: 3
Pain or other discomfort (i.e., aching, heaviness, fatigue, soreness, burning) Presumes venous origin		Occasional pain or other discomfort (i.e., not restricting regular daily activity)	Daily pain or other discomfort (i.e., interfering with but not preventing regular daily activities)	Daily pain or discomfort (i.e., limits most regular daily activities)
Varicose veins "Varicose" veins must be ≥3 mm in diameter to qualify in the standing position		Few: scattered (i.e., isolated branch varicosities or clusters); also includes corona phlebectatica (ankle flare)	Confined to calf or thigh	Involves calf and thigh
Venous edema Presumes venous origin		Limited to foot and ankle area	Extends above ankle but below knee	Extends to knee and above
Skin pigmentation Presumes venous origin Does not include focal pigmentation over varicose veins or pigmentation due to other chronic diseases (e.g., vasculitis purpura)	None or focal	Limited to perimalleolar area	Diffuse over lower third of calf	Wider distribution above lower third of calf
Inflammation More than just recent pigmentation (e.g., erythema, cellulitis, venous eczema, dermatitis)		Limited to perimalleolar area	Diffuse over lower third of calf	Wider distribution above lower third of calf
Induration Presumes venous origin of secondary skin and subcutaneous changes (i.e., chronic edema with fibrosis, hypodermitis) Includes white atrophy and lipodermatosclerosis		Limited to perimalleolar area	Diffuse over lower third of calf	Wider distribution above lower third of calf
Active ulcer number	0	1	2	≥3
Active ulcer duration (longest active)	N/A	<3 mo	>3 mo but <1 y	Not healed for >1 y

Continued

TABLE 21–1 Revised Venous Clinical Severity Score—cont'd

	None: 0	Mild: 1	Moderate: 2	Severe: 3
Active ulcer size (largest active)	N/A	Diameter <2 cm	Diameter 2-6 cm	Diameter >6 cm
Use of compression therapy	0	1	2	3
	Not used	Intermittent use of stockings	Wears stockings most days	Full compliance: stockings

Instructions for Using the Revised Venous Clinical Severity Score

On a separate form, the clinician will be asked:

"For each leg, please check 1 box for each item (symptom and sign) that is listed below."

Pain or Other Discomfort (i.e., Aching, Heaviness, Fatigue, Soreness, Burning)

The clinician describes the four categories of leg pain or discomfort that are outlined below to the patient and asks the patient to choose, separately for each leg, the category that best describes the pain or discomfort the patient experiences.

None = 0:   None

Mild = 1:   Occasional pain or discomfort that does not restrict regular daily

Moderate = 2:   Daily pain or discomfort that interferes with, but does not prevent, regular daily activities

Severe = 3:   Daily pain or discomfort that limits most regular daily activities

Varicose Veins

The clinician examines the patient's legs and, separately for each leg, chooses the category that best describes the patient's superficial veins. The standing position is used for varicose vein assessment. Veins must be ≥3 mm in diameter to qualify as "varicose veins."

None = 0:   None

Mild = 1:   Few, scattered varicosities that are confined to branch veins or clusters. Includes "corona phlebectatica" (ankle flare), defined as >5 blue telangiectases at the inner or sometimes the outer edge of the foot

Moderate = 2:   Multiple varicosities that are confined to the calf or the thigh

Severe = 3:   Multiple varicosities that involve both the calf and the thigh

Venous Edema

The clinician examines the patient's legs and, separately for each leg, chooses the category that best describes the patient's pattern of leg edema. The clinician's examination may be supplemented by asking the patient about the extent of leg edema that is experienced.

None = 0:   None

Mild = 1:   Edema that is limited to the foot and ankle

Moderate = 2:   Edema that extends above the ankle but below the knee

Severe = 3:   Edema that extends to the knee or above

Skin Pigmentation

The clinician examines the patient's legs and, separately for each leg, chooses the category that best describes the patient's skin pigmentation. Pigmentation refers to color changes of venous origin and not secondary to other chronic diseases (i.e., vasculitis purpura).

None = 0:   None or focal pigmentation that is confined to the skin over varicose veins

Mild = 1:   Pigmentation that is limited to the perimalleolar area

Moderate = 2:   Diffuse pigmentation that involves the lower third of the calf

Severe = 3:   Diffuse pigmentation that involves more than the lower third of the calf

TABLE 21–1 Revised Venous Clinical Severity Score—cont'd

Inflammation

The clinician examines the patient's legs and, separately for each leg, chooses the category that best describes the patient's skin inflammation. Inflammation refers to erythema, cellulitis, venous eczema, or dermatitis, rather than just recent pigmentation.

None = 0:   None

Mild = 1:   Inflammation that is limited to the perimalleolar area

Moderate = 2:   Inflammation that involves the lower third of the calf

Severe = 3:   Inflammation that involves more than the lower third of the calf

Induration

The clinician examines the patient's legs and, separately for each leg, chooses the category that best describes the patient's skin induration. Induration refers to skin and subcutaneous changes such as chronic edema with fibrosis, hypodermitis, white atrophy, and lipodermatosclerosis.

None = 0:   None

Mild = 1:   Induration that is limited to the perimalleolar area

Moderate = 2:   Induration that involves the lower third of the calf

Severe = 3:   Induration that involves more than the lower third of the calf

Active Ulcer Number

The clinician examines the patient's legs and, separately for each leg, chooses the category that best describes the number of active ulcers.

None = 0:   None

Mild = 1:   1 Ulcer

Moderate = 2:   2 Ulcers

Severe = 3:   ≥3 Ulcers

Active Ulcer Duration

If there is at least one active ulcer, the clinician describes the four categories of ulcer duration that are outlined below to the patient and asks the patient to choose, separately for each leg, the category that best describes the duration of the longest unhealed ulcer.

None = 0:   No active ulcers

Mild = 1:   Ulceration present for <3 mo

Moderate = 2:   Ulceration present for 3-12 mo

Severe = 3:   Ulceration present for >12 mo

Active Ulcer Size

If there is at least one active ulcer, the clinician examines the patient's legs, and separately for each leg, chooses the category that best describes the size of the largest active ulcer.

None = 0:   No active ulcer

Mild = 1:   Ulcer <2 cm in diameter

Moderate = 2:   Ulcer 2-6 cm in diameter

Severe = 3:   Ulcer >6 cm in diameter

Use of Compression Therapy

Choose the level of compliance with medical compression therapy.

None = 0:   Not used

Mild = 1:   Intermittent use

Moderate = 2:   Wears stockings most days

Severe = 3:   Full compliance: stockings

PEARLS AND PITFALLS

Chronic venous disease is a complex condition with numerous possible presentations and manifestations. Diagnosis is not always straightforward, generally requiring the application of clinical experience and diagnostic testing. Recently, physician- and patient-based survey instruments have been used to assess and quantify the disease. While these surveys are not in themselves diagnostic, they may provide valuable information about the most beneficial therapeutic direction to take.

Such surveys must be carefully chosen to address specific elements of the disease state in question. A generic measure such as the SF-36 may not address the specific elements of venous disease that are important to the clinician and patient, while an ulcer-specific survey such as the Charing Cross Venous Ulceration Questionnaire may not reflect the severity of other elements of venous disease. It is more relevant to have assessment instruments that are based on the specific language of venous disease.[4] A carefully designed and chosen survey can initially aid in diagnosis and treatment planning. If it is serially applied throughout the treatment process, it can add valuable data on outcomes. When analyzed for a significant relevant population, these outcomes data add to the combined body of knowledge and clinical experience, providing evidence for the best practice treatment of chronic venous disease.[26]

The selection of outcomes variables to study and report is crucial. Clinical outcomes measure improvement in survival, symptoms, or quality of life as a result of therapy. Surrogate outcomes include diagnostic test results, physical signs, or physiologic variables. Examples include vein occlusion rates following ablation or venous stent patency rates. These often provide quantifiable results during a limited follow-up period. However, it is important to note that surrogate outcomes should not be held to the same standards as clinical outcomes. While the change in response to treatment should still be predictive of benefit to the patient, the relationship between the two outcomes should be clear and well defined. Surrogate outcomes should not simply be correlated with clinical outcomes but should be predictive.[26] In our practice, a combination of clinical examination, duplex Doppler study, and the revised VCSS is used to diagnose chronic venous disease and to plan therapeutic intervention. Any of these elements on its own would most likely provide insufficient information to plan a treatment strategy. By integrating all three, a more complete picture is obtained of the clinical severity of the venous disease and the elements that are most important to the patient. This three-spoke strategy helps to guide therapy to achieve a successful outcome for the patient.

Holding assessment instruments to the standard of psychometric analysis ensures the value of tests and their results. Psychometric standards have been used for years to apply standard practices to the development of tests in education, personality analysis, and skill assessment. The benchmarks for a good test are feasibility (whether the test is practical to administer and score), reliability (whether a score can be replicated when the same tester readministers the test), and validity (whether the scores are responsive to change).[27]

Several generic and disease-specific instruments have been validated psychometrically. The physical and mental health summary measures of the SF-36 are based on the use of psychometric tests, and the instrument itself has been validated in large populations.[12] The VEINES instrument has been psychometrically tested in the areas of diagnostic elements (exclusion of classification of anatomic and physiologic variables that might aid choice of treatment) and outcomes scores (whether they could they be scaled and if they accurately delineate clinical significance and degree of change over time).[20] The CIVIQ evaluates physical, psychological, social, and pain dimensions and has been validated in large investigations.[12] The Aberdeen Varicose Vein Questionnaire also measures physical symptoms and social issues but is specific to varicose veins. It has been used with the SF-36 and the VCSS in large studies to assess quality of life at specific intervals following intervention.[12] The Charing Cross Venous Ulceration Questionnaire is specific to ulcers and has been used with the SF-36 to measure quality of life in patients with ulcers.[12]

We have reported on the VCSS as a valuable measure of objective and subjective outcomes in treating chronic venous disease. Others have evaluated the VCSS in large populations, finding it generally useful. Some deficiencies were noted, including the scope of the clinical descriptors used. Because a large part of the VCSS depends on patient responses to physician queries, the ability to interpret the description of symptoms and to match them to a category in the VCSS is crucial in generating accurate data. Can the revised VCSS meet the standard of psychometric evaluation as a valid and reliable assessment tool?[12,19,28,29] The VCSS is generated by the clinician on the basis of straightforward questions asked of the patient during examination. There is a combination focus to the instrument. Several categories, including inflammation, induration, pigmentation, ulcers, and veins, are objective and are scored by the physician on the basis of clinical evidence. At the same time, other categories, including pain, edema, and the use of compression hose, are scored based on the subjective responses of the patient. The range of categories covered by the VCSS is representative of chronic venous disease and compiles a more complete picture of quality of life than specialized instruments.[12]

One of the advantages of the revised VCSS is its ability to provide visual scoring data in chronic venous insufficiency. With the use of revised clinical descriptors, patient-reported symptoms can be combined with physician assessment to more accurately translate the picture of venous disease (Fig. 21-2). This may help to bridge the gap between physician-scored assessment instruments and patient-reported tools and to transport surveys farther into the land of science with standardized language, reliability, and validity.

The visual advantage of a survey like the revised VCSS can be illustrated in three of the common pitfalls in treating chronic venous disease. These include refractory unilateral leg swelling, chronic venous insufficiency without varicose veins, and venous ulcers resulting from complex venous insufficiency at multiple levels.

Refractory unilateral leg swelling can be the result of many factors, including compromise of the muscle pump, venous outflow obstruction, or reflux of the deep, superficial, or perforator systems.[30] In conjunction with clinical examination and appropriate testing, the revised VCSS can help to track changes associated with therapy. Unilateral leg swelling that remains after an initial treatment can be further evaluated to rule out other causes and to guide future interventions.

Chronic venous insufficiency without varicose veins may be difficult to discern on initial examination. The use of a survey like the revised VCSS can help to elucidate patient symptoms consistent with underlying venous insufficiency and to guide the rest of the diagnostic process (Fig. 21-3).

Venous ulcers resulting from complex venous insufficiency at multiple levels can be difficult to manage, even with a staged approach to treatment. The revised VCSS can track changes with each therapeutic intervention and provide specific information on the ulcers, including number, size, and duration. This helps to maintain a record of the progress of ulcer healing over time (Fig. 21-4).

Evidence-based medicine and outcomes assessment are critical tools for vascular surgery. The results of high-volume procedures should be followed up with a validated instrument. We found the VCSS and each of its components to be useful, significant, and easily applicable for the assessment of outcomes after radiofrequency ablation in limbs with symptomatic venous insufficiency.[29]

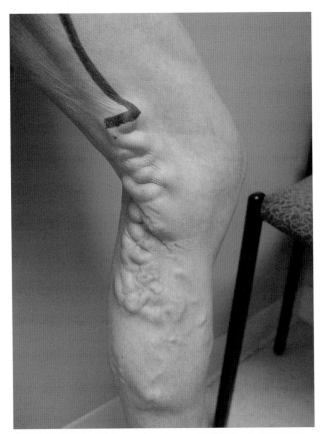

A

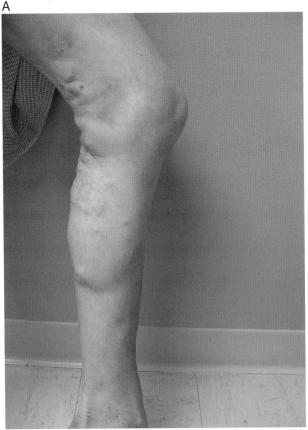

B

■ **Fig 21–2** The language of revised VCSS. Simplified clinician scoring and reporting allows for a common language of venous disease. **A,** Pretreatment score, Clinical CEAP 3–VCSS 8. **B,** Posttreatment score, CEAP 3–VCSS 4.

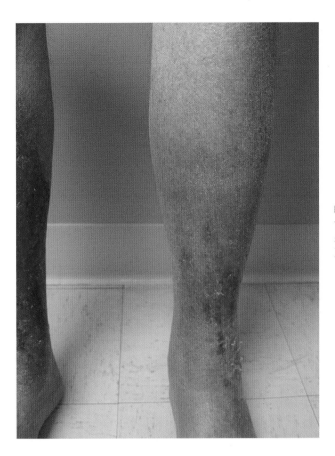

■ **Fig 21–3** Chronic venous insufficiency without visible varicosities. Use of the VCSS allowed patient symptoms to be followed, and helped guide diagnostic decision making.

COMPARATIVE EFFECTIVENESS OF EXISTING TREATMENTS

Surgical procedures for varicosities have been practiced for centuries, beginning with interventions for ulcers and progressing to surgery on venous valves as understanding about the vascular system grew.[4] In 1916, Homans wrote about the relationship between varicose veins and ulcers, at a time when surgical excision of the saphenous vein was being practiced; 20 years later, Linton demonstrated decreased ambulatory venous pressure after ligation of perforating veins, and the widespread treatment of venous disease was under way.[4]

The movement toward less invasive therapeutic techniques has affected venous surgery. Modern surgical methods for treatment of chronic venous disease include superficial venous ablation, deep venous reconstruction, injection of sclerosing foam, and percutaneous ablation of perforator veins. While these methods have largely replaced saphenous vein stripping, the use of outcomes assessment instruments will help to determine their long-term efficacy and address any shortcomings.

Great saphenous vein stripping was considered the standard of care for chronic venous disease for many years. Removing the saphenous vein from the circulation virtually ensured resolution of any symptoms attributed to it. However, recurrent symptoms were seen when all levels of underlying disease were not addressed. The existence of deep or perforator vein reflux or the failure to completely eradicate sources of venous hypertension led to recurrent symptoms, sometimes necessitating additional invasive procedures.

Endovascular venous ablation is proving to be effective in the long term as part of a strategy to address superficial veins, tributaries, and perforators. Recurrence of clinical symptoms and emergence of new veins are rare in patients treated with ablation, and evaluations performed on the procedure over 5 or more years indicate that it provides a standard of care comparable to saphenous vein stripping.[31]

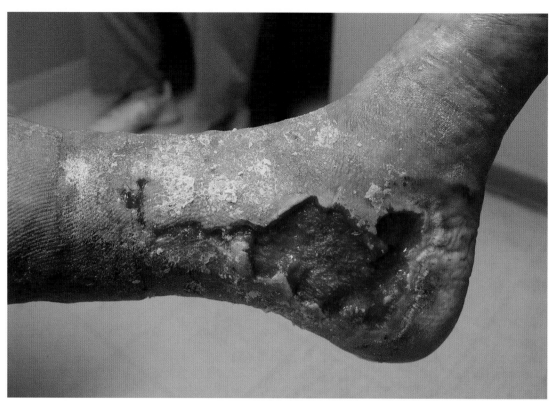

■ **Fig 21–4** A complex ulcer such as this may be the result of numerous factors. Using VCSS to track changes after each intervention helps guide the staging of therapy.

The goal of treating venous disease can be very different for the physician versus the patient. While useful, morbidity and mortality statistics report only the direct clinical outcome of an intervention, failing to consider other factors of potential importance to others. For an outcome to be fully evaluated, its effect on the physician, patient, and community must be considered.[32] In a quotation attributed to Phaedrus, "Every one is bound to bear patiently the results of his own example." The physician who is willing to adopt a habit of outcomes assessment and to share those results will be empowered to provide qualified and compassionate care.

REFERENCES

1. Gloviczki P. Presidential address: Venous surgery: from stepchild to equal partner. J Vasc Surg 2003;38:871-878.
2. Yao JST. Presidential address: Venous disorders: reflections of the past three decades. J Vasc Surg 1997;26:727-735.
3. Scultetus AH, Villavicencio JL, Rich NM. Facts and fiction surrounding the discovery of the venous valves. J Vasc Surg 2001;33:435-441.
4. Vasquez MA, Munschauer CE. The importance of uniform venous terminology in reports on varicose veins. Semin Vasc Surg 2010;23:70-77.
5. Mozes G, Gloviczki P. New discoveries in anatomy and new terminology of leg veins: clinical implications. Vasc Endovasc Surg 2004;38:367-374.
6. Dayal R, Kent KC. Standardized reporting practices. In: Rutherford RB, editor. Vascular Surgery. 6 ed. Philadelphia: WB Saunders; 2005:41-52.

7. Rutherford RB. Presidential address: Vascular surgery: comparing outcomes. J Vasc Surg 1996;23:5-17.

8. Meissner MH, Moneta G, Burnand K, et al. The hemodynamics and diagnosis of venous disease. J Vasc Surg 2007;46:4S-24S.

9. Rutherford RB, Moneta GL, Padberg FT, Meissner MH. Outcome assessment in chronic venous disease. In: Gloviczki P, editor. Handbook of Venous Disorders. London: Hodder Arnold; 2009:684-693.

10. White JV, Jones DN, Rutherford RB. Integrated assessment of results: standardized reporting of outcomes and the computerized vascular registry. In: Rutherford RB, editor. Vascular Surgery. 6 ed. Philadelphia: WB Saunders; 2005:20-37.

11. Rutherford RB, Flanigan DP, Gupta SK, et al; Ad Hoc Committee on Reporting Standards, Society for Vascular Surgery/North American Chapter, International Society for Cardiovascular Surgery. Suggested standards for reports dealing with lower extremity ischemia [published correction appears in J Vasc Surg 1986;4:350]. J Vasc Surg 1986;4:80-94.

11a. Maurins U, Hoffmann BH, Lösch C, et al. Distribution and prevalence of reflux in the superficial and deep venous system in the general population—results from the Bonn Vein Study, Germany. J Vasc Surg 2008;48:680-687.

12. Vasquez MA, Munschauer CE. Venous Clinical Severity Score and quality-of-life assessment tools: application to vein practice. Phlebology 2008;23:259-275.

13. Davies AH, Rudarakanchana N. Quality of life and outcome assessment in patients with varicose veins. In: Davies AH, Lees TA, Lane IF, editors. Venous Disease Simplified. Shropshire, England: TFM Publishing Ltd; 2006.

14. US Department of Health and Human Services. Guidance for Industry: Patient-Reported Outcome Measures: Use in Medical Product Development to Support Labeling Claims. Rockville, MD: Food and Drug Administration; December 2009.

15. Jantet G. Chronic venous insufficiency: worldwide results of the RELIEF study: reflux assessment and quality of life improvement with micronized flavonoids. Angiology 2002;53:245-256.

16. Garratt AM, Macdonald LM, Ruta DA, et al. Towards measurement of outcome for patients with varicose veins. Qual Health Care 1993;2:5-10.

17. Smith JJ, Guest MG, Greenhalgh RM, Davies AH. Measuring the quality of life in patients with venous ulcers. J Vasc Surg 2000;31:642-649.

18. Guex JJ, Zimmet SE, Boussetta S, et al. Construction and validation of a patient-reported outcome dedicated to chronic venous disorders: SQOR-V (Specific Quality of Life and Outcome Response–Venous). J Mal Vas 2007;32:135-147.

19. Vasquez MA, Rabe E, McLafferty RB, et al. Revision of the Venous Clinical Severity Score: Venous outcomes consensus statement: special communication of the American Venous Forum Ad Hoc Outcomes Working Group. J Vasc Surg 2010;52:1387-1396.

20. Padberg F. Regarding "Evaluating outcomes in chronic venous disorders of the leg: Development of a scientifically rigorous, patient-reported measure of symptoms and quality of life." J Vasc Surg 2003;37:911-912.

21. Lamping DL, Schroter S, Kurz X, et al. Evaluation of outcomes in chronic venous disorders of the leg: Development of a scientifically rigorous, patient-reported measure of symptoms and quality of life. J Vasc Surg 2003;37:410-419.

22. Smith JJ, Garratt AM, Guest M, et al. Evaluating and improving health-related quality of life in patients with varicose veins. J Vasc Surg 1999;30:710-719.

23. Meissner MH, Natiello C, Nicholls SC. Performance characteristics of the Venous Clinical Severity Score. J Vasc Surg 2002;36:889-895.

24. Kundu S, Lurie F, Millward SF, et al. Recommended reporting standards for endovenous ablation for the treatment of venous insufficiency: joint statement of the American Venous Forum and the Society of Interventional Radiology. J Vasc Surg 2007;46:582-589.

25. White JV. Proper outcomes assessment: patient based and economic evaluations of vascular interventions. In: Rutherford RB, editor. Vascular Surgery. 6 ed. Philadelphia: WB Saunders; 2005:35-41.

26. Meissner MH. "I enjoyed your talk, but …": Evidence-based medicine and the scientific foundation of the American Venous Forum. J Vasc Surg 2009;49:244-248.

27. Revicki DA, Cella D, Hays RD, et al. Responsiveness and minimal important differences for patient reported outcomes. Health Qual Life Outcomes 2006;4:e70-e74.

28. Vasquez MA. Editor's corner. AVForum Spring 2007;1:6-7.

29. Vasquez MA, Wang J, Mahathanaruk M, et al. The utility of the Venous Clinical Severity Score in 682 limbs treated by radiofrequency saphenous vein ablation. J Vasc Surg 2007;45: 1008-1015.

30. Eberhardt RT, Raffetto JD. Chronic venous insufficiency. Circulation 2005;111:2398-2409.

31. Merchant RF, Pichot O. Long-term outcomes of endovenous radiofrequency obliteration of saphenous reflux as a treatment for superficial venous insufficiency. J Vasc Surg 2005;42: 502-509.

32. Vasquez MA, Munschauer CE. Clinical and surrogate outcomes from the new radiofrequency catheter: an experience of 700 limbs. In: Greenhalgh R, editor. Vascular and Endovascular Challenges Update. Bodmin, Cornwall, England: MPG Books Ltd; 2010:425-433.

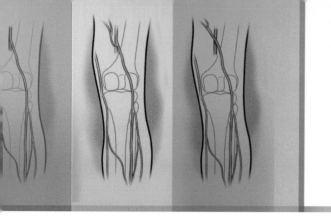

CHAPTER 22

Evidence-Based Summary of Guidelines from the American Venous Forum and the Society for Vascular Surgery

Mark H. Meissner and Peter Gloviczki

Chronic venous disorders are among the world's oldest afflictions and are responsible for substantial socioeconomic morbidity in the Western world. Varicose veins are the most common clinical manifestation of chronic venous disease, occurring in one fourth to one third of Western adult populations,[1,2] while severe chronic venous insufficiency with skin changes and ulceration is present in 2% to 5% of Western populations.[3] There have been many technological advances in the management of venous disease over the past decade, and many of these have had substantial benefits for afflicted patients. Unfortunately, many of these treatments are quite costly and are often approved, marketed, and adopted by clinicians without solid evidence supporting their use.

Although the current federal regulatory processes are effective in encouraging the development of new technology and do provide some mechanism for ensuring safety, they do not favor proof of clinically relevant efficacy.[4,5] It is therefore becoming increasingly important for the clinician to have the skills to evaluate the clinical evidence and recommend the best treatment for their patients. The American Venous Forum has taken the lead in providing the clinical data clinicians require in caring for patients with venous disease and have published, together with the Society for Vascular Surgery, the most up-to-date practice guidelines for the care of patients with venous disorders.[6]

EVIDENCE-BASED MEDICINE AND PRACTICE GUIDELINES

Evidence-based medicine is perhaps best defined as "the conscientious, explicit, and judicious use of the current best evidence in making decisions about the care of individual patients."[7] This specifically involves integrating clinical expertise, the patient's individual values and preferences, and the *best available* clinical evidence. Older approaches to evaluating clinical evidence relied primarily on a hierarchy of study methodology, a system that provides little guidance to physicians in daily practice. While randomized clinical trials are usually less prone to bias and are less likely to lead to false-positive conclusions, it is unrealistic to expect data from rigorously conducted trials to guide every clinical question that arises. Furthermore, they may not be appropriate for all diseases and interventions.[8] Randomized trials are difficult to justify when interventions are clearly harmful or show a large beneficial treatment effect (risk ratio <0.4) in observational studies or when the treatment effect is so small (risk ratios 0.9 to 1.0) that sample size requirements preclude adequately powered randomized trials. Perhaps most importantly, clinicians are less interested in the precise study methodology than they are in reliable estimates of the benefits and harms associated with a therapy.[9] For high-quality evidence, the effects of therapy are precise, and further research is unlikely to change our confidence in the estimate of effect. In contrast, the estimated effect provided by poor-quality evidence may be unclear and subject to change as better-quality evidence becomes available.

Current approaches to the evaluation of clinical evidence account for these concerns and are based largely on an assessment of the estimate of effect (beneficial or ill) associated with a treatment. The approach developed by the Grading of Recommendations, Assessment, Development, and Evaluation (GRADE) working group[9] has been adopted by the American Venous Forum in developing practice guidelines.[9] According to this system, there are two components to any treatment recommendation—the first a designation of the strength of the recommendation (1 or 2) based upon the degree of confidence that the recommendation will do more good than harm, the second an evaluation of the strength of the evidence (A to D) based upon the confidence that the estimate of effect is correct. (Table 22-1).

The strength of a recommendation (1 or 2) reflects the balance of benefits and risks, as well as cost to the health care system. Grade 1 recommendations are those in which the benefits of intervention clearly outweigh its risk and burdens. All well-informed patients would choose such a treatment and the physician, often without a detailed knowledge of the underlying data, can securely recommend it. Grade 2 recommendations are weaker and reflect therapies in which the benefits and risks are either uncertain or more closely balanced. For such interventions, patients may choose different options based upon their underlying values.

TABLE 22–1 GRADE Approach to Treatment Recommendations

Recommendation	Benefit Versus Risk	Quality of Evidence	Comment
1A	Clear	**High:** Consistent results from RCTs or observational studies with large effects	Strong recommendation, generalizable
1B	Clear	**Moderate:** RCTs with limitations and very strong observational studies	Strong recommendation; may change with further research
1C	Clear	**Low:** Observational studies **Very Low:** Case series, descriptive reports, expert opinion	Intermediate recommendation; likely to change with further research
2A	Balanced or Unclear	**High:** Consistent results from RCTs or observational studies with large effects	Intermediate recommendation: may vary with patient values
2B	Balanced or Unclear	**Moderate:** RCTs with limitations and very strong observational studies	Weak recommendation; may vary with patient values
2C	Balanced or Unclear	**Low:** Observational studies **Very Low:** Case series, descriptive reports, expert opinion	Weak recommendation; alternative treatments may be equally valid

Adapted from Guyatt G, Schunemann HJ, Cook D, et al. Applying the grades of recommendation for antithrombotic and thrombolytic therapy. Chest 2004;126:179S-187S.
RCTs, Randomized control trials.

The grade system recommends four levels (A to D) of methodological quality, which reflects the degree of confidence in the strength of a recommendation. High-quality, or grade A, evidence usually comes from well-executed randomized trials yielding consistent results and occasionally from observational studies with significant effects. Further research is unlikely to change our confidence in the estimate of effect derived from Grade A evidence. Moderate-quality evidence (Grade B) comes from randomized clinical trials with important limitations and strong observational studies. Low-quality evidence (Grade C) includes flawed randomized trials and most observational studies. Very low-quality evidence, which the guidelines committee has collapsed into Grade C, includes data from case reports, descriptive studies, and expert opinion.

In accordance with the American College of Chest Physicians (ACCP) guidelines for the antithrombotic treatment of venous thromboembolic disease,[10] the American Venous Forum has adopted the language of "recommending" the use of strong Grade 1 guidelines and "suggesting" the use of weaker Grade 2 guidelines. These guidelines should be viewed as a summary of the best available clinical evidence to guide the management of patients with chronic venous disease. However, consistent with the goals of evidence-based medicine, they are subject to the physician's clinical judgment, resources, and expertise and the patient's individual values and preferences. They should not be interpreted as a rigid "standard of care." The key elements of the evidence-based guidelines are outlined in Table 22-2.

TABLE 22–2 Key Treatment Recommendations for Chronic Venous Disease

Guideline	Grade of Recommendation
Diagnosis of Chronic Venous Disease	
We recommend initial clinical evaluation including a thorough history, focusing on the underlying etiology (congenital, primary, or secondary), symptoms, and risk factors for venous disease.	1A
We recommend duplex ultrasonography, including an evaluation of reflux in the upright position, as the initial diagnostic test in patients with CVD.	1A
We recommend threshold values for reflux of >500 ms for reflux in the saphenous, deep femoral, tibial, and perforating veins and >1 s in the femoral and popliteal veins.	1B
We recommend adjunctive studies including plethysmography, CT/MR venography, and IVUS in selected patients in whom the pathophysiology is incompletely defined by ultrasound or in whom a surgical or endovenous intervention is planned.	1B
Management of C1-C3 Chronic Venous Disease	
We suggest the use of venoactive drugs such as horse chestnut seed extract for amelioration of the symptoms of pain and swelling.	**2B**
We suggest the use of 20–30 mm Hg compression stockings for patients with symptomatic varicose veins who are not candidates for superficial venous intervention.	2C
We recommend stripping or ablation of the saphenous vein in preference to compression stockings in patients who are suitable candidates.	1B
We recommend endothermal venous ablation in preference to high ligation and stripping or foam sclerotherapy for the management of saphenous vein incompetence.	1B
We recommend sclerotherapy for the treatment of reticular veins, telangiectasias, and recurrent varicose veins.	1B
We recommend phlebectomy over sclerotherapy for the treatment of tributary varicosities once axial reflux has been addressed.	1B
We recommend against the treatment of incompetent perforating veins in patients with C2 CVD.	1B
Management of C4-C6 Chronic Venous Disease	
We recommend compression therapy for the treatment of venous leg ulcers.	1A
We suggest pentoxifylline as an adjunct for the healing of venous leg ulcers.	2B
We recommend sharp debridement of venous ulcers associated with significant slough and nonviable tissue.	1C
Depending on the specific agent, specialized wound dressings can be only weakly suggested.	2 B/C
We recommend the treatment of saphenous incompetence to reduce the recurrence of venous leg ulcers.	1A
We suggest the treatment of pathologic perforating veins—defined as incompetent perforating veins ≥3.5 mm in diameter with outward flow ≥500 ms in duration and located beneath a healed or open venous ulcer.	2B
The benefit of deep venous valvular reconstruction is poorly established and is suggested only in centers with substantial experience and after failure of treatments supported by more substantial data.	2C

CT/MR, Computed tomography/magnetic resonance; *CVD*, chronic venous disease; *IVUS*, intravascular ultrasound.

EVIDENCE-BASED MANAGEMENT OF VENOUS DISEASE

Evaluation and Follow-up of the Patient with Chronic Venous Disease

Evaluation of the patient with venous disease should include a thorough history, focusing on the underlying etiology (congenital, primary, or secondary), symptoms, and risk factors for venous disease (Grade 1A). This should include an assessment of the degree of disability and effect on the patient's quality of life. Physical examination should focus on specific features of venous disease and exclusion of other etiologies of the patient's signs and symptoms. In clinical practice, every patient should be characterized using both the basic CEAP classification and the Venous Clinical Severity Score (VCSS).[11,12]

Duplex ultrasonography, including an evaluation of reflux in the upright position, should be the initial diagnostic test in patients with suspected venous disease (Grade 1A). Threshold values of greater than 500 milliseconds are recommended for reflux in the saphenous, deep femoral, tibial, and perforating veins and greater than 1 second in the femoral and popliteal veins (Grade 1B). Pathologic perforating veins should be differentiated from "incompetent perforating veins." Pathologic perforating veins are those 3.5 mm or grater in diameter with outward flow of 500 milliseconds or greater located beneath an open or a healed venous ulcer.

The use of adjunctive studies including plethysmography, computed tomography (CT)/magnetic resonance (MR) venography, and intravascular ultrasound (IVUS) is recommended for selected patients in whom the pathophysiology is incompletely defined by ultrasound or in whom a surgical or endovenous intervention is planned (Grade 1B).

For research investigations, the use of patient-important outcomes is strongly recommended, while the use of technical or surrogate outcome measures should be restricted to early feasibility studies. Several disease-specific quality of life measures are available for this purpose.[13-15]

Treatment of Mild (C2-C3) Chronic Venous Disease

The treatment of varicose veins has rapidly evolved over the past several years, largely due to the advent of endovenous technologies. Current management options for symptomatic varicose veins include conservative management with compression hosiery and leg elevation, pharmacologic interventions, and superficial venous surgery. Unfortunately, the evidence supporting many of these treatments is sparse and heavily reliant on short-term outcomes and surrogate markers such as rates of saphenous vein closure.

Compression Therapy

Despite the absence of methodologically sound data, compression stockings are often considered first-line therapy for mild to moderate chronic venous disorders. The majority of comparative studies of compression stockings have evaluated surrogate hemodynamic parameters rather than patient-important outcomes, and it does appear that stockings improve a variety of hemodynamic measurements.[16] However, the clinical benefits are less clear. Comparisons to placebo are very limited but do suggest some improvement in symptoms with the use of compression stockings.[16] Others have reported improvement in up to one third of patients with compression stockings.[17] Definitive data regarding the optimal degree of compression are lacking. However, symptomatic improvement is clearly less than after surgical treatment of varicose veins,[17] and the authors of one systematic review concluded that the benefits of compression as a first-line treatment are limited.[16] Although 20 to 30 mm Hg compression stockings are suggested for patients with symptomatic varicose veins (Grade 2C), the American Venous Forum recommends against their use as the primary treatment in patients who are candidates for superficial venous intervention (Grade 1B). Compression stockings should be considered only after a thorough history and measurement of the ankle-brachial index to exclude arterial disease and should be fitted by appropriately trained personnel.[16]

Pharmacologic Therapy

Phlebotonic agents have been used to address many of the symptoms of chronic venous disorders, including leg pain, swelling, and pruritus. These include a heterogeneous group of plant extracts (rutosides, hidrosmine, diosmine, and others) as well as synthetic drugs with similar properties. A systematic review of 44 randomized, placebo-controlled trials evaluating oral phlebotonics suggested efficacy for some signs such as edema, although the global evidence for their efficacy was insufficient to recommend routine use.[18] While other preparations are available abroad, horse chestnut seed extract is the most studied preparation available in the United States. A systematic review of 17 randomized, controlled trials of horse chestnut seed extract suggests significant benefits with respect to leg pain, edema, and pruritus.[19] Two of these trials demonstrated similar improvements with horse chestnut seed extract and compression. Although the data are somewhat heterogeneous and the consequences of long-term use are poorly documented, there is at least a suggestion that the venoactive drugs may have some benefit in patients with C2-C3 disease (Grade 2B).

Surgical Management

The surgical management of varicose veins has evolved over the past century, with high ligation and stripping of the great saphenous vein being the standard approaches in recent decades. High ligation alone fails to control reflux in a high proportion of patients. In comparison to high ligation alone, high ligation and stripping reduced the need for reoperation by two thirds after 5 years of follow-up.[20] Surgical treatment of varicose veins has been shown to be more efficacious and cost-effective than management with compression stockings. The REACTIV trial[17] randomized 246 patients to conservative management (lifestyle advice and compression hosiery) versus surgery (saphenous ligation, stripping, and phlebectomy). There was significantly greater improvement in symptoms and quality of life in the surgical group and surgery was cost-effective with an incremental cost-effectiveness of £1936 per quality-adjusted life year (QALY) over a 10-year period. Notably 31% of patients did have some improvement in symptoms with compression hosiery alone, although 51.6% of patients assigned to conservative management crossed over to surgical treatment by the third year of follow-up. These data are supported by a Markov model demonstrating a variety of interventions for varicose veins, including surgical stripping, ultrasound-guided foam sclerotherapy and endovenous thermal ablation, to be more cost effective than conservative management.[21] Based upon this reasonably compelling evidence, surgical management of saphenous vein incompetence is recommended over compression stockings in suitable patients (Grade 1B).

An array of endovenous techniques, including thermal and chemical ablation, has largely replaced high ligation and stripping for the management of saphenous reflux. A recent meta-analysis that included all available evidence (randomized trials, observational studies, cases series) and used saphenous obliteration as a weak surrogate outcome concluded that ultrasound-guided foam sclerotherapy was equivalent to and the endovenous techniques superior to saphenous vein stripping.[22] With respect to the endovenous techniques, initial closure rates (92.9% versus 88.8%) and intermediate-term durability (94.5% versus 79.9% at 5 years) were better for laser ablation than for the first-generation radiofrequency (RF) device (ClosurePLUS [VNUS Medical

Technologies, San Jose, CA]). Among larger studies, the EVOLVes trial randomized 85 patients to high ligation and stripping or endovenous RF ablation of the great saphenous vein. Early follow up demonstrated a more rapid return to usual activities and work among patients undergoing RF ablation. This is supported by smaller trials demonstrating less pain,[23,24] edema,[25] and bruising[23-25] after endovenous ablation. However, Rasmussen[26] randomized 121 patients to high ligation and stripping of the saphenous veins or endovenous laser ablation (EVLA) and found the procedures to be equally efficacious at 6 months. Despite slightly greater pain over the first 7 days after surgical treatment (high ligation and stripping), there was no difference in analgesic requirements or return to normal activities or work. Based on the evidence that the early efficacy and safety of the endovenous techniques are at least equivalent to high ligation and stripping, with potential advantages with respect to early postoperative pain and pending long-term studies evaluating clinically relevant outcome measures (e.g., recurrence, quality of life), the endovenous techniques can be recommended over saphenous vein stripping (Grade 1B).

Appropriately conducted trials comparing the different endovenous modalities are beginning to appear. In a randomized comparison of the first-generation ClosurePLUS device and the 810-nm laser, RF ablation was associated with less perioperative bruising and discomfort, but greater 1-year anatomic failure, than laser ablation.[27] Closure rates appear to have been improved with the second generation ClosureFAST (VNUS Medical Technologies) device. Two randomized trials and one cohort study have compared ClosureFAST RF ablation to 980-nm laser ablation. In a cohort study,[28] RF ablation was associated with significantly less pain (median pain scores 13 mm versus 23.3 mm, $p = .014$) and more rapid return to work (median 5 versus 9 days, $p = .022$) in comparison to EVLA. Among 87 limbs randomized to RF or EVLA, venous occlusion was achieved in all patients at 1 month.[29] However, RF ablation was associated with significantly less pain, fewer complications, and improved quality of life at 1 and 2 weeks but not at 4 weeks. A second randomized trial demonstrated significantly less pain and analgesic use at 3 days with RF in comparison to EVLA, although this did not translate into more rapid recovery or improved quality of life at 6 weeks.[30]

Several new fiber designs, including radially firing fibers and those with wavelengths (1320 and 1470 nm) targeting water rather than hemoglobin, are now available.[31,32] Reduced hemoglobin absorption may theoretically be associated with less vein wall perforation and fewer complications such as pain and bruising.[32] Although early data with these fibers suggest excellent efficacy with reduced postprocedural pain,[32] robust data comparing these fiber designs to either older designs or RF ablation are lacking, and these fibers can be only weakly suggested over those with hemoglobin-specific wavelengths (Grade 2C).

Sclerotherapy has previously been considered an alternative to surgery for varicose veins. Several randomized trials have directly compared liquid sclerotherapy to surgery, with the results suggesting that although sclerotherapy is effective in early follow-up, the 5-year results substantially favor surgery.[33] Despite these findings, foam sclerotherapy has been demonstrated to be more efficacious than liquid and has emerged as an alternative to foam elsewhere in the world. Three-month GSV occlusion rates were significantly higher among veins randomized to treatment with polidocanol foam (54%) in comparison to veins treated with liquid polidocanol (17%).[34] Even higher occlusion rates have been reported in single-center studies using different protocols. A meta-analysis of 69 studies including over 9000 patients reported venous occlusion in a mean of 87% of patients (range 60% to 98.2%).[35] Among randomized trials evaluating venous occlusion as an outcome, foam sclerotherapy was more effective than liquid sclerotherapy (relative risk [RR] 1.39; 95% confidence interval [CI] 0.91 to 2.11) but less effective than surgery (RR 0.86, 95% CI 0.67 to 1.10). Serious complications of foam sclerotherapy included DVT in 0.02% to 0.7%, ulceration in 0% to 4%, arterial events in 0% to 2.1%, and rare case reports of stroke and myocardial infarction. Other adverse events included matting or pigmentation in 17.8%, thrombophlebitis in 4.7%, visual disturbances in 1.4%, headache in 4.2%, and cough, chest tightness, and vasovagal events in 0% to 2.8% of patients. It is clear that this is a high maintenance procedure, with occlusion rates declining to 35% at 5 years and reintervention rates ranging from 6.7% to 16.5% per year.[36] Although initial costs of ultrasound-guided foam sclerotherapy are lower than other treatment strategies, the need for retreatment is likely associated with reduced quality of life and increased costs. Despite somewhat higher costs, Gohel et al. concluded that other treatment strategies might in fact be associated with better value.[21] Based upon currently available evidence, endovenous thermal ablation of the incompetent saphenous vein is recommended over foam sclerotherapy (Grade 1B).

Once saphenous reflux has been eliminated, the most widely used options for the management of tributary varicosities include sclerotherapy and ambulatory phlebectomy. A systematic review of the sclerotherapy literature found the data to be of marginal quality but to generally support the current role of sclerotherapy in treating reticular veins, telangiectasias, and recurrent varicose veins[37] (Grade 1B). There are little robust data to guide sclerosant choice, type of compression, or length of compression. Data directly comparing ambulatory phlebectomy to sclerotherapy for varicose veins are also sparse. One randomized trial demonstrated significantly higher 2-year recurrence rates for liquid sclerotherapy (37.5%) in comparison to ambulatory phlebectomy (2.1%).[38] A further small randomized trial suggested that phlebectomy performed at the time of ablation is associated with early improvements in quality of life in comparison to sequential phlebectomy.[39] Based upon the results of these trials, which did have reasonable methodology, phlebectomy is recommended over sclerotherapy for the treatment of tributary varicosities once saphenous reflux has been addressed (Grade 1B).

The incidence of deep venous thrombosis (DVT) detected by routine ultrasound imaging after saphenous vein surgery has been reported to be 5.3%, with the vast majority of these cases having been asymptomatic and isolated to the calf veins.[40] The incidence of DVT was not influenced by a single preoperative dose of low-molecular-weight heparin. Others have shown rates of symptomatic venous thromboembolism to be as low as 0.18% after varicose vein surgery, with perioperative prophylaxis having no effect on VTE rates in low-risk patients.[41] In a study of 460 limbs treated with EVLA, rates of true DVT, pulmonary embolism, and saphenofemoral thrombus extension were 0.7%, 0.2%, and 7.2%, respectively.[42] These rates were not influenced by institution of a risk-based thromboprophylaxis policy. These data tend to support the general ACCP guidelines recommending no specific thromboprophylaxis other than early ambulation in patients without thromboembolic risk factors (Grade 2B) and consideration of prophylaxis with unfractionated heparin, low-molecular-weight heparin, or fondaparinux in patients with additional thromboembolic risk factors (Grade 1C).

Class 4 to 6 Chronic Venous Disease

Given the socioeconomic consequences of venous ulceration, it is not surprising that there are several approaches to the management of advanced chronic venous disease. These include various types of compression dressings; adjuvants to compression including skin substitutes, biological agents, and wound dressings; drugs; and surgical procedures directed toward the superficial, perforator, and deep venous systems. Ulcer healing and ulcer recurrence rates are the most relevant clinical outcomes, and the various therapeutic options often have differential effects on these two measures.

Compression

Although imperfect, treatment of venous ulcers with compression dressings represents the "gold standard" to which all other therapy must be compared. Proposed mechanisms include a reduction in ambulatory venous pressure, improvements in skin and subcutaneous tissue microcirculation, and augmented diffusion of nutrients and oxygen secondary to edema reduction. There are several options for active and maintenance treatment including the "Unna" boot, the multilayer compression bandage, compression stockings, and devices such as the CircAid (CircAid Medical Products, Inc., San Diego, CA). A systematic review of 23 randomized and controlled clinical trials concluded that compression clearly increases healing rates in comparison to no compression and that high compression is more efficacious than low compression.[43] However, it is not clear that there are substantial differences between the high compression alternatives. Compression is the most widely validated treatment for venous ulcers and can be considered a Grade 1A recommendation for ulcer healing.

Compression is, however, limited by substantial rates of recurrence. Although there are no randomized trials comparing ulcer recurrence with and without compression, there is strong observational evidence of higher recurrence rates without compression. The available data suggest recurrence rates of 32% to 64% without compression in comparison to 19% to 34% among compliant patients.[44] Based on strong observational evidence, the use of compression stockings for the prevention of ulcer recurrence is a Grade 1B recommendation.

Adjuncts to Compression

At least one observational study has suggested that sharp debridement of chronic ulcers with significant slough and nonviable tissue accelerates wound healing, and this is a Grade 1C recommendation. Although there does appear to be a correlation between bacterial density and delayed wound healing, the data regarding the use of systemic or topical antibiotics are poor and provide few solid conclusions. Based on the lack of any clear benefit and an association with bacterial resistance, current evidence argues *against* the use of systemic antibiotics in the absence of clinically significant infection[45] (Grade 1B). Among topical preparations, only cadexomer iodine has been associated with significantly improved rates of complete wound healing (RR 6.72; 95% CI 1.56 to 28.95)[45] and can be considered a Grade 2B recommendation. One randomized trial has demonstrated a larger reduction in wound area with a sustained-release silver foam dressing in comparison to a hydrocellular dressing.[46] However, area reduction is a surrogate measure of unclear clinical significance, and such dressings can be only weakly recommended (Grade 2C) based on the current evidence.

There are few pharmacologic agents available for the treatment of venous ulcers and none are as efficacious as high-level compression. Pentoxifylline is the only agent available in the United States and is postulated to act through the suppression of tumor necrosis factor alpha and leukocyte adhesion molecules.[47,48] Among five trials comparing pentoxifylline to placebo with background compression, patients in the treatment group were 30% more likely to completely heal their ulcer than were those receiving placebo.[47] Unfortunately, none of these trials were of sufficient duration to address their role in preventing ulcer recurrence. Randomized trials have similarly shown micronized purified flavanoid fraction, which is unavailable in the United States, to increase the odds of ulcer healing by 32% in comparison to compression and local wound care alone.[48] Despite the efficacy of theses pharmacologic adjuncts, they are probably indicated in only selected patients (with large or long-standing ulcers) and are therefore a Grade 2B recommendation.

A number of wound dressings are available as adjuncts to compression therapy. These include nonocclusive and semiocclusive/occlusive dressings, growth factors, and human skin equivalents. A recent meta-analysis suggests that although most of these dressings afford little advantage over compression alone, five (zinc oxide paste–impregnated bandage, Tegasorb, perilesional injection of granulocyte-macrophage colony-stimulating factor, porcine small-intestinal submucosa, and cultured human skin equivalent) did show statistically significant benefits.[49] However, given the modest benefits and variation in wound characteristics, drainage capabilities, ease of application, and cost, even those dressings that may be efficacious are at best a Grade 2A or 2B recommendation.

Surgery

The ESCHAR trial[50] has provided that most definitive evidence regarding the role of superficial venous surgery in the management of venous ulcers. Five hundred patients with healed (C5) or open (C6) ulcers were randomized to compression, using a multilayer bandage for those with open ulcers, or surgery, which included great or small saphenous vein stripping and phlebectomy. Although there was no difference in 24-week healing rates, which were 65% in both arms, patients randomized to surgery had significantly lower 12-month recurrence rates (12% versus 28%). These results were durable through 4 years of follow-up, at which point ulcer recurrence rates were significantly lower among patients randomized to compression plus surgery (31% versus 56%).[51] After 3 years, patients randomized to surgery had 15 weeks more ulcer-free time than those receiving compression alone. Although superficial venous surgery is of questionable value in ulcer healing, it can be considered a Grade 1A recommendation for the prevention of ulcer recurrence.

Most of the data supporting the use of endovenous ablation in the management of venous ulceration are indirect, extrapolated from the results in patients with mild to moderate venous disease. However, one small randomized trial has demonstrated that in comparison to compression alone, laser ablation of the great and/or small saphenous veins was associated with higher 12-month healing rates (24% versus 81.5%) and lower recurrence rates.[52] The reason for the discrepancy in wound healing between the ESCHAR trail and this study are unclear, although the 12-month ulcer healing rate with compression alone was remarkably low and should be questioned. However, based on weak indirect data and pending further direct evidence, endovenous ablation for the treatment of saphenous reflux associated with ulceration should be considered equivalent to stripping for the prevention of recurrence (Grade 1C).

Unfortunately, the data supporting the use of surgery for deep venous and perforator incompetence are substantially weaker. A variety of minimally invasive techniques, including subfascial endoscopic perforator surgery, thermal ablation, and sclerotherapy are available for the treatment of perforating veins. One systematic review of subfascial endoscopic perforator surgery (SEPS),[53] with or without saphenous extirpation, reported a recurrence rate of 13% after a mean follow-up of 29 months. This is close to the 12-month recurrence rate of 12% reported in the ESCHAR trial with superficial venous surgery alone. In a small randomized trial that specifically excluded patients with ulcers, the addition of SEPS to high ligation, stripping, and phlebectomy decreased the number of perforators present at 12 months but was not associated with significant differences in the clinically important measures of pain, mobility, cosmetic appearance, or quality of life.[54] One other trial randomized 200 ulcerated legs to compression alone or compression with SEPS and, when indicated, surgery of the superficial system.[55] Unfortunately, this trial used ulcer-free period, a composite of ulcer healing and recurrence, as the primary endpoint. As demonstrated by the ESCHAR trial,[50] surgical intervention may have different effects on the components of this composite measure. In comparing conservative therapy with SEPS, no significant differences were noted in the primary endpoint, ulcer-free period (53% versus 72%), or in the secondary endpoints of ulcer healing (73% versus 83%) and recurrence (23% versus 22%). Based on the currently available data, perforator interruption cannot be recommended in the treatment of C2 disease (Grade 2B). However, because the data remain flawed and could change if better evidence becomes available, the potential value of interruption of pathologic perforators (>3.5 mm, reflux ≥0.5 second, located near the ulcer bed) in C5-C6 disease cannot be excluded and can be weakly suggested in appropriate patients (Grade 2B).

Finally, the benefits of deep venous reconstruction (valve repair, transposition, transplantation) have not been evaluated outside of case series from highly specialized centers, and no estimated effect can be inferred. These procedures can be considered at best a very weak Grade 2C recommendation.

SUMMARY

Although many aspects of the treatment of chronic venous disorders have remained the same for almost a century, several recent advances have provided new and beneficial treatment opportunities for patients with chronic venous disorders. Unfortunately, the current regulatory environment does not favor proof of clinically relevant efficacy prior to widespread adoption of new technology. The efficient use of limited health care resources therefore demands that the clinician have some ability to interpret the clinical evidence. Fortunately, methods of evaluating clinical evidence based solely on a hierarchy of study design have been replaced by more clinically relevant systems using an assessment of risk versus benefit, the degree of confidence in the estimate of effect, and the likelihood that recommendations will change with future research. Unfortunately, much of the evidence in venous disease continues to rely on case series and the use of irrelevant and possibly misleading surrogate outcome measures. Optimal care of our patients and the health care system requires that we understand both the strengths and weakness of the evidence surrounding any clinical question and effectively apply it to the care of our patients. Clinical practice guidelines must continually evolve with the development of new technology and generation of new evidence, but the guidelines jointly published by the American Venous Forum are based on the best evidence currently available.[6] Consistent with the goals of evidence-based medicine, they should be appropriately influenced by the physician's expertise and individual patient's values and preferences.

REFERENCES

1. Fowkes FG, Lee AJ, Evans CJ, et al. Lifestyle risk factors for lower limb venous reflux in the general population: Edinburgh Vein Study. Int J Epidemiol 2001;30:846-852.
2. Bradbury A, Evans CJ, Allan P, et al. The relationship between lower limb symptoms and superficial and deep venous reflux on duplex ultrasonography: The Edinburgh Vein Study. J Vasc Surg 2000;32:921-931.
3. Krijnen RMA, de Boer EM, Bruynzeel DP. Epidemiology of venous disorders in the general and occupational populations. Epidemiol Rev 1997;19:294-309.
4. Newburger AE. Cosmetic medical devices and their FDA regulation. Arch Dermatol 2006;142: 225-228.
5. Nygaard I. What does "FDA Approved" mean for medical devices? Obstet Gynecol 2008;111: 4-6.
6. Gloviczki P, Comerota AJ, Dalsing MC, et al. The care of patients with varicose veins and associated chronic venous diseases: clinical practice guidelines of the Society for Vascular Surgery and the American Venous Forum. J Vasc Surg 2011;53(5 Suppl):2S-48S.
7. Sackett DL. Evidence-based medicine. Spine 1998;23:1085-1086.
8. Ioannidis JPA, Haidich AB, Lau J. Any casualties in the clash of randomised and observation evidence? BMJ 2001;322:879-880.
9. Group GW. Grading quality of evidence and strength of recommendation. BMJ 2004;328: 1490-1494.
10. Kearon C, Kahn SR, Agnelli G, et al. Antithrombotic therapy for venous thromboembolic disease: American College of Chest Physicians Evidence-Based Clinical Practice Guidelines (8th Edition). Chest 2008;133(6 Suppl):454S-545S.
11. Eklof B, Rutherford RB, Bergan JJ, et al. Revision of the CEAP classification for chronic venous disorders: consensus statement. J Vasc Surg 2004;40:1248-1252.

12. Rutherford RB, Padberg FT, Comerota AJ, et al. Venous severity scoring: An adjunct to venous outcome assessment. J Vasc Surg 2000;31:1307-1312.

13. Garratt AM, Ruta DA, Abdalla MI, et al. Responsiveness of the SF-36 and a condition-specific measure of health for patients with varicose veins. Qual Life Res 1996;5:223-234.

14. Lamping DL, Schroter S, Kurz X, et al. Evaluation of outcomes in chronic venous disorders of the leg: development of a scientifically rigorous, patient-reported measure of symptoms and quality of life. J Vasc Surg 2003;37:410-419.

15. Launois R, Reboul-Marty J, Henry B. Construction and validation of a quality of life questionnaire in chronic lower limb venous insufficiency (CIVIQ). Qual Life Res 1996;5:539-554.

16. Palfreyman SJ, Michaels JA. A systematic review of compression hosiery for uncomplicated varicose veins. Phlebology 2009;24(Suppl 1):13-33.

17. Michaels JA, Campbell WB, Brazier JE, et al. Randomised clinical trial, observational study and assessment of cost-effectiveness of the treatment of varicose veins (REACTIV trial). Health Technol Assess 2006;10:1-196, iii-iv.

18. Martinez MJ, Bonfill X, Moreno RM, et al. Phlebotonics for venous insufficiency. Cochrane Database Syst Rev 2005;(3):CD003229.

19. Pittler MH, Ernst E. Horse chestnut seed extract for chronic venous insufficiency. Cochrane Database Syst Rev 2006;(1):CD003230.

20. Dwerryhouse S, Davies B, Harradine K, et al. Stripping the long saphenous vein reduces the rate of reoperation for recurrent varicose veins: five-year results of a randomized trial. J Vasc Surg 1999;29:589-592.

21. Gohel MS, Epstein DM, Davies AH. Cost-effectiveness of traditional and endovenous treatments for varicose veins. Br J Surg 2010;97:1815-1823.

22. van den Bos R, Arends L, Kockaert M, et al. Endovenous therapies of lower extremity varicosities: A meta-analysis. J Vasc Surg 2009;49:230-239.

23. Hinchliffe RJ, Ubhi J, Beech A, et al. A prospective randomised controlled trial of VNUS closure versus surgery for the treatment of recurrent long saphenous varicose veins. Eur J Vasc Endovasc Surg 2006;31:212-218.

24. Stotter L, Schaaf I, Bockelbrink A. Comparative outcomes of radiofrequency ablation, invagination stripping, and cryostripping in the treatment of great saphenous vein insufficiency. Phlebology 2006;12:60-64.

25. de Medeiros CA, Luccas GC. Comparison of endovenous treatment with an 810 nm laser versus conventional stripping of the great saphenous vein in patients with primary varicose veins. Dermatol Surg 2005;31:1685-1694.

26. Rasmussen LH, Bjoern L, Lawaetz M, et al. Randomized trial comparing endovenous laser ablation of the great saphenous vein with high ligation and stripping in patients with varicose veins: short-term results. J Vasc Surg 2007;46:308-315.

27. Gale SS, Lee JN, Walsh ME, et al. A randomized, controlled trial of endovenous thermal ablation using the 810-nm wavelength laser and the ClosurePLUS radiofrequency ablation methods for superficial venous insufficiency of the great saphenous vein. J Vasc Surg 2010;52:645-650.

28. Shepherd AC, Gohel MS, Lim CS, et al. Pain following 980-nm endovenous laser ablation and segmental radiofrequency ablation for varicose veins: a prospective observational study. Vasc Endovascular Surg 2010;44:212-216.

29. Almeida JI, Kaufman J, Gockeritz O, et al. Radiofrequency endovenous ClosureFAST versus laser ablation for the treatment of great saphenous reflux: a multicenter, single-blinded, randomized study (RECOVERY study). J Vasc Interv Radiol 2009;20:752-759.

30. Shepherd AC, Gohel MS, Brown LC, et al. Randomized clinical trial of VNUS ClosureFAST radiofrequency ablation versus laser for varicose veins. Br J Surg 2010;97:810-818.

31. Pannier F, Rabe E, Rits J, et al. Endovenous laser ablation of great saphenous veins using a 1470 nm diode laser and the radial fibre: follow-up after six months. Phlebology 2011;26:35-39.

32. Proebstle TM, Moehler T, Gul D, et al. Endovenous treatment of the great saphenous vein using a 1,320 nm Nd:YAG laser causes fewer side effects than using a 940 nm diode laser. Dermatol Surg 2005;31:1678-1683; discussion 1683-1684.

33. Rigby KA, Palfreyman SJ, Beverley C, et al. Surgery versus sclerotherapy for the treatment of varicose veins. Cochrane Database Syst Rev 2004(4):CD004980.

34. Rabe E, Otto J, Schliephake D, et al. Efficacy and safety of great saphenous vein sclerotherapy using standardised polidocanol foam (ESAF): a randomised controlled multicentre clinical trial. Eur J Vasc Endovasc Surg 2008;35:238-245.

35. Jia X, Mowatt G, Burr JM, et al. Systematic review of foam sclerotherapy for varicose veins. Br J Surg 2007;94:925-936.

36. Chapman-Smith P, Browne A. Prospective five-year study of ultrasound-guided foam sclerotherapy in the treatment of great saphenous vein reflux. Phlebology 2009;24:183-188.

37. Tisi PV, Beverley C, Rees A. Injection sclerotherapy for varicose veins. Cochrane Database Syst Rev 2006(4):CD001732.

38. de Roos KP, Nieman FH, Neumann HA. Ambulatory phlebectomy versus compression sclerotherapy: results of a randomized controlled trial. Dermatol Surg 2003;29:221-226.

39. Carradice D, Mekako AI, Hatfield J, et al. Randomized clinical trial of concomitant or sequential phlebectomy after endovenous laser therapy for varicose veins. Br J Surg 2009;96:369-375.

40. van Rij AM, Chai J, Hill GB, et al. Incidence of deep vein thrombosis after varicose vein surgery. Br J Surg 2004;91:1582-1585.

41. Enoch S, Woon E, Blair SD. Thromboprophylaxis can be omitted in selected patients undergoing varicose vein surgery and hernia repair. Br J Surg 2003;90:818-820.

42. Knipp BS, Blackburn SA, Bloom JR, et al. Endovenous laser ablation: venous outcomes and thrombotic complications are independent of the presence of deep venous insufficiency. J Vasc Surg 2008;48:1538-1545.

43. Cullum N, Nelson EA, Fletcher AW, et al. Compression for venous leg ulcers. Cochrane Database Syst Rev 2001;Issue 2:Art No.:CD000265. doi:10.1002/14651858.CD000265.

44. Nelson EA, Bell-Syer SE, Cullum NA. Compression for preventing recurrence of venous ulcers. Cochrane Database Syst Rev 2000(4):CD002303.

45. O'Meara S, Al-Kurdi D, Ovington LG. Antibiotics and antiseptics for venous leg ulcers. Cochrane Database Syst Rev 2008(1):CD003557.

46. Jorgensen B, Price P, Andersen KE, et al. The silver-releasing foam dressing, Contreet Foam, promotes faster healing of critically colonised venous leg ulcers: a randomised, controlled trial. Int Wound J 2005;2:64-73.

47. Jull AB, Waters J, Arroll B. Pentoxifylline for treating venous leg ulcers. Cochrane Database Syst Rev 2002(1):CD001733.

48. Meissner MH, Eklof B, Smith PC, et al. Secondary chronic venous disorders. J Vasc Surg 2007;46(Suppl S):68S-83S.

49. O'Donnell TF Jr, Lau J. A systematic review of randomized controlled trials of wound dressings for chronic venous ulcer. J Vasc Surg 2006;44:1118-1125.

50. Barwell JR, Davies CE, Deacon J, et al. Comparison of surgery and compression with compression alone in chronic venous ulceration (ESCHAR study): randomised controlled trial. Lancet 2004;5(363):1854-1859.

51. Gohel MS, Barwell JR, Taylor M, et al. Long term results of compression therapy alone versus compression plus surgery in chronic venous ulceration (ESCHAR): randomised controlled trial. BMJ 2007;335:83.

52. Viarengo LM, Poterio-Filho J, Poterio GM, et al. Endovenous laser treatment for varicose veins in patients with active ulcers: measurement of intravenous and perivenous temperatures during the procedure. Dermatol Surg 2007;33:1234-1242.

53. Tenbrook JA Jr, Iafrati MD, O'Donnell TF Jr, et al. Systematic review of outcomes after surgical management of venous disease incorporating subfascial endoscopic perforator surgery. J Vasc Surg 2004;39:583-589.

54. Kianifard B, Holdstock J, Allen C, et al. Randomized clinical trial of the effect of adding subfascial endoscopic perforator surgery to standard great saphenous vein stripping. Br J Surg 2007;94:1075-1080.

55. van Gent WB, Hop WC, van Praag MC, et al. Conservative versus surgical treatment of venous leg ulcers: a prospective, randomized, multicenter trial. J Vasc Surg 2006;44:563-571.

INDEX

Page numbers followed by *b* indicate boxes; *f*, figures; *t*, tables.

487